Most Commons in
Pathology and
Laboratory Medicine

Most Commons in
Pathology and
Laboratory Medicine

■ **Edward F. Goljan, MD**
Professor and Chairman of Pathology
Oklahoma State University
College of Osteopathic Medicine
Tulsa, Oklahoma

W.B. SAUNDERS COMPANY
A Division of Harcourt Brace & Company
Philadelphia ■ London ■ Toronto ■ Montreal ■ Sydney ■ Tokyo

W.B. SAUNDERS COMPANY
A Division of Harcourt Brace & Company

The Curtis Center
Independence Square West
Philadelphia, Pennsylvania 19106

Library of Congress Cataloging-in-Publication Data

Most commons in pathology and laboratory medicine / Edward F. Goljan—
1st ed.

p.   cm.

ISBN 0–7216–7992–7

1. Pathology—Outlines, syllabi, etc.   2. Diagnosis, Laboratory—Outlines,
syllabi, etc.   3. Pathology—Examinations, questions, etc.
4. Diagnosis, Laboratory—Examinations, questions, etc.   I. Goljan,
Edward F.   [DNLM: 1. Pathology.   2. Laboratory Techniques and
Procedures.   QZ 4 G626m 1999]

RB120.G65 1999   616.07′02′02—dc21

DNLM/DLC   98-38024

MOST COMMONS IN PATHOLOGY AND LABORATORY
MEDICINE   ISBN 0–7216–7992–7

Printed in the United States of America.

Last digit is the print number: 9   8   7   6   5   4   3   2   1

This book is dedicated to my second grandson,
Dylan Alexander, whose recent entry into
this world, as quoted in James 1:17,
is yet another "good and perfect gift from above
that comes down from the Father of lights."

◼ PREFACE

This pocket-sized, highly factual, table-formatted, book covers the "most commons" in pathology and laboratory medicine. Excerpted from material discussed more thoroughly in a larger text in pathology (*Pathology*, part of the Saunders Text and Review Series, 1998), it provides the student with the following benefits:

- A two-column table format for ease in reviewing key points in disease processes and laboratory test interpretation.
- A USMLE style question at the end of each table, followed by a brief discussion of the correct and incorrect choices.
- An integrated approach with correlations connecting concepts learned in basic science with clinical disorders commonly encountered in clinical practice.
- A heavy emphasis on pathophysiology and mechanisms of disease.
- Key points that are commonly asked on examinations in pathology, introduction to clinical medicine, and laboratory medicine and as "pimp questions" on clinical rotations in medicine, pediatrics, surgery, and obstetrics and gynecology.

It is my opinion, based on 16 years of teaching pathology and 6 years of teaching part 1 and 2 USMLE board reviews around the country, that knowing the "most commons" of every disease (common or uncommon) and laboratory test result represents one of the most important initial steps in clinical decision making. The thought of writing a "Most Commons" series of books was based on my own use of the concept in teaching medical students, my observation that students who extracted out the "most commons" from my notes in final preparation for the USMLE step 1 and 2 exams successfully completed the exams, and my amazement that very few book series were available for medical students that used the concept of "most commons" in covering the major specialties. Additional books following this approach are already scheduled in the near future for medicine, pediatrics, surgery, and obstetrics and gynecology.

I would like to express my heartfelt thanks to my darling wife, Joyce; our three children, Keith, Lauren, and Renee; and my two grandsons, Austin and Dylan, who have all been my emotional and spiritual support throughout the writing of this book as well as others over the last few years.

Edward F. Goljan, M.D.

NOTICE

Medicine is an ever-changing field. Standard safety precautions must be followed, but as new research and clinical experience broaden our knowledge, changes in treatment and drug therapy become necessary or appropriate. The author of this work has carefully checked the generic and trade drug names and verified drug dosages to ensure that the dosage information in this work is accurate and in accord with the standards accepted at the time of publication. Readers are advised, however, to check the product information currently provided by the manufacturer of each drug to be administered to be certain that changes have not been made in the recommended dose or in the contraindications for administration. This is of particular importance in regard to new or infrequently used drugs. It is the responsibility of the treating physician, relying on experience and knowledge of the patient, to determine dosages and the best treatment for the patient. The editors cannot be responsible for misuse or misapplication of the material in this work.

THE PUBLISHER

◼ CONTENTS

CHAPTER

CONCEPTS IN LABORATORY MEDICINE

CONTENTS

Table 1–1. OPERATING CHARACTERISTICS OF LABORATORY TESTS

Most Common...	Answer and Explanation
reasons for ordering lab tests	*screen asymptomatic people* (e.g., newborn screen for PKU), *screen symptomatic people* (e.g., stress ECG in suspected angina), *confirm disease* (e.g., serum CK-MB in AMI), *monitor disease* (e.g., HbA_{1c} for glycemic control in DM)
STAT tests [STAT: immediate results; life-threatening situation]	**CBC**, *UA, glucose, electrolytes, ABGs, Gram stain, amylase, drug screen*
types of lab test results in people with and without disease	*true positive* (TP; positive test result in patient with disease), *false negative* (FN; normal test result in a patient with disease), *true negative* (TN; normal test result in a person without disease), *false positive* (FP; positive test result in person without disease)
use of a test with 100% sensitivity [sensitivity = chance test is positive in disease; TP ÷ (TP + FN) × 100]	*screen for disease* (e.g., serum ANA for SLE) [A test with 100% sensitivity has no FNs. A negative test result must be a TN (disease is excluded). A positive test result may be a TP (disease is included) or an FP.]
use of a test with 100% specificity [specificity = chance test is normal in someone without disease; TN ÷ (TN + FP) × 100]	*distinguish a TP from an FP, hence confirming disease* (e.g., anti-Smith antibody in SLE) [A test with 100% specificity has no FPs. A positive test result must be a TP (confirms disease); a normal test result is an FP.]

Table continued on following page

Table 1-1. OPERATING CHARACTERISTICS OF LABORATORY TESTS *Continued*

Most Common...	Answer and Explanation
cause of an FP test result	*low prevalence of disease* [Prevalence is the total number of people with disease in the population being studied ([TP + FN] ÷ [TP + FN + TN + FP] × 100). A positive test result (predictive value of a positive test result: [PV+ = (TP ÷ TP + FP) × 100]) in a population with low prevalence of disease is more likely an FP than a TP (low PV+). A test with 100% specificity always has a PV+ of 100% (confirms disease).]
cause of an FN test result	*low prevalence of disease* [A negative test result (predictive value of a negative test result: [PV− = (TN ÷ TN + FN) × 100]) in a population with low prevalence of disease is more likely a TN than an FN (high PV−). A test with 100% sensitivity always has a PV− of 100% (excludes disease).]
effect of increasing duration of a disease on the prevalence and incidence of disease	*P (prevalence) = I (incidence) × D (duration of disease)* [Incidence is the number of new cases of disease over a set period of time and is not affected by the duration of disease. Prevalence increases or decreases with an increase or decrease in duration of the disease.]
statistical method that expresses the precision (i.e., reliability) of a test	*standard deviation* (SD) [Precision represents how close the test results are to each other after repetitive measurements. The lower the SD, the greater the precision, and vice versa. Accuracy reflects how close the test results are to the true value of the test.]
effect of increasing the upper limit of normal for fasting glucose for diagnosing DM from 115 mg/dL to 140 mg/dL	*increase the specificity and PV+ test result* [fewer FPs] *and decrease the sensitivity and PV− test result* [more FNs]
effect of decreasing the upper limit of normal for fasting glucose for diagnosing DM from 140 mg/dL to 126 mg/dL	*increase the sensitivity and PV− test result* [fewer FNs] *and decrease the specificity and PV+ test result* [more FPs]

Table 1–1. OPERATING CHARACTERISTICS OF LABORATORY TESTS *Continued*

Most Common...	Answer and Explanation
method of establishing the reference interval for a test	*2 SDs from the mean of the test established after performing the test on a population of normal people* [Two SDs includes 95% of the normal population; hence, 5% (1 : 20) normal people are outside the reference interval (FP test result). **Example:** mean of a test is 100 mg/dL, 1 SD = 10 mg/dL); reference interval = 80–120 mg/dL (2 SD = 20 mg/dL); 100 − 20 = 80 and 100 + 20 = 120.]

Question: A patient has a positive RPR serologic test for syphilis and a negative FTA-ABS. The RPR is **MOST LIKELY** a/an:
- (A) TP
- (B) TN
- (C) FP
- (D) FN

Answer: (C): An FTA-ABS is the confirmatory test for a positive RPR. A positive test result indicates that the RPR is a TP rather than an FP, while a negative test result indicates that the RPR is an FP.

ABGs = arterial blood gases, AMI = acute myocardial infarction, ANA = antinuclear antibody, CBC = complete blood cell count, CK-MB = creatine kinase MB, DM = diabetes mellitus, ECG = electrocardiogram, FN = false negative, FP = false positive, FTA-ABS = fluorescent treponemal antibody-absorption, HbA$_{1c}$ = glycosylated hemoglobin, PKU = phenylketonuria, PV− = predictive value of a negative test result, PV+ = predictive value of a positive test result, RPR = rapid plasma reagin, SD = standard deviation, SLE = systemic lupus erythematosus, TN = true negative, TP = true positive, UA = urinalysis.

Table 1–2. VARIABLES AFFECTING LABORATORY TEST RESULTS

Most Common...	Answer and Explanation
anticoagulants utilized to prevent clotting in test tubes in order to harvest plasma	*heparin* (enhances AT III activity, which neutralizes certain clotting factors), *EDTA* (binds calcium, hence preventing clotting), *citrate* (binds calcium) [Plasma contains all the coagulation factors.]

Table continued on following page

Table 1–2. **VARIABLES AFFECTING LABORATORY TEST RESULTS** *Continued*

Most Common...	Answer and Explanation
coagulation factors used up in a clot tube	*allowing blood to clot harvests serum, which lacks fibrinogen (I), prothrombin (II), factor V, factor VIII, and platelets* after the specimen is centrifuged
cause of a turbid blood sample	*an increase in triglycerides (TGs) in a patient who was not fasting* [The TG comes from saturated fats in the diet that are packaged into chylomicrons.]
tests requiring a fasting sample	*lipid profile (CH, TG, HDL, calculated LDL)* [Fasting eliminates the effect of saturated fats in the diet (TG, not CH or HDL), which falsely increase the total TG concentration (see above) and lower the calculated LDL (LDL = CH − HDL − ↑**TG**/5).] *fasting glucose* [Fasting glucose level is used in diagnosing DM (≥126 mg/dL on two separate occasions).]
medically significant lab test alterations in a hemolyzed blood sample	*increase in potassium* (pseudohyperkalemia), *lactate dehydrogenase* (LDH), *aspartate aminotransferase* (AST)
effect of drugs that enhance the liver cytochrome system on lab values	*drugs like alcohol and barbiturates cause hyperplasia of the SER* (houses the cytochrome system) *leading to an increased synthesis of GGT and increased metabolism of drugs metabolized in the liver* (lowers their concentration)
effect of drugs that inhibit the liver cytochrome system on lab values	*drugs like cimetidine block the cytochrome system and cause potentially dangerous elevations in drugs normally metabolized by the liver*
newborn lab test alterations that differ from children and adults	*high hemoglobin* (Hb; mean 18.5 g/dL) [This is due to HbF, which left-shifts the oxygen dissociation curve, hence stimulating erythropoietin and subsequent RBC synthesis.]
lab test alterations in children that differ from adults	*increased serum alkaline phosphatase* (3–5 times higher than adults; increased osteoblast activity from active bone growth), *increased serum phosphate* (driving force for depositing calcium in bone), *lower Hb* (11–12 g/dL)

Table 1–2. VARIABLES AFFECTING LABORATORY TEST RESULTS *Continued*

Most Common...	Answer and Explanation
lab test alterations in women that significantly differ from men	*lower serum iron, total iron binding capacity, percent saturation,* and *ferritin* owing to menses, less testosterone than men, and childbearing
lab test alterations in a normal pregnancy that differ from non-pregnant women	*greater increase in plasma volume than in RBC mass decreases Hb* (dilutional effect) and *increases creatinine clearance* (effect of increased plasma volume) leading to *lower serum BUN, uric acid,* and *creatinine concentrations* (all cleared more rapidly) [Additional differences: *increased alkaline phosphatase* (placental origin), *respiratory alkalosis* (progesterone effect on respiratory center), *increased total T_4 and cortisol* (estrogen increases synthesis of binding proteins without altering free hormone levels), *mild glucose intolerance* (effect of hPL), *glucosuria* (lower renal threshold for glucose; normal blood glucose).]
lab alterations in the elderly population	*decreased creatinine clearance* (low GFR, problem with renal excretion of drugs), *Hb concentration in men* (drop in testosterone reduces erythropoiesis), *CD8 suppressor cells* (increased autoantibodies) See Chapter 7 for additional changes.

Question: Which of the following tests has the same reference intervals in adult men, adult non-pregnant women, and pregnant women?
- (A) Serum Hb
- (B) Serum BUN
- (C) Serum creatinine
- (D) Serum AST
- (E) Serum ferritin

Answer: (D): Serum AST is not altered by pregnancy, sex, or age of the patient. Hb, creatinine, and ferritin are higher in men than in women and lower in pregnant than non-pregnant women. Serum BUN is similar in men and women and lower in pregnant than non-pregnant women.

AST = aspartate aminotransferase, AT III = antithrombin III, BUN = blood urea nitrogen, CH = cholesterol, DM = diabetes mellitus, EDTA = ethylenediaminetetraacetic acid, GFR = glomerular filtration rate, GGT = γ-glutamyltransferase, Hb = hemoglobin, HDL = high density lipoprotein, hPL = human placental lactogen, LDH = lactate dehydrogenase, LDL = low density lipoprotein, RBC = red blood cell, SER = smooth endoplasmic reticulum, T_4 = thyroxine, TG = triglyceride.

CHAPTER

2

CELL INJURY

CONTENTS

Table 2–1. TISSUE HYPOXIA

Most Common...	Answer and Explanation
causes of tissue hypoxia [inadequate oxygenation of tissue]	**ischemia**, *hypoxemia, Hb-related problems, defective or uncoupled oxidative phosphorylation*
sites in the CNS most susceptible to tissue hypoxia	**neurons in the hippocampus**, *Purkinje cells in the cerebellum, neurons in layers 3, 5, and 6 of the cerebral cortex*
cause of ischemia [reduction of arterial blood flow to tissue]	**atherosclerosis** [*less common causes:* vessel compression (e.g., expanding mass), torsion of vessels (e.g., volvulus [twisting of bowel around mesentery]), decreased cardiac output (e.g., LHF)]
consequences of ischemia	**infarction** [localized cell necrosis], *atrophy* [reduction in cell/tissue mass], *organ dysfunction*
causes of hypoxemia [low partial pressure of oxygen in plasma; PaO_2]	*respiratory acidosis* [hypoventilation; increased $PaCO_2$], *ventilation defect* (e.g., atelectasis [collapse of alveoli]), *perfusion defect* (e.g., pulmonary embolus), *diffusion defect* (e.g., interstitial fibrosis)
causes of Hb-related problems	**anemia**, *metHb* [heme iron in ferric condition], *CO poisoning, left-shifted ODC* [Hb with a high affinity for oxygen]
alterations in O_2 content in anemia [O_2 content = (1.34 × Hb) × O_2 saturation + PaO_2]	*decreased O_2 content* owing to a reduction in Hb concentration; SaO_2 [percentage of heme groups occupied by O_2] and PaO_2 are normal

Table continued on following page

Table 2–1. TISSUE HYPOXIA *Continued*

Most Common...	Answer and Explanation
alterations in O_2 content in respiratory acidosis	*decreased O_2 content* owing to a reduction in SaO_2 and PaO_2.
alterations in O_2 content in methemoglobinemia and CO poisoning	*decreased O_2 content* owing to a reduction in SaO_2; Hb concentration and PaO_2 are normal
causes of a left-shifted ODC	*CO poisoning, metHb, alkalosis, HbF, hypo-thermia*
treatment for methemoglobinemia	**methylene blue**, which activates a normally inactive metHb reductase system that converts ferric to ferrous ions [*Ascorbic acid* is used as an ancillary treatment, since it reduces ferric to ferrous ions.]
treatment for CO poisoning	*oxygen*, which displaces CO from the heme group
causes of uncoupled oxidative phosphorylation [uncoupling: increased permeability of the inner mitochondrial membrane to protons]	*block of cytochrome oxidase* (e.g., cyanide, CO), *uncoupling agents* (e.g., salicylates, alcohol, dinitrophenol)
organelle and biochemical process altered in tissue hypoxia	*mitochondria* and generation of ATP by oxidative phosphorylation
biochemical consequence of tissue hypoxia	*decrease in ATP synthesis*
initial light microscopic finding in tissue hypoxia	*cellular swelling due to loss of the sodium/potassium ATPase pump*
reversible consequences of reduction in ATP	**cellular swelling due to loss of the sodium/potassium ATPase pump** (correlates with dilatation of endoplasmic reticulum), *detachment of ribosomes* leading to decreased protein synthesis (fatty liver from decreased apolipoproteins), increased *anaerobic glycolysis*

Table 2–1. TISSUE HYPOXIA *Continued*

Most Common...	Answer and Explanation
causes of enhanced anaerobic glycolysis in tissue hypoxia	*allosteric enhancement of PFK:* increased AMP and decreased citrate
irreversible consequences of reduction in ATP	**cell membrane** and *mitochondrial injury* due to FR injury and increase in cytosolic calcium [*Nuclear pyknosis* is the most common light microscopic change.]
effects of calcium in tissue hypoxia	*activates phospholipase in the cell membrane, endonuclease in the nucleus; enters the mitochondria to produce large amorphous densities that are visible with EM*
lab marker of tissue injury	*serum enzymes* (e.g., CK in AMI, transaminases in hepatitis)
lab finding indicating anaerobic glycolysis	*increased anion gap metabolic acidosis due to lactic acidosis* from anaerobic glycolysis

Question: Which of the following causes tissue hypoxia without altering the oxygen content of blood?
  (A) Respiratory acidosis
  (B) CO poisoning
  (C) MetHb
  (D) Cyanide poisoning
  (E) Anemia

Answer: (D): Cyanide blocks cytochrome oxidase. MetHb and CO lower the SaO_2, anemia lowers the Hb concentration, and respiratory acidosis lowers both SaO_2 and PaO_2.

AMI = acute myocardial infarction, AMP = adenosine monophosphate, ATP = adenosine triphosphate, CK = creatine kinase, CNS = central nervous system, CO = carbon monoxide, EM = electron microscopy, FR = free radical, Hb = hemoglobin, LHF = left-sided heart failure, metHb = methemoglobin, ODC = oxygen dissociation curve, $PaCO_2$ = partial pressure of arterial CO_2, PaO_2 = partial pressure of arterial O_2, PFK = phosphofructokinase, SaO_2 = oxygen saturation.

Table 2–2. CELL INJURY

Most Common...	Answer and Explanation
free radicals [FRs; unpaired electron in outer orbit]	*superoxide, hydroxyl ions, drugs* (e.g., acetaminophen, CCl_4), *hydrogen peroxide*

Table continued on following page

Table 2–2. CELL INJURY *Continued*

Most Common...	Answer and Explanation
sources for FRs	*ionizing radiation, damaged mitochondria, oxidase reactions* (e.g., xanthine oxidase), *drugs, chemicals, granulocytes/macrophages*
metal associated with generation of FRs	*iron* [The Fenton reaction generates hydroxyl free radicals, which are the mechanism of injury in iron overload diseases (e.g., hemochromatosis and hemosiderosis).]
site for generation of drug/chemical FRs	*cytochrome P450 system in the liver*
injuries associated with FRs	*lipid peroxidation of cell membranes, reperfusion injury* (e.g., post-infusion tPA), *retinopathy of prematurity* (superoxide FRs), *bronchopulmonary dysplasia* (superoxide FRs), *cancer* (FR-induced point mutations)
antioxidants that neutralize FRs	*SOD* (superoxide), *catalase* (peroxide), *GSH* (peroxide, acetaminophen), *vitamin E* (cell membrane lipid peroxidation), *selenium* (cofactor in glutathione peroxidase), *ascorbic acid* (FR scavenger), β-*carotenes.*
cause of individual cell necrosis [cell death]	*apoptosis* [Apoptosis is important in programmed cell death, involution of wolffian and müllerian duct remnants, atrophy, toxin-induced injury, cell death by cytotoxic T cells (e.g., Councilman bodies in viral hepatitis).]
cause of coagulation necrosis [necrotic tissue with cell structures intact]	*ischemia secondary to atherosclerosis* [Less common causes include *radiation* and *heavy metals* (e.g., lead).]
site of coagulation necrosis	*heart* [AMI is the leading cause of death in the United States.]
sites of pale infarctions [localized areas of tissue necrosis without hemorrhage]	**heart**, *kidneys, liver* (least likely to infarct owing to a dual blood supply), *spleen, brain* (atherosclerotic stroke; liquefactive not coagulative necrosis)
sites of hemorrhagic (red) infarctions [localized areas of tissue necrosis with hemorrhage]	**lungs**, *bowel, ovaries, testicles, brain* (embolic stroke)

Table 2–2. CELL INJURY *Continued*

Most Common...	Answer and Explanation
cause of gangrene in the toes of a diabetic	*atherosclerotic peripheral vascular disease* [Dry gangrene is primarily coagulative necrosis (no infection). Wet gangrene begins as coagulative necrosis, but superimposed infection results in liquefactive necrosis.]
sites for watershed infarcts [infarctions in areas between two overlapping blood supplies]	*cerebral cortex and splenic flexure* (overlap area between the superior and inferior mesenteric arteries)
mechanism of liquefactive necrosis	*destructive effect of proteolytic enzymes* (neutrophils, macrophages, cells in the CNS)
cause of enzymatic fat necrosis	*acute pancreatitis* [It is most commonly secondary to alcoholism and biliary tract disease. Fatty acids and calcium combine (saponification) and form chalky white areas in the tissue.]
cause of calcifications in the LUQ on a radiograph	*dystrophic calcification* [calcification of damaged tissue] *in a patient with recurrent pancreatitis*
site of traumatic fat necrosis	*pendulous breast tissue* [It is often confused with cancer owing to calcifications and induration of the tissue.]
tissue manifestation of caseous necrosis [combination of coagulative and liquefactive necrosis]	*granulomas* [Granulomas are a localized collection of activated macrophages (epithelioid cells) and CD$_4$ T helper cells (type IV cellular immune reaction). Caseation (cheesy appearance) is from lipids released from the cell walls of dead organisms (TB, systemic fungi).]
causes of caseation necrosis	**tuberculosis**, *systemic fungal infections* (**histoplasmosis**)
causes of noncaseating necrosis	**sarcoidosis**, *Crohn's disease*
cause of fibrinoid necrosis [eosinophilic staining fibrin-like material]	*immune complex vasculitis* (e.g., HSP) [*other examples:* vegetations in rheumatic fever, rheumatoid nodules]

Table continued on following page

Table 2–2. CELL INJURY *Continued*

Most Common...	Answer and Explanation
cause and sites of gummatous necrosis [granulomatous variant of caseous necrosis]	*tertiary syphilis with the skin and bone representing the most common sites* [Gummas have a rubbery consistency and have a necrotic center surrounded by macrophages.]

Question: Which of the following is an example of liquefactive necrosis?
- (A) Myocardial infarction
- (B) Cerebral infarction
- (C) Apoptosis
- (D) Acute tubular necrosis
- (E) Gummatous necrosis

Answer: (B): A and C are coagulation necrosis, D is individual cell necrosis, E is a variant of caseous necrosis.

AMI = acute myocardial infarction, CCl₄ = carbon tetrachloride, CNS = central nervous system, FR = free radical, GSH = glutathione, LUQ = left upper quadrant, HSP = Henoch-Schönlein purpura, SOD = superoxide dismutase, TB = tuberculosis, tPA = tissue plasminogen activator.

Table 2–3. CELL ACCUMULATIONS

Most Common...	Answer and Explanation
lipid accumulation	*cholesterol* (CH) in an atherosclerotic plaque
cause of a fatty liver	*alcohol* [Substrates from alcohol metabolism that increase VLDL synthesis (lipid of fatty change) include NADH (increases production of DHAP in the glycolytic cycle → glycerol 3-PO₄, the CHO backbone of VLDL), acetate (fatty acid), AcCoA (substrate for fatty acid synthesis).]
cause of hepatomegaly in kwashiorkor	*fatty change* [A decreased protein intake decreases apoprotein synthesis and secretion of VLDL from the liver (VLDL must be coated by protein to be soluble in plasma).]
skin lesions associated with CH accumulation	*xanthelasma* (yellow patches on eyelids; type II hyperlipidemia), *tendon xanthomas* (familial hypercholesterolemia)
protein associated with amyloid formation	**light chains in primary amyloidosis due to plasma cell dyscrasias** (e.g., multiple myeloma). See Chapter 8.

Table 2–3. CELL ACCUMULATIONS *Continued*

Most Common...	Answer and Explanation
examples of protein accumulations in tissue	**hyaline arteriolosclerosis** (small vessel disease of DM and hypertension), *amyloid*, *Ig* (e.g., red globules in reactive plasma cells)
lesions with melanin accumulation	**nevocellular nevi**, *malignant melanoma*
causes of excess melanin deposition in skin	*increased release of ACTH from hypocortisolism:* Addison's disease, adrenogenital syndrome (enzyme deficiencies) *increased production of ACTH:* ectopic Cushing's syndrome (small cell carcinoma of lung)
disorders with absence of melanin	**vitiligo** (autoimmune destruction of melanocytes), *albinism* (AR; deficiency of tyrosinase), *PKU* (decreased production of tyrosine → decreased melanin)
disorders associated with melanin look-alikes	**CWP** (anthracotic pigment), *melanosis coli* (pigment from laxatives discolors colon), *alcaptonuria* (AR; deficiency of homogentisate oxidase; accumulation of homogentisate)
pigments derived from Hb	**bilirubin**, *hemosiderin* (packets of ferritin), *hematin* (oxidized heme that has a black color; melena in stools [acid pH in the stomach converts Hb into hematin])
disorders associated with glycogen accumulation	**DM** (deposition in renal tubules called Armanni-Epstein anomaly; deposition in the nuclei of hepatocytes), *glycogen storage diseases* (e.g., von Gierke's [hepatorenomegaly], Pompe's disease [restrictive cardiomyopathy], McArdle's disease [absence of muscle phosphorylase with accumulation of glycogen in muscle])
mechanism of dystrophic calcification	*calcification of damaged tissue in the presence of a normal serum calcium level* (e.g., atherosclerotic plaque)
mechanism of metastatic calcification	*calcification of tissue secondary to an increase in calcium or phosphate* (e.g., primary hyperparathyroidism)

Table continued on following page

Table 2–3. CELL ACCUMULATIONS *Continued*

Most Common...	Answer and Explanation
pigment associated with FR injury and atrophy	*lipofuscin*, which is a brown pigment representing the undigestible end-product of lipid peroxidation
cause of GAG accumulations	**mucopolysaccharidoses**, which are predominantly AR lysosomal storage diseases (e.g., Hurler's disease)

Question: Which of the following materials other than bilirubin accumulates in blood or tissue in intrahepatic obstruction to bile flow?
(A) Hematin
(B) Lipofuscin
(C) Cholesterol
(D) Triglyceride
(E) Melanin

Answer: (C): Bile contains conjugated bilirubin and cholesterol (hypercholesterolemia, skin eruptions).

AcCoA = acetyl CoA, ACTH = adrenocorticotropic hormone, AR = autosomal recessive, CH = cholesterol, CHO = carbohydrate, CWP = coal worker's pneumoconiosis, DHAP = dihydroxyacetone phosphate, DM = diabetes mellitus, FR = free radical, GAG = glycosaminoglycan, Hb = hemoglobin, Ig = immunoglobulin, NADH = nicotinamide adenine dinucleotide, PKU = phenylketonuria, VLDL = very low density lipoprotein.

Table 2–4. GROWTH ALTERATIONS

Most Common...	Answer and Explanation
cell cycle regulators in cell growth	*cyclins and kinases* [Cyclins are proteins that activate kinases, which regulate the progression from one phase of the cycle to the next (G1 → S → G2 → M → G1 with repeat of the cycle or from G1 to G0 [resting phase]).]
suppressor gene controlling cell growth	*p53 suppressor gene* [This gene produces a protein that controls kinase activity.]
cell cycle phase that controls whether the cell divides again or terminally differentiates itself	*G1 phase* [This is also the most variable phase of the cycle (all the other phases remain constant).]

Table 2–4. GROWTH ALTERATIONS *Continued*

Most Common...	Answer and Explanation
cell cycle phase for chromosomal replication	*S phase* [DNA and organelles double in this phase.]
cell cycle phase for synthesis of components required for mitosis	*G2 phase*
cell cycle phase blocked by vinca alkaloids	*M phase* (mitosis) [Vinca alkaloids (e.g., vincristine, vinblastine) bind to tubulin (protein forming the mitotic spindle), hence disrupting the spindle apparatus in mitosis.]
cell cycle phase blocked by antimetabolites interfering with DNA synthesis	*S phase* (e.g., methotrexate)
growth alteration	*atrophy* [reduced cell/tissue mass]
causes of atrophy	**normal aging**, *ischemia* (e.g., cerebral atrophy), *disuse* (e.g., decreased muscle workload), *loss of trophic stimulation* (e.g., denervation of muscle), *malnutrition* (e.g., marasmus), *compression* (e.g., renal cortex in hydronephrosis)
cell alterations in atrophy	*destruction of cell organelles and structural proteins* (called autophagy; leaves lipofuscin behind)
underdevelopment of an organ	*hypoplasia*, where there is incomplete or partial development of an organ or tissue (e.g., hypoplasia of the left ventricle) [*Agenesis* is absence of the primordial tissue (no organ). *Aplasia* is presence of primordial tissue without any further development.]
type of tissue containing stem cells	*labile tissue*, where >1.5% of the cells are in active mitosis [Stem cells rather than all the cells in the tissue are involved in mitosis. *Examples*: basal cells in the skin, bone marrow stem cells, cells in the intestinal crypts, lymphoid tissue.]

Table continued on following page

Table 2–4. GROWTH ALTERATIONS *Continued*

Most Common...	Answer and Explanation
theory for cell hypertrophy [increase in cell size]	*block prior to the G2 phase of the cell cycle by transforming growth factor-β*
theory for cell hyperplasia [increase in cell number]	*block after mitosis causing cells to remain in the cell cycle and not enter the G0 phase*
types of tissue capable of undergoing both hyperplasia and hypertrophy	*labile (see above) and stable cells* [Stable cells are normally in the G0 phase of the cycle and do not have stem cells. They must be stimulated (e.g., hormones, growth factors) to enter the G1 phase of the cell cycle (e.g., smooth muscle, hepatocytes).]
muscle types that undergo only hypertrophy	*cardiac and skeletal muscle* [These are permanent cells (cannot enter the cell cycle), hence they cannot divide. Smooth muscle cells undergo hypertrophy and hyperplasia.]
examples of permanently differentiated tissue	*skeletal and cardiac muscle, neurons*
cause of left ventricular hypertrophy (LVH)	*essential hypertension* [Increased peripheral resistance increases the afterload the muscle must contract against.]
example of equal proportions of hypertrophy and hyperplasia	*gravid uterus*, where there is both smooth muscle hyperplasia (estrogen-induced) and hypertrophy
cause of bone marrow erythroid hyperplasia	*hypoxemia* [A reduced PaO_2 is a stimulus for erythropoietin release, which stimulates the erythroid stem cell to undergo mitosis.]
growth alteration predisposing to endometrial cancer	*endometrial hyperplasia*, which may progress into carcinoma in situ, and invasive adenocarcinoma [Endometrial hyperplasia is due to unopposed estrogen.]

Table 2–4. GROWTH ALTERATIONS *Continued*

Most Common...	Answer and Explanation
cause of squamous metaplasia of the respiratory tract [metaplasia: replacement of one adult cell type by another]	*smoking* [Both the true vocal cords and the mainstem bronchus are lined by ciliated pseudostratified columnar epithelium. Toxins in smoke cause irritation, leading to squamous metaplasia.]
cause of glandular metaplasia of the distal esophagus	*GERD* [A relaxed LES leads to acid injury of squamous epithelium and subsequent glandular metaplasia (Barrett's esophagus), which predisposes to adenocarcinoma.]
cause of intestinal metaplasia in the stomach	*chronic atrophic gastritis secondary to Helicobacter pylori.* [Intestinal metaplasia refers to the presence of goblet cells and Paneth cells in the stomach.]
infectious agent causing squamous metaplasia in the bladder	*Schistosoma hematobium* [The eggs deposited by adult worms in the venous plexus of the bladder cause inflammation and squamous metaplasia of the overlying transitional epithelium. Squamous cancer may also occur.]
vitamin deficiency producing squamous metaplasia	*vitamin A deficiency* [Vitamin A normally prevents squamous metaplasia.]
growth alteration predisposing to cancer	*dysplasia* (atypical hyperplasia), which, in mild cases, may regress with removal of the offending agent. [Irreversible lesions progress into carcinoma in situ and then invasive cancer.]
cause of squamous dysplasia of the cervix [dysplasia: atypical hyperplasia]	*HPV type 16*, which produces squamous metaplasia that may progress into dysplasia, carcinoma in situ, and invasive cancer

Table continued on following page

Table 2–4. GROWTH ALTERATIONS *Continued*

Question: An increase in goblet cells in the nonrespiratory terminal bronchioles is an example of which of the following?

    (A) Metaplasia
    (B) Hyperplasia
    (C) Hypertrophy
    (D) Dysplasia
    (E) Mesenchymal metaplasia

Answer: (A): Goblet cells are not normally in the nonrespiratory bronchioles. They are increased in smokers. Goblet cell increase in the mainstem bronchus is an example of hyperplasia, since they are normally present in this tissue.

GERD = gastroesophageal reflux disease, HPV = human papilloma virus, LES = lower esophageal sphincter, LVH = left ventricular hypertrophy, PaO_2 = partial pressure of arterial oxygen.

CHAPTER

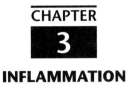

INFLAMMATION

CONTENTS

Table 3–1. Acute inflammation (AI).
Table 3–2. Chronic inflammation (CI).
Table 3–3. Laboratory test abnormalities in acute and chronic inflammation.

Table 3–1. ACUTE INFLAMMATION (AI)

Most Common...	Answer and Explanation
cause of rubor [redness] in AI	*arteriolar vasodilatation*, due to histamine release from tissue mast cells
cause of tumor [swelling] in AI	*increased venular permeability* primarily due to histamine
cause of calor [heat] in AI	*arteriolar vasodilatation* with increased blood flow due to histamine
cause of dolor [pain] in AI	*bradykinin, prostaglandin G_2*
cause of functio laesa [loss of function] in AI	*swelling, pain*
histamine-mediated vascular events in AI	*arteriolar vasodilatation* → *endothelial cell contraction in venules* [BM exposed] → *increased vessel permeability*
cause of the stroke line, flare, and wheal in the Lewis triple response [dull object is drawn across the skin surface]	*stroke line*: histamine-mediated capillary dilatation; *flare at the periphery*: neurogenic-induced arteriolar dilatation; *wheal of the stroke line*: histamine-mediated increase in vessel permeability

Table continued on following page

Table 3–1. ACUTE INFLAMMATION (AI) *Continued*

Most Common...	Answer and Explanation
sequential neutrophil events in AI	*margination* [neutrophils pushed to the side in small vessels] → *neutrophil adhesion* to venular endothelium [due to adhesion molecule synthesis by neutrophils and endothelial cells] → *emigration* out of venules [neutrophil collagenases dissolve type IV collagen in exposed BM] → *directed chemotaxis* [neutrophils have G protein receptors, Gαp, causing them to move to the area of infection] → *opsonization* of bacteria [bacteria coated by IgG and C3b] → *phagocytosis* of opsonized bacteria [internalization of bacteria] → *killing* of bacteria
chemical mediators responsible for neutrophil synthesis of adhesion molecules [CD11/ CD18 complex with glycoproteins and β_1-β_2 integrins] and endothelial cell leukocyte and intercellular adhesion molecules	*C5a and LTB$_4$* (neutrophils only), *IL-1* and *TNF* (neutrophils and endothelial cell synthesis of adhesion molecules) [ELAM-1 synthesized in endothelial cells binds to neutrophil receptors. ICAM-1 adheres to neutrophil and lymphocyte receptors.]
clinical findings in β_2 integrin deficiency	*failure of separation of the umbilical cord in the newborn and absence of acute inflammatory cells in the umbilical cord*
chemical mediators serving as chemotactic agents	**C5a, LTB$_4$**, *IL-8*, *bacterial products*
causes of decreased adhesion molecule synthesis	**corticosteroids**, *catecholamines*, *lithium* [This increases the total neutrophil count by releasing the marginating pool.]
pathologic cause of increased adhesion molecule synthesis	*endotoxemia* in gram-negative sepsis [This lowers the total neutrophil count (absolute neutropenia).]
cause of the low total WBC count in black people	*increased marginating pool of neutrophils*, due to increased neutrophil adhesion [Normally, the peripheral circulating pool of neutrophils (pool counted in a CBC) and marginating pool are about equal.]

Table 3-1. ACUTE INFLAMMATION (AI) *Continued*

Most Common...	Answer and Explanation
type of interstitial fluid accumulation in AI	*exudate* containing neutrophils, RBCs, fibrin, and digested debris
O_2-dependent bactericidal systems in neutrophils and monocytes	*oxygen-dependent MPO system* (most potent system), *generation of superoxide FRs* [The MPO system requires O_2, NADPH oxidase (converts O_2 to superoxide), NADPH (cofactor), SOD (converts superoxide into peroxide), and chloride ions (MPO catalyzes the reaction between chloride ions and peroxide to form bleach, which kills bacteria.]
O_2-independent bactericidal systems in neutrophils, monocytes, and macrophages	*pH changes in phagolysosomes, lysosomal enzymes*
source of NADPH in the O_2-dependent MPO system	*the pentose phosphate shunt* [glucose 6-phosphate dehydrogenase is the key enzyme] is the major source of NADPH in the body
disease associated with deficiency of NADPH oxidase	*chronic granulomatous disease (CGD) of childhood* [It is an SXR disease. Deficiency of the enzyme leads to absence of peroxide and inability to form bleach, even though chloride ions and MPO are present in the phagolysosome.]
screening test for CGD	*Nitroblue tetrazolium (NBT) test* [Normally, conversion of molecular O_2 into superoxide FRs emits energy (called the respiratory burst). When colorless NBT is added to a test tube containing neutrophils, it is phagocytosed and superoxide converts NBT into a colored dye. In CGD, the respiratory burst is absent.]
COD in CGD	*sepsis due to catalase-positive bacteria* (e.g., *Staphylococcus aureus*) [Catalase from the bacteria destroys the peroxide generated by the organism, hence neutrophils are deprived of peroxide to synthesize bleach necessary to kill the bacteria.]

Table continued on following page

Table 3–1. ACUTE INFLAMMATION (AI) *Continued*

Most Common...	Answer and Explanation
genetic disease associated with a defect in microtubule polymerization	*Chédiak-Higashi syndrome* [It is an AR disease. Inability to polymerize microtubules impairs leukocyte motility (defective chemotaxis) and also results in delayed fusion of lysosomes with phagosomes to form phagolysosomes (responsible for the giant lysosomes noted in the peripheral blood leukocytes).]
cells involved in AI associated with bacteria, viruses, and allergic reactions	*neutrophils, lymphocytes,* and *eosinophils,* respectively
vasoactive amines	*histamine* and *serotonin* [Histamine is preformed in the granules of mast cells and basophils. Serotonin is present in the dense bodies of platelets. Both are vasodilators and increase vessel permeability.]
plasma-derived proteases	*coagulation factors, kinins* [These proteases (and complement) have a cascade type of system, in which one activated product activates the next product.]
complement factors involved in AI	*C3a* [anaphylatoxin; direct stimulation of mast cell release of histamine], *C3b* [opsonization], *C5a* [adhesion molecule synthesis, chemotactic agent, anaphylatoxin]
plasma-derived protease that activates the intrinsic clotting system, kinin system [source of bradykinin], and the fibrinolytic system [source of plasmin]	*Hageman factor XII*
drug that blocks the synthesis of both prostaglandins and leukotrienes	*corticosteroids* [They block phospholipase, which prevents cell membrane release of arachidonic acid. In AI, prostaglandins are vasodilators and increase vessel permeability. LTB_4 enhances adhesion molecule synthesis in neutrophils and is a chemotactic agent. $LTC_4,$-$D_4,$-E_4 are potent vaso- and bronchoconstrictors and increase vessel permeability.]

Table 3–1. ACUTE INFLAMMATION (AI) *Continued*

Most Common...	Answer and Explanation
drugs that block cyclooxygenase and the formation of prostaglandins	*aspirin* and *NSAIDs*
sources of IL-1 and TNF	*macrophages* and *endothelial cells*
site for synthesis of acute phase reactants	*liver* [IL-1 and TNF stimulate hepatocytes to synthesize various proteins (fibrinogen, CRP, complement, coagulation factors) and reduce synthesis of transferrin and albumin.]
stimulus for fever in AI	*IL-1* and *TNF* [They stimulate the synthesis of prostaglandin in the hypothalamus, which in turn activates the thermoregulatory center.]
benefits of fever	*it right-shifts the O_2 dissociation curve* (releases more O_2 to tissue) and *hinders viral and bacterial reproduction*
expression of serous inflammation [thin, watery exudate]	*blister fluid* (second-degree burn)
expression of catarrhal (phlegmonous) inflammation [excessive mucous secretions]	*runny nose* in the common cold
expression of fibrinous inflammation [exudate rich in fibrin, producing a "bread and butter" appearance of a serosal surface]	*fibrinous pericarditis* (rheumatic fever, uremia, SLE)
expression of suppurative inflammation [collection of pus in a localized area]	*abscess* (most commonly *Staphylococcus aureus*) [Abscesses are most commonly located on the skin.]

Table continued on following page

Table 3–1. ACUTE INFLAMMATION (AI) *Continued*

Most Common...	Answer and Explanation
expression of cellulitis [thin exudate that spreads in subcutaneous tissue]	*cellulitis due to Streptococcus pyogenes*
disorder associated with pseudo-membranous inflammation [toxin-induced membrane along a mucosal surface]	*pseudomembranous colitis due to Clostridium difficile* [Pseudomembranes also occur in diphtheria.]
outcome of AI	*organization and repair with scar tissue formation* [*Resolution* (restoration back to normal without scar formation) and *CI* are less frequent outcomes].
sequential reactions in healing by primary intention [wound edges are apposed]	wound fills with blood clot → neutrophils emigrate into wound (24 hours) → squamous cells migrate below clot and form a continuous lining (1–2 days) → macrophages replace neutrophils in wound; granulation tissue begins forming (vascular tissue with fibroblasts; 3 days) → granulation tissue peaks (5 days) → tensile strength of wound from type III collagen 10% (7–10 days) → maximal tensile strength of 80% (3 months; type III collagen replaced by type I collagen)
differences between secondary and primary intention wounds	secondary intention wounds are *not apposed* and *myofibroblasts* bring the wound edges together [Myofibroblasts have contractile properties.]
cell types involved in wound repair	*macrophages* (growth factors, phagocytosis of debris), *fibroblasts* (collagen synthesis in granulation tissue), *endothelial cells* (vessels in granulation tissue)
chemical mediators involved in wound repair	*fibronectin* (chemotactic for above cell types; molecular glue; promotes angiogenesis) and *basic fibroblast growth factor* (major promoter of angiogenesis)

Table 3–1. ACUTE INFLAMMATION (AI) *Continued*

Most Common...	Answer and Explanation
cause of poor wound repair	**infection** [Other causes: *malnutrition, scurvy, zinc deficiency* (zinc is a cofactor in collagenase in remodeling of collagen), *copper deficiency* (copper is a cofactor in lysyl oxidase involved in forming cross-links in collagen), *corticosteroids* (interfere with collagen synthesis), *DM* (glucose is a culture medium for bacteria; ischemia; impaired chemotaxis), *Ehlers-Danlos syndrome* (defect in collagen), *Marfan's syndrome* (defect in fibrillin in elastic tissue).]
source of collagen in organization and repair of liver tissue	*Ito cell* [It normally serves as a storage depot for retinoic acid, but in liver injury, it synthesizes collagen.]
site injured in the kidney	*renal medulla* [Only 10% of the 20–25% of the cardiac output devoted to the kidneys is directed to the medulla (cortex receives 90%), hence it lacks O_2 for effective repair of tissue.]
reserve cell responsible for organization and repair in the lungs	*type II pneumocyte* [This cell replaces type I pneumocytes and synthesizes surfactant.]
type of tissue involved in cardiac muscle repair	*scar tissue* [Cardiac muscle is permanent tissue, hence it is replaced with scar tissue.]
type of organization and repair in injury of the CNS	*gliosis* [Gliosis is equivalent to scar tissue formation outside the CNS. Astrocytes are analogous to fibroblasts. Astrocyte proliferation and extension of their protoplasmic processes provide support to the tissue.]
type of organization and repair of peripheral nerves	*Wallerian degeneration* [Axonal regeneration (axonal sprouts from the proximal end of the nerve) and myelination (from Schwann cells) occur after transection of a nerve.]

Table continued on following page

Table 3–1. ACUTE INFLAMMATION (AI) *Continued*

Question: Which of the following cells or chemical mediators has the **LEAST** significant role in the first 24 hours of AI?
  (A) Neutrophils
  (B) Histamine
  (C) C5a
  (D) Monocytes
  (E) Bradykinin

Answer: (D): In AI, neutrophils are the primary effector cell. Histamine is the key chemical mediator of AI and is a vasodilator and increases vessel permeability. C5a enhances adhesion molecule synthesis, is a chemotactic agent, and is an anaphylatoxin. Bradykinin is a vasodilator, increases vessel permeability, and produces pain.

AI = acute inflammation, AR = autosomal recessive, BM = basement membrane, CBC = complete blood cell count, CGD = chronic granulomatous disease, CI = chronic inflammation, CNS = central nervous system, COD = cause of death, CRP = C-reactive protein (nonspecific activator of the complement system and opsonizing agent), DM = diabetes mellitus, ELAM = endothelial cell leukocyte adhesion molecule, FR = free radical, ICAM-1 = intercellular adhesion molecule, IL = interleukin, MPO = myeloperoxidase, NADPH = nicotinamide adenine dinucleotide phosphate, NBT = nitroblue tetrazolium, NSAID = nonsteroidal anti-inflammatory drug, RBC = red blood cell, SLE = systemic lupus erythematosus, SOD = superoxide dismutase, SXR = sex-linked recessive, TNF = tumor necrosis factor, WBC = white blood cell.

Table 3–2. CHRONIC INFLAMMATION (CI)

Most Common...	Answer and Explanation
cause of CI	*AI*
types of diseases that are chronic at their inception	*autoimmune disease, granulomatous inflammation*
immunoglobulin (Ig) associated with CI	*IgG* [IgM is the most common Ig associated with AI before isotype switching after a week to 10 days.]
cell type in CI	*monocyte*

Table 3–2. **CHRONIC INFLAMMATION (CI)** *Continued*

Most Common...	Answer and Explanation
functions of monocyte	*transforms into a macrophage* (fixed or wandering), *contains growth factors, secretes IL-1 and TNF, synthesizes complement and nitric oxide* (potent vasodilator), *kills microbial pathogens* (O_2-dependent MPO system), *processes antigen, key cell in delayed hypersensitivity reactions, destroys intracellular microbial pathogens* [e.g., TB, systemic fungi, *Legionella*), *reservoir cells for HIV* [Other cell types in CI include lymphocytes, fibroblasts, endothelial cells, plasma cells.]
cell type in syphilis	*plasma cells* surrounding inflamed arterioles (called endarteritis obliterans)
cell type responsible for producing epithelioid and multinucleated giant cells in a granuloma	*macrophage* [Activated macrophages resemble epithelial cells (epithelioid). Epithelioid cells fuse together to form multinucleated giant cells when they die.]
cause of a sinus tract [communication with the skin surface]	*skin abscess* due to *Staphylococcus aureus*
cause of fistula in the GI tract [communication between two hollow organs]	**diverticulosis**, *Crohn's disease*
type of repair in CI	*fibrosis* (scar tissue formation)

Table continued on following page

Table 3–2. CHRONIC INFLAMMATION (CI) *Continued*

Question: Which of the following is more likely to represent chronic rather than AI?
(A) Rheumatoid arthritis
(B) Appendicitis
(C) *Streptococcus pneumoniae* pneumonia
(D) Rhinitis in a common cold
(E) Bee sting site

Answer: (A): rheumatoid arthritis is a chronic inflammatory condition that begins in the synovial tissue and eventually involves the destruction of articular cartilage. The other choices listed are acute inflammatory reactions.

AI = acute inflammation, CI = chronic inflammation, GI = gastrointestinal, HIV = human immunodeficiency virus, Ig = immunoglobulin, IL = interleukin, MPO = myeloperoxidase, TB = tuberculosis, TNF = tumor necrosis factor.

Table 3–3. LABORATORY TEST ABNORMALITIES IN ACUTE AND CHRONIC INFLAMMATION

Most Common...	Answer and Explanation
neutrophil response in AI	*absolute neutrophilic leukocytosis* [increased neutrophil count in a CBC], *left shift* [≥10 band neutrophils in a 100 WBC differential count], *toxic granulation* [prominence of azurophilic granules containing MPO in neutrophils], *phagolysosomes* [evidence of phagocytosis], *Döhle bodies* [dull gray cytoplasmic inclusions representing dilated endoplasmic reticulum]
CBC finding in viral infections	*absolute lymphocytosis* [increased number of lymphocytes in a 100 cell differential count] [Some infections produce normal-appearing lymphocytes (e.g., infectious lymphocytosis), while others produce antigenically stimulated (atypical) lymphocytes (e.g., infectious mononucleosis, viral hepatitis). Some bacterial infections produce a lymphocytosis, particularly those due to *Bordetella pertussis*.]

Table 3–3. LABORATORY TEST ABNORMALITIES IN ACUTE AND CHRONIC INFLAMMATION *Continued*

Most Common...	Answer and Explanation
CBC finding in type I hypersensitivity reactions and invasive helminthic infections	*eosinophilia* [Protozoal infections do not produce eosinophilia. Pinworm infections do not produce eosinophilia, since they are noninvasive. Strongyloidiasis, hookworm infections, etc., do produce eosinophilia.]
CBC finding in CI	*monocytosis* [Monocytes are the primary cell of CI.]
anemia in CI	*anemia of chronic inflammation* [Iron is delivered to macrophages by neutrophil-derived lactoferrin, where it is blocked from being used for erythropoiesis. This lowers the serum iron. Increased iron stores reduce liver synthesis of transferrin (binding protein for iron); hence the total iron-binding capacity (TIBC) is also decreased.]
factors increasing/ decreasing the ESR	*fibrinogen* and *gamma globulins* [Both of these produce rouleaux ("stack of coins" effect), which increases the rate of settling of RBCs in a test tube over a 1-hour period. Inflammation and anemia increase the ESR. In sickle cell anemia and polycythemia, the ESR is zero, since abnormally shaped RBCs and excess numbers of RBCs do not settle well.]
reason for ordering a SPE	*rule out a monoclonal gammopathy* (MG; e.g., multiple myeloma) [MGs are spikes in the γ-globulin region that are due to synthesis of a single Ig from a single clone of plasma cells.]
peaks identified in a routine SPE	in sequential order from anode to cathode: *prealbumin, albumin,* α_1-globulins (contain AAT), α_2-globulins (contain haptoglobin, α_2-macroglobulin), β-*globulins* (contain transferrin, complement, LDL), γ-*globulins* (contain IgG, IgA, IgM, IgD, IgE), and *CRP*
functions of prealbumin (transthyretin)	*complexes with retinol-binding protein to bind both thyroxine and retinoic acid*

Table continued on following page

Table 3–3. LABORATORY TEST ABNORMALITIES IN ACUTE AND CHRONIC INFLAMMATION *Continued*

Most Common...	Answer and Explanation
functions of albumin	*due to a strong negative charge, it avidly binds cations (calcium, magnesium), drugs, fatty acids, and UCB; it is also responsible for 80% of the oncotic pressure in plasma (keeps fluid in vessels)*
cause of hypocalcemia	*hypoalbuminemia* [Albumin binds 40% of the calcium. Measured total calcium is calcium bound to albumin, calcium bound to phosphate/sulfate (13%), and free, ionized calcium (47%). To correct the total calcium for the degree of hypoalbuminemia, the following formula is useful: corrected calcium = total calcium − serum albumin + 4.]
function of AAT	*an antiprotease that neutralizes elastase in tissue* [Genetic deficiency of AAT or inactivation of AAT by cigarette smoke allows elastases from neutrophils in the lung to destroy the elastic tissue support of the airways, leading to COPD.]
SPE finding in AAT deficiency	*flat α_1-peak* [AAT deficiency is an AR disease that may produce liver disease in children or panacinar emphysema in adults that is limited to the lower lobes.]
function of haptoglobin	*binds to Hb to form a Hb-haptoglobin complex that is phagocytosed by macrophages* [This salvages the amino acids and iron that would be lost by eliminating Hb in the urine. Low haptoglobin levels are an excellent marker of intravascular hemolysis.]
location on a SPE for IgA	*the junction of the β and γ peaks* [IgA is increased in alcoholic cirrhosis, hence filling in the valley between the two peaks results in a single β-γ peak.]
Ig responsible for the size of the γ-globulin peak	*IgG* [The concentration of Igs in descending order are IgG, IgA, IgM, IgD, and IgE. Hence, an increase in IgG automatically increases the size of the γ-globulin peak.]
cause of a polyclonal gammopathy	*CI with an increase in IgG* [IgG is the primary Ig of CI, hence its increase by multiple clones of plasma cells results in a diffuse increase in the size of the γ-globulin peak.]

Table 3–3. LABORATORY TEST ABNORMALITIES IN ACUTE AND CHRONIC INFLAMMATION *Continued*

Most Common...	Answer and Explanation
cause of a flat γ-globulin peak	*decreased concentration of IgG* [Hypogammaglobulinemia, which includes low IgG levels, is noted in Bruton's agammaglobulinemia, nephrotic syndrome, CLL.]
clinical usefulness of CRP	*marker of bacterial infection versus viral infection* [CRP is only increased in bacterial infections and conditions with excessive necrosis (e.g., AMI).]

Question: Which of the following would more likely be noted in an acute rather than chronic bacterial infection?
(A) Polyclonal gammopathy
(B) Left-shifted smear
(C) Monocytosis
(D) Macrophage blockade of iron
(E) Increased ESR

Answer: (B): A left-shifted smear means a band neutrophil count ≥10% in a 100 WBC differential count. Neutrophils are the dominant cells in AI. Monocytes (choice C) and anemia of CI (choice D) are more common in CI. Polyclonal gammopathy implies an increase in IgG, which is a feature of CI. The ESR is increased in both AI and CI.

AAT = α₁-antitrypsin, AI = acute inflammation, AMI = acute myocardial infarction, AR = autosomal recessive, CBC = complete blood cell count, CI = chronic inflammation, CLL = chronic lymphocytic leukemia, COPD = chronic obstructive pulmonary disease, CRP = C-reactive protein, ESR = erythrocyte sedimentation rate, Hb = hemoglobin, Ig = immunoglobulin, LDL = low density lipoprotein, MG = monoclonal gammopathy, MPO = myeloperoxidase, RBC = red blood cell, SPE = serum protein electrophoresis, TIBC = total iron binding capacity, UCB = unconjugated bilirubin, WBC = white blood cell.

CHAPTER

IMMUNOPATHOLOGY

CONTENTS

Table 4–1. HEREDITARY AND ACQUIRED IMMUNODEFICIENCIES

Most Common...	Answer and Explanation
components of natural immunity	*physicochemical barriers* (e.g., skin), *complement system, interferons, phagocytic cells* (e.g., neutrophils, monocytes/macrophages), *acute phase reactants* (e.g., coagulation factors), *macrophage cytokines* (e.g., IL-1), *natural killer (NK)* cells
NK cell functions	*antibody-mediated cellular cytotoxicity (type II hypersensitivity) reactions, graft-versus-host reactions*, and *destruction of tumor and virus-infected cells*
morphologic appearance of NK cells in the PB	*large granular lymphocytes*
components of specific immunity	*B cells* (humoral immunity with antibody production) and *T cells* (cellular immunity)
B cell functions	*Ig synthesis* (G, A, M, D, E), *defense against encapsulated organisms, neutralization of bacterial and chemical toxins, mucosal defense against pathogens and pollens* (e.g., secretory IgA)

Table continued on following page

Table 4–1. HEREDITARY AND ACQUIRED IMMUNODEFICIENCIES *Continued*

Most Common...	Answer and Explanation
T cell functions	*defense against intracellular pathogens, DHRs, regulation of B lymphocytes* (CD8 suppressor T cells), and *lymphokine production* (e.g., IL-2)
lymphocyte in the PB	*CD4 helper T cells* [T cells account for 60% of the PB lymphocytes. The normal ratio of CD4 to CD8 T cells is 2 : 1; therefore, CD4 cells are the most abundant cells.]
B cell tests	*Ig concentration, marker studies* (presence of surface μ heavy chains [antigen recognition site] connotes mature B cells, intracytoplasmic μ heavy chains, a pre-B cell), *presence of isohemagglutinins* (e.g., anti-A [IgM antibody] in a blood group B individual; simplest screening test), *B cell count* (10–20% of lymphocytes), *B cell mitogen stimulation* (functional test; use staphylococcal A antigen and pokeweed), *lymph node biopsy* (B cells present in follicles, presence of plasma cells)
T cell tests	*T cell count* (flow cytometry), *marker studies* (identify T cell subsets [CD_4 helper cells, CD_8 cytotoxic/suppressor cells, TdT [indicates immature T cell]), *mitogen stimulation* (PHA, con A), *intradermal skin testing with common antigens* (functional T cell test; use streptokinase/streptodornase, *Candida* [most cost-effective test], mumps antigens (no reaction indicates anergy), *lymph node biopsy* (T cells present in paracortical areas)
predisposing causes of ID	**infections** (e.g., AIDS), *prematurity, autoimmune disease, lymphoproliferative disease* (e.g., CLL), *immunosuppressive therapy* (e.g., corticosteroids)
complication associated with ID	*infections* [B cell deficiencies have problems with defense against encapsulated pathogens (e.g., *Streptococcus pneumoniae*), whereas T cell deficiencies have problems with intracellular pathogens (e.g., TB, fungi, viruses). Other problems include an increase in leukemia/lymphoma and autoimmune disease.]

Table 4–1. HEREDITARY AND ACQUIRED
IMMUNODEFICIENCIES Continued

Most Common...	Answer and Explanation
source of IgG in a newborn's blood	*transplacental passage of maternal IgG*
cause of increased IgM in a newborn's blood	*congenital infection* (CMV is the most common infection)
site of isohemagglutinin synthesis in an infant	*Peyer's patches in the small intestine* [A and B antigens in food are the stimulus for antibody production.]
source of IgA in a newborn	*colostrum in breast milk*
cause of Bruton's agammaglobulinemia	*failure of pre-B cells to differentiate into mature B cells* [Bruton's agammaglobulinemia is an SXR disease. Absence of mature B cells connotes absence of plasma cells, resulting in hypogammaglobulinemia.]
genetic ID	*IgA deficiency* [It occurs in 1 in 500 individuals. It is an intrinsic defect in the differentiation of B cells committed to synthesizing IgA.]
complications associated with IgA deficiency	**sinopulmonary disease**, *diarrhea* (giardiasis), *allergies, autoimmune disease, anaphylactic reaction if infused with blood products containing IgA*
cause of ID in common variable ID	*defect in the maturation of mature B cells into plasma cells*
ID associated with EBV	*sex-linked lymphoproliferative syndrome* [It is associated with hypogammaglobulinemia and malignant lymphoproliferative disease.]
ID associated with an IgG_2 and IgG_4 subclass deficiency	*IgA deficiency*
cause of ID in DiGeorge syndrome	*failure of the third* (inferior parathyroids/thymus) *and fourth* (superior parathyroids) *pharyngeal pouches to develop* [It presents with tetany and absence of the thymic shadow on a chest radiograph.]

Table continued on following page

Table 4–1. HEREDITARY AND ACQUIRED IMMUNODEFICIENCIES *Continued*

Most Common...	Answer and Explanation
immunologic complication and infection associated with blood transfusion in T cell–deficient patients	*graft-versus-host reaction* (see below) and *CMV, respectively* [CMV is present in donor lymphocytes. Donor transfusions should be irradiated prior to transfusion to prevent both complications.]
enzyme deficiency that is present in severe combined B and T cell ID (SCID)	*deficiency of adenine deaminase* [This enzyme is necessary to degrade adenine, which is toxic to both B and T lymphocytes.]
genetic ID treated by gene therapy	*SCID* [Reported cures have been documented with gene therapy.]
S/S of Wiskott-Aldrich syndrome	*combined B and T cell ID associated with a triad of eczema, thrombocytopenia, and recurrent sinopulmonary infections* [It is an SXR disease with a characteristic failure of an Ig response to polysaccharide antigens. Bone marrow transplantation may be curative].
S/S of ataxia telangiectasia	*AR disease with combined B and T cell ID, characterized by cerebellar ataxia and arteriolar telangiectasias around the eyes and on the skin* [Owing to chromosome instability, there is an increased incidence of leukemia/lymphoma. It is also associated with an elevated serum AFP.]

Question: Which of the following immunodeficiencies would **MOST LIKELY** be complicated by *Pneumocystis carinii* pneumonia and cyanotic congenital heart disease?
(A) Bruton's agammaglobulinemia
(B) Common variable immunodeficiency
(C) Wiskott-Aldrich syndrome
(D) Ataxia telangiectasia
(E) DiGeorge syndrome

Answer: (E): DiGeorge syndrome is a T cell ID, hence PCP is a common finding. It is also associated with truncus arteriosus, which is a cause of cyanotic CHD. Choices C and D also have T cell deficiency, but they are not associated with CHD. Choices A and B represent B cell ID states, so PCP is not likely to be a complication.

AIDS = acquired immunodeficiency syndrome, AFP = alpha-fetoprotein, AR = autosomal recessive, CHD = congenital heart disease, CLL = chronic lymphocytic leukemia, CMV = cytomegalovirus, con A = concanavalin A, DHR = delayed hypersensitivity reaction, EBV = Epstein-Barr virus, ID = immunodeficiency, Ig = immunoglobulin, IL = interleukin, NK = natural killer, PB = peripheral blood, PCP = *Pneumocystis carinii* pneumonia, PHA = phytohemagglutinin, SCID = severe combined immunodeficiency, S/S = signs and symptoms, SXR = sex-linked recessive, TB = tuberculosis, TdT = terminal deoxynucleotidyltransferase.

Table 4–2. ACQUIRED IMMUNODEFICIENCY SYNDROME (AIDS)

Most Common...	Answer and Explanation
acquired immunodeficiency (ID) in the United States	*AIDS*
etiologic agent in the United States	*human immunodeficiency virus* (HIV)-1 (RNA retrovirus) [HIV-2 is the most common cause in West and Central America.]
cause of death in women and black men between 25 and 44 years of age	*AIDS* [Accidents (usually motor vehicle) are now the most common cause of death in white men in this age bracket.]
incidence of AIDS, by racial group	**whites** 47%, *blacks 35%, Hispanics 18%, Asians <1%, Native Americans <1%*
attachment site on a helper T cell of viral gp120 [viral envelope protein]	*CD4 molecule* [It also attaches to CD4 molecules on monocytes, macrophages, dendritic cells, astrocytes, and microglial cells (CNS macrophage). It requires a coreceptor for fusion to the host cell membrane.]
protein surrounding viral genomic RNA	*p24 core protein* [It is increased in serum at two times: at the initial infection and when the patient develops AIDS.]
cell that is lysed by the virus	*CD4 T helper cell* [It is lysed by apoptosis, NK cells, ADCC, direct HIV cytotoxicity, or HIV-specific cytolytic T lymphocytes.]
reservoir cell for viral replication	*monocyte lineage cells* (macrophage, dendritic cells) [Viruses replicate in these cells without killing them.]

Table continued on following page

Table 4–2. ACQUIRED IMMUNODEFICIENCY
SYNDROME (AIDS) *Continued*

Most Common...	Answer and Explanation
role of reverse transcriptase	*converts genomic RNA into proviral double-stranded DNA* (integrated into target cell's DNA with virally encoded integrase enzyme)
HIV genome site encoding envelope proteins gp120 and gp41, reverse transcriptase and integrase, and p24 core antigen	*env*, *pol*, and *gag*, respectively
body fluids containing the virus	*blood* (most infective body fluid), *saliva, semen, amniotic fluid, breast milk, spinal fluid, urine, tears,* and *bronchoalveolar lavage material*
mode of transmission in the United States	*intimate sexual contact between men* [Blood is the second most common mode (intravenous drug abuse and sharing needles). Heterosexual transmission is the most common mode of transmission worldwide.]
mode of sexual transmission in the United States	*receptive anal intercourse between men* [This is followed in descending order by *vaginal intercourse male to female* and *vaginal intercourse female to male.*]
mode of transmission in women	*heterosexual transmission in minority females who are IV drug abusers* (sharing contaminated needles and/or vaginal intercourse with males who are HIV positive)
mechanism of transmission by anal intercourse	*direct inoculation into the blood from mucosal trauma or an open wound* (e.g., syphilitic chancre)
blood product containing virus	*whole blood/packed red blood cells* (1 in 676,000 risk of transmission per unit)
mode of transmission in health care workers	*accidental needle stick* (0.3% risk)
mode of transmission in children	*vertical transmission* (mother to fetus) *from an infected mother* (90%) [Most cases are transplacental, followed by breast feeding.]

Table 4–2. ACQUIRED IMMUNODEFICIENCY SYNDROME (AIDS) *Continued*

Most Common...	Answer and Explanation
treatment of pregnant women who are HIV positive	*AZT* [It has reduced the rate of newborns' developing AIDS from ~25–30% to 7.6%.]
cause of a positive EIA test for HIV in a newborn	*transplacental transmission of the IgG antibody from the infected mother*
tests to document HIV infection in a newborn	**detection of HIV RNA by PCR** *(best test), culture of HIV from lymphocytes, p24 antigen capture assay*
antibody detected by EIA	*anti-gp120 antibody* [Sensitivity of EIA is 99.5–99.8% but the specificity is poor owing to the low prevalence of HIV positivity in the general population. EIA is positive in 4–8 weeks.]
test performed if the EIA is indeterminate or positive	*Western blot assay* [A positive test result is the presence of p24 and gp41 antibodies and either gp120 or gp160 antibodies. The combined positive predictive value of a positive EIA and Western blot is 99.5%.]
tests performed to screen for HIV in blood banks	*p24 capture assay, EIA for HIV-1 and HIV-2*
test used to monitor the current immune status of an HIV-positive patient	*CD4 T helper cell count* [For example, a count <200 cells/μL implies an increased risk for PCP and the need for prophylaxis (trimethoprim) against *Pneumocystis carinii* and also against *Toxoplasma*.]
test to monitor viral burden in an HIV-positive patient	*HIV RNA by PCR*
immunologic abnormalities	*lymphopenia, anergy to skin testing, hypergammaglobulinemia* (polyclonal stimulation of B cells by EBV and CMV), *decreased mitogen blastogenesis of T cells, decreased production of cytokines, dysfunctional NK cells, increased p24 antigens, CD4:CD8 ratio <1*

Table continued on following page

Table 4–2. ACQUIRED IMMUNODEFICIENCY SYNDROME (AIDS) Continued

Most Common...	Answer and Explanation
PPD skin test value that is considered positive	*>5 mm induration* (set for highest sensitivity)
initial presentation of HIV infection	*mononucleosis-like syndrome 3–6 weeks after contracting the virus*
phase following the acute HIV syndrome	*asymptomatic, clinically latent phase* [Viral replication is occurring in dendritic cells in lymph nodes.]
phase following the asymptomatic latent phase	*early symptomatic phase* [This phase is marked by non–AIDS-defining infections, generalized lymphadenopathy, and hematologic abnormalities.]
non–AIDS-defining infections in the early symptomatic phase	**oral thrush**, *oral hairy leukoplakia* (EBV infection of the tongue), *recurrent herpes simplex or herpes genitalis, condyloma acuminata (HPV), shingles (herpes zoster),* and *molluscum contagiosum* (poxvirus)
hematologic abnormality in the early symptomatic phase	*thrombocytopenia* [Possible mechanisms include immunocomplex destruction (type III hypersensitivity) and antibodies directed against platelet antigens (type II hypersensitivity).]
AIDS-defining conditions: HIV positive plus	*CD4 T helper cell count <200 cells/µL, specific malignancies* (e.g., Kaposi's sarcoma), *specific infections* (e.g., PCP)
AIDS-defining malignancies	**Kaposi's sarcoma**, *Burkitt's lymphoma, invasive cervical cancer, primary CNS malignant lymphoma*
AIDS-defining opportunistic bacterial infections	**MAI (disseminated or extrapulmonary)**, *Mycobacterium kansasii* (disseminated or intrapulmonary), *Mycobacterium tuberculosis* (any site), *recurrent pneumonia, Salmonella septicemia*
AIDS-defining opportunistic fungal infections	**PCP**, *candidiasis* (airways, esophagus), *coccidioidomycosis* (disseminated or extrapulmonary), *cryptococcosis* (extrapulmonary), *histoplasmosis* (disseminated or extrapulmonary)

Table 4–2. ACQUIRED IMMUNODEFICIENCY SYNDROME (AIDS) *Continued*

Most Common...	Answer and Explanation
systemic fungal infection	*candidiasis*
CNS systemic fungal infection	*cryptococcosis* [It commonly produces meningitis.]
opportunistic viral infections	**CMV** (involving tissues other than liver, lymph nodes, and spleen), *CMV retinitis with visual loss*, *H. simplex* (with chronic ulcers, esophagitis, bronchitis, pneumonia), *HIV-related encephalopathy* (AIDS dementia), *HIV-related wasting syndrome*, *progressive multifocal leukoencephalopathy* (papovavirus)
opportunistic parasitic viral infections	**CNS toxoplasmosis**, *cryptosporidiosis* (chronic intestinal >1 month), *isosporiasis* (chronic intestinal >1 month)
target organ involved	*lungs (PCP)*
cause of fever, night sweats, and weight loss	*MAI*
cause of lymphoid interstitial pneumonia in children	*EBV*
fungal organism involving the GI tract	*Candida*
protozoan that is acid-fast positive and a cause of diarrhea	*Cryptosporidium*
infectious cause of a Whipple-like syndrome	*MAI* [The organisms infect the macrophages in the lamina propria of the small bowel, which in turn block off lymphatic drainage from the intestinal cell.]
cause of anal squamous cancer	*HPV* [This complication is related to anal intercourse.]

Table continued on following page

Table 4–2. ACQUIRED IMMUNODEFICIENCY SYNDROME (AIDS) *Continued*

Most Common...	Answer and Explanation
cause of viral hepatitis	*HBV*
cause of Kaposi's sarcoma	*herpesvirus 8*
disease that simulates Kaposi's sarcoma	*bacillary angiomatosis due to Bartonella henselae*
cutaneous lesion in AIDS	*Kaposi's sarcoma* [It is a vascular malignancy.]
malignant lymphoma in AIDS	*B cell immunoblastic lymphoma* [It is a high-grade malignancy.]
malignant lymphoma in AIDS that is related to EBV	*Burkitt's lymphoma*
cause of primary CNS malignant lymphoma	*HIV in association with EBV*
extranodal site for malignant lymphoma in AIDS	*CNS*
drug-induced cause of marrow suppression in AIDS	*AZT*
nutritional cause of anemia in AIDS	*vitamin B_{12} deficiency*
cause of neutropenia in AIDS	*marrow suppression from AZT*
renal disease	*focal segmental glomerulosclerosis* [It produces the nephrotic syndrome.]
drugs that produce nephrotoxic damage	*amphotericin* (treatment of systemic fungal infections), *pentamidine* (treatment of PCP), *foscarnet* (treatment of disseminated CMV)

Table 4–2. ACQUIRED IMMUNODEFICIENCY SYNDROME (AIDS) *Continued*

Most Common...	Answer and Explanation
cause of weight loss of >10%, fever, chronic diarrhea >1 month, and fatigue	*HIV-related wasting syndrome* [It is one of the top three causes of death in AIDS.]
source of entry of HIV into the CNS	*monocytes*
reservoir cell in the CNS	*microglial cell (CNS macrophage)*
CNS disease in AIDS associated with multinucleated giant cells	*HIV-encephalopathy (AIDS dementia complex)* [The multinucleated giant cells are fused microglial cells. This concentrates the virus to localized areas in the brain.]
HIV-related CNS disease	*HIV encephalopathy* (60%) [It is characterized by motor impairment, cognitive deficits, neurologic deficits, and behavioral impairment.]
type of HIV-related spinal cord lesion	*vacuolar myelopathy* (20–30%) [It is similar to vitamin B_{12} deficiency, mainly subacute combined degeneration (posterior column and lateral corticospinal tract).]
type of HIV-related peripheral neuropathy	*ascending type of paralysis reminiscent of Guillain-Barré syndrome*
cause of a space-occupying lesion in the CNS	*toxoplasmosis*
cause of focal epileptic seizures	*toxoplasmosis*
cause of blindness	*CMV retinitis* [Treat with ganciclovir.]
mechanism of action of dideoxynucleoside drugs	*block reverse transcriptase*
recommendation to prevent AIDS	*sexual abstinence* [In lieu of this, latex condoms with non–oxynol-9 viral spermicide is recommended.]

Table continued on following page

Table 4–2. ACQUIRED IMMUNODEFICIENCY
SYNDROME (AIDS) *Continued*

Most Common...	Answer and Explanation
type of polio vaccine that should be given to HIV-positive patients	*Salk* (killed) *vaccine*
live viral vaccine permitted in HIV-positive patients	*measles/mumps/rubella* [The natural infection is worse than the potential infection from the vaccination.]

Question: Arrange the following modes of transmission of HIV in descending order of infectivity: 1. male to female by vaginal intercourse, 2. female to male by vaginal intercourse, 3. male to male by anal intercourse.
(A) 3-2-1
(B) 2-3-1
(C) 3-1-2
(D) 2-1-3
(E) 1-3-2

Answer: (C): The incidence of male homosexual transmission is decreasing, but it still leads the list for transmission.

ADCC = antibody-dependent cell-mediated cytotoxicity, AIDS = acquired immunodeficiency syndrome, AZT = azidothymidine, CMV = cytomegalovirus, CNS = central nervous system, EBV = Epstein-Barr virus, EIA = enzyme immunoassay, GI = gastrointestinal, HBV = hepatitis B, HIV = human immunodeficiency virus, HPV = human papillomavirus, ID = immunodeficiency, IV = intravenous, MAI = *Mycobacterium avium-intracellulare*, NK = natural killer, PCP = *Pneumocystis carinii* pneumonia, PCR = polymerase chain reaction, PPD = purified protein derivative (tuberculin).

Table 4–3. COMPLEMENT SYSTEM AND QUALITATIVE
PHAGOCYTIC DISORDERS

Most Common...	Answer and Explanation
site for complement synthesis	*liver*
function of complement	*enhance natural immune host defenses*

**Table 4–3. COMPLEMENT SYSTEM AND QUALITATIVE
PHAGOCYTIC DISORDERS** *Continued*

Most Common...	Answer and Explanation
host defense activities	*opsonization* (C3b), *anaphylatoxins* (C3a and C5a; stimulate histamine release from mast cells), *chemotactic agents* (C5a), *synthesis of neutrophil adhesion molecules* (C5a), *cytotoxic immune reactions* (type II hypersensitivity), *immune complex reactions* (type III hypersensitivity)
activators of the classical pathway	**IgM** (most potent), *IgG* (requires two molecules), *immune complexes* (e.g., SLE)
activators of the alternative pathway	*endotoxin* (most potent), *IgA*, *immune complexes* (e.g., group A streptococcal GN)
factor inactivating C3 convertase (C4b2a) on cell membranes	*decay accelerating factor (DAF)* [It is deficient in paroxysmal nocturnal hemoglobinuria.]
inhibitor of C1 esterase	*C1 esterase inhibitor* [It is deficient in the AD disease hereditary angioedema.]
complement factors used to identify classical pathway, alternative pathway, and both pathway dysfunction	*C2 or C4, factor B, C3*, respectively
test to assess functional activity of the complement system	CH_{50} *total hemolytic complement assay* [It tests the ability of the complement system to lyse sheep RBCs coated with rabbit IgG antibodies against sheep RBC antigens. Low values indicate low complement levels.]
cause of complement deficiency	*consumption of complement in immune complex disease*
S/S of C1 esterase inhibitor deficiency	*an AD disease* (unusual for an AD disease to be an enzyme deficiency) *with increased production of C2-derived kinins that produce increased vessel permeability and edema, leading to recurrent swelling of the face and/ or oropharynx*

Table continued on following page

Table 4–3. COMPLEMENT SYSTEM AND QUALITATIVE PHAGOCYTIC DISORDERS *Continued*

Most Common...	Answer and Explanation
screening test for hereditary angioedema (C1 esterase inhibitor deficiency)	*C4 levels (low concentration)* [In addition, C2 is low and C3 is normal. The enzyme assay is the confirmatory test. Androgens are used in therapy.]
hereditary complement deficiency	*C2 deficiency* [It is associated with SLE in children.]
hereditary complement deficiency associated with severe infections	*C3 deficiency* [C3b is an important opsonin.]
complement deficiencies in disseminated gonococcemia	*C5 through C8 deficiency* [These components are necessary for phagocytosis of the organism.]
cause of NADPH oxidase deficiency	*chronic granulomatous disease of childhood* (see Table 3–1)
genetic defect involving defective microtubule polymerization	*Chédiak-Higashi syndrome* (see Table 3–1)
defect seen in newborns	*phagocytic dysfunction, particularly chemotactic dysfunction*
phagocytic defects in DM	*impaired chemotaxis, phagocytosis, intracellular killing,* and *cell-mediated immunity*

Table 4–3. COMPLEMENT SYSTEM AND QUALITATIVE PHAGOCYTIC DISORDERS *Continued*

Question: In a patient with recurrent attacks of laryngeal edema and laboratory evidence of low C4 levels, normal C3, and normal factor B, the pathogenesis is most closely related to which of the following?
(A) Endotoxemia
(B) Immunocomplex disease
(C) C1 esterase inhibitor deficiency
(D) Hereditary deficiency of C4
(E) Activation of the classical pathway by IgM

Answer: (C): The patient has hereditary angioedema, an AD disease characterized by a deficiency of the inhibitor for C1 esterase. Lab findings include low C2, low C4, normal C3, normal factor B, and low enzyme levels. Factor B and C3 are low in endotoxemia, since it activates the alternative pathway. Immune complexes that activate either pathway should have low C3 levels as well as activation of the classical pathway by IgM.

AD = autosomal dominant, DM = diabetes mellitus, GN = glomerulonephritis, Ig = immunoglobulin, RBC = red blood cell, SLE = systemic lupus erythematosus, S/S = signs and symptoms.

Table 4–4. MAJOR HISTOCOMPATIBILITY (HLA) COMPLEX AND TRANSPLANTATION

Most Common...	Answer and Explanation
chromosome site of the HLA system	*chromosome 6*
membrane glycoproteins synthesized	*HLA-A, -B, -C, -D* (and their subdivisions)
function of the HLA system	*marker of identity* [HLA antigens are usually different in each person.]
sites for synthesis of class I antigens	*HLA-A, -B, -C* [Class I antigens are recognized by CD8 cytotoxic T cells.]
site for synthesis of class II antigens	*HLA-D loci* [Class II antigens are located on antigen-presenting cells (macrophages, dendritic cells, B cells, activated T cells) and interact with CD4 T helper cells.]
method of inheritance of HLA antigens	*co-dominant inheritance* [Co-dominance means that the haplotypes inherited from both the mother and father are able to express themselves.]

Table continued on following page

Table 4–4. MAJOR HISTOCOMPATIBILITY (HLA)
COMPLEX AND TRANSPLANTATION *Continued*

Most Common...	Answer and Explanation
cell type lacking HLA antigens	*mature RBCs*
non-nucleated hematopoietic cell with HLA antigens	*platelets*
transplantation test utilized to identify the HLA antigens in a patient	*lymphocyte microcytotoxicity test* [Specific antibodies against HLA antigens plus complement are mixed together with patient lymphocytes. Lysis of the lymphocytes indicates a match. This test is good for identifying HLA-A, -B, and some -D antigens.]
transplantation test utilized to detect preformed anti-HLA antibodies in a patient's serum	*lymphocyte cross-match* [The patient's serum plus complement is mixed with donor lymphocytes. Lysis of the donor lymphocytes indicates that anti-HLA antibodies are present. The exact antibodies are then determined by reacting them with a panel of lymphocytes with known HLA antigens.]
transplantation test utilized to test for compatibility between the class II (D antigens) of a patient and a donor	*mixed lymphocyte reaction* [The patient's lymphocytes are functional and donor lymphocytes are inactivated. They are mixed together in a test tube with tritiated thymidine. An increased radioactive count indicates dissimilar D antigens to which the patient's lymphocytes are reacting. No reaction indicates identity of the D loci.]
type of transplant with the best graft survival	**autograft** [transfer of tissue from self to self] [Other graft types include *isograft* (between identical twins), *allograft* (between two unrelated individuals of the same species), *xenograft* (between two different species; e.g., pig heart in a human).]
source for finding compatible donors for transplantation	*siblings* [In a family with four children, there is a 25% chance of an identical two-haplotype match, 50% chance of a one-haplotype match, and 25% chance of no haplotype match. A parent is automatically a one-haplotype match.]

Table 4–4. MAJOR HISTOCOMPATIBILITY (HLA)
COMPLEX AND TRANSPLANTATION *Continued*

Most Common...	Answer and Explanation
factors that improve graft survival	**ABO compatibility**, absence of *anti-HLA antibodies*, and *HLA compatibility between D loci*
cause of a hyper-acute rejection	*ABO incompatibility* or the *presence of anti-HLA antibodies* against donor tissue [This is a type II hypersensitivity reaction leading to immediate thrombosis of donor vessels and death of donor tissue.]
type of transplant rejection	*acute rejection* [It usually occurs within 3 months (most commonly between 10 and 14 days). It is a combination of cell-mediated immunity with cytotoxic CD8 T cells producing parenchymal damage and humoral immunity, where antibodies produce vessel thickening and ischemic damage.]
cell types involved in acute rejection	*donor macrophages*, whose class I antigens interact with *host CD8 cytotoxic T cells* and whose class II antigens interact with *host CD4 T helper cells* [Helper T cells release IL-2, which increases host CD4 and CD8 proliferation and B cell production of antibodies. CD8 cytotoxic cells attack class I antigens in the graft and antibodies attack vessel endothelium.]
drugs used to prevent acute rejection	*cyclosporine* (inhibits CD4 T helper release of IL-2), *corticosteroids* (suppresses host immune response), *OKT₃* (monoclonal antibody directed against host T cell antigen recognition sites)
immune reactions in chronic rejection	*possibly recurrent antibody-mediated damage to vessels leading to intimal fibrosis and ischemic damage to the parenchyma with subsequent atrophy and fibrosis*
transplants associated with GVH	**bone marrow** *and liver*
cell types involved in GVH	*donor T lymphocytes* and *NK cells* [Cytokines released by donor T cells damage host tissue and stimulate proliferation of CD8 cytotoxic T cells, which also attack host tissue. IL-2 released from donor CD4 T cells activates host NK, which become lymphokine-activated killer cells, which lyse normal host cells.]

Table continued on following page

Table 4–4. MAJOR HISTOCOMPATIBILITY (HLA) COMPLEX AND TRANSPLANTATION *Continued*

Most Common...	Answer and Explanation
target tissues involved in GVH	*bile duct epithelium* (epithelial cell necrosis of small bile ducts leading to jaundice), *skin* (maculopapular rash), and *GI tract* (mucosal ulceration with bloody diarrhea)
tissue transplant with the best overall survival	*corneal transplant* [The cornea is avascular.]
type of renal transplant with the best survival	*transplant between living donors with a two-haplotype match* (90–95%; e.g., sibling, identical twin) [Cadaver transplants have ~80% 5-year survival.]
malignancy associated with immunosuppressive therapy in transplant patients	*squamous cell carcinoma of the skin* [Other types include *cervical cancer*, *malignant lymphomas*, and *basal cell carcinoma* of the skin.]
HLA-associated disease with the highest relative risk for developing disease	*ankylosing spondylitis* (~80% relative risk)

Question: A 23-year-old woman with postpartum congestive cardiomyopathy receives an ABO compatible heart transplant. Coronary vessel thrombosis in the transplanted heart occurs the moment blood flow is restored to the heart. The mechanism responsible for this reaction is most closely related to which of the following?
  (A) Natural killer cells
  (B) CD8 cytotoxic T cells
  (C) Anti-HLA cytotoxic antibodies
  (D) GVH
  (E) Improper matching of HLA-D antigen sites

Answer: (C): The patient has a hyperacute transplant rejection because of the presence of anti-HLA cytotoxic antibodies, which react against the donor endothelial cells causing thrombosis of the vessels. This is a type II hypersensitivity reaction, hence excluding choice B and E (no time for HLA matching). NK cells are involved in GVH (choice D), which is more likely to occur in bone marrow transplants.

GI = gastrointestinal, GVH = graft-versus-host reaction, HLA = human leukocyte antigen, IL = interleukin, NK = natural killer, RBC = red blood cell.

Table 4–5. HYPERSENSITIVITY DISEASES

Most Common...	Answer and Explanation
effector cells and antibody involved in type I hypersensitivity reactions (HRs)	*mast cells/basophils* and *IgE*, respectively
T cell subtype involved in type I HRs	*CD4⁺ Th1* [Antigen-presenting cells (macrophages/dendritic cells in skin) present allergens to Th2 subclass cells, with subsequent release of IL-4, which causes B cells to switch from IgM to IgE synthesis.]
causes of mast cell/basophil degranulation (release reaction) in type I HRs	*cross-bridging of IgE antibodies by pollens* [Other causes include *food allergens* (peanuts), *anaphylatoxins* (C3a, C5a), *temperature changes, pressure.* Drugs can also produce type I HRs (e.g., penicillin rash).]
preformed chemicals released with mast cell/basophil degranulation	**histamine** (most important), *eosinophil and neutrophil chemotactic factors, heparin, proteases*
secondary mediators released from activated mast cells/basophils	*prostaglandins, leukotrienes,* and *platelet activating factor* [Synthesis occurs directly after the release reaction and enhances the inflammatory reaction.]
term used to describe an allergic individual	*atopic*
physical finding of type I HR in newborns/infants	*atopic dermatitis (eczema) on the face and extensor surfaces, mouth breathing*
physical findings in allergic rhinitis	**pale boggy nasal mucosa,** *allergic shiner, allergic crease; allergic polyps* in adults
physical findings in allergic conjunctivitis	**pruritus,** *redness of the conjunctiva, tearing, normal vision*
COD from a venomous bite	*bee sting with an anaphylactic reaction* (type I HR)
COD in anaphylaxis	*laryngeal obstruction by edema followed by cardiovascular collapse*

Table continued on following page

Table 4–5. HYPERSENSITIVITY DISEASES *Continued*

Most Common...	Answer and Explanation
initial treatment for an anaphylactic reaction with respiratory compromise	*subcutaneous administration of aqueous epinephrine 1:1000*
test used to measure the total IgE concentration	*PRIST* (**p**aper-based **r**ad**i**o**i**mmun**o**sorbent **t**est) [It is not a very sensitive test.]
test used to evaluate type I HRs	*prick (scratch) skin testing* [It is the best all-around test for type I HRs. Positive test result is a wheal and flare reaction.]
serum test used to measure specific IgE antibodies	*RAST* (**r**adi**o**a**l**lerg**o**sorbent **t**est)
finding in a CBC in type I HRs	*eosinophilia*
screening test for allergic rhinitis	*nasal smear for eosinophils*
mediators of type II HRs	*antibodies, complement, NK cells, macrophages, eosinophils*
type II HRs associated with autoantibodies against receptors	**Graves' disease** and *myasthenia gravis*, the former with IgG thyroid-stimulating antibodies and the latter with IgG antibodies against acetylcholine receptors
cell type associated with ADCC	*NK cells* [NK cells have low affinity Fc receptors for IgG. Complement is not necessary for lysis of the target cell.]
test utilized in diagnosing a group of hemolytic anemias associated with type II HRs	*Coombs' test* [This test detects the presence of IgG and/or C3 on the surface of RBCs (direct Coombs') or antibodies causing hemolysis in the serum (indirect Coombs').]
type of type II HR associated with destruction of invasive helminths	*ADCC* [IgE antibodies attach to the surface of the helminth and eosinophils with Fc receptors for IgE hook into the antibodies and release major basic protein, which kills the helminth.]

Table 4–5. HYPERSENSITIVITY DISEASES *Continued*

Most Common...	Answer and Explanation
mediators of type III HRs	*antigens, antibodies* (IgG, IgM; must be complement fixing antibodies), *neutrophils, macrophages, complement*
cause of inflammatory reaction related to type III HRs	*IC activation of the complement system with production of C5a, which is chemotactic to neutrophils,* which damage the target tissue containing the ICs
term applied to a localized (noncirculating ICs) type III HR	*Arthus reaction*
site of a type III HR	*small blood vessel vasculitis* (e.g., venules in Henoch-Schönlein purpura)
site of an Arthus reaction	*lungs* (e.g., farmer's lung: antigen is thermophilic actinomycetes + antibodies + complement).
mediators of type IV HRs	*CD4 T helper cells, CD8 cytotoxic T cells, macrophages, dendritic cells in the skin* (Langerhans' cells), *antigens, pathogens*
types of DHR (type IV HR)	*granuloma formation* (e.g., TB), *allergic contact dermatitis, types of autoimmune disease* (e.g., destruction of islet cells, type I DM), *skin tests for anergy*
test utilized to document allergic contact dermatitis	*patch test* [The suspected irritant is placed on a patch and applied to the skin to see if an eczematous reaction occurs.]
cell types involved in granuloma formation (e.g., in TB)	*macrophages, CD4 helper T cells* [Th1 subclass also formed when macrophages secrete IL-12 after interacting with CD4 helper T cells; this subclass retains memory of the antigen exposure], *epithelioid cells* (activated macrophages [activated by γ-IF from CD4 T cells; MIF keeps macrophages localized], *multinucleated giant cells* (fused activated macrophages)

Table continued on following page

Table 4–5. HYPERSENSITIVITY DISEASES *Continued*

Most Common...	Answer and Explanation
functions of CD8 cytotoxic T cells in type IV HRs	*kill tumor cells, kill virally infected cells, transplant rejection* [They interact with class I antigens on the target cell (e.g., donor tissue). Neoplastic cells and virally infected cells frequently have altered class I antigens to which the cytotoxic T cells react.]

Question: Which of the following disorders is a different type of HR from the others listed?
  (A) Serum sickness
  (B) Goodpasture's syndrome
  (C) Graves' disease
  (D) Warm autoimmune hemolytic anemia
  (E) ABO incompatibility

Answer: (A): Serum sickness is a type III IC disease often accompanying the treatment of snake envenomations with horse antiserum. All the other choices are examples of type II HRs.

ADCC = antibody-dependent cell-mediated cytotoxicity, CBC = complete blood cell count, COD = cause of death, DHR = delayed hypersensitivity reaction, DM = diabetes mellitus, HRs = hypersensitivity reactions, IC = immune complex, γ-IF = gamma interferon, Ig = immunoglobulin, IL = interleukin, MIF = macrophage inhibitory factor, NK = natural killer, RBC = red blood cell, TB = tuberculosis.

Table 4–6. AUTOIMMUNE DISEASES (ADs)

Most Common...	Answer and Explanation
cause of AD in rheumatic fever	*cross-reactivity with other antigens* (e.g., group A streptococcal antigens)
cause of AD in SLE	*polyclonal activation of B lymphocytes*
organ-specific AD	*Hashimoto's thyroiditis*
systemic AD	*rheumatoid arthritis*
test utilized in screening for ADs	*serum ANA* [Antibodies detected are against DNA (double- and single-stranded), histones, acidic proteins (anti-Sm, anti-RNP), nucleolar antigens.]
serum ANA pattern	*speckled* [It is a common pattern found in PSS (anti-Scl antibody), MCTD (anti-RNP), and Sjögren's syndrome (anti-SS-A [Ro], -SS-B [La])].

Table 4-6. AUTOIMMUNE DISEASES (ADs) *Continued*

Most Common...	Answer and Explanation
cause of a rim pattern on a serum ANA	*anti–double-stranded DNA in a patient with SLE and renal disease*
cause of a positive LE prep	*SLE* [An LE cell is a neutrophil that has phagocytosed DNA that has been altered by anti-DNA antibodies. A positive LE is not pathognomonic of SLE.]
mechanism of destruction of articular cartilage in RA	*pannus* [hyperplastic synovial tissue that grows over articular cartilage in a joint and destroys it and the underlying bone (erosions)] [Reactive fibrosis in the repair process causes fusion of the joint (ankylosis). Most patients with RF have an HLA-Dr4 haplotype.]
antibody synthesized by synovial tissue lymphocytes in RA	*RF (positive in 70%)* [It is an IgM antibody against IgG. It forms complexes with itself that activate the complement system, producing chemotactic factors that attract neutrophils and macrophages into the joint.]
cell type that phagocytoses RF to form a ragocyte	*neutrophil*
joints involved in RA	*symmetric involvement of the **second** and third MCP joints and PIP joints* [It produces ulnar deviation of the hands, morning stiffness, and carpal tunnel syndrome. Other joints: knees, feet, elbows, shoulders, jaw.]
lung disease in RA	*chronic pleuritis* [Other findings include *rheumatoid nodules, diffuse interstitial lung disease, Caplan's syndrome* (RA plus a pneumoconiosis [e.g., pneumoconiosis of the lung, coal worker's, silicosis]), *pseudochylous effusions* (milky-white effusion of inflammatory cells plus cholesterol; low PF glucose is characteristic).]
hematologic disease in RA	*anemia of chronic disease* [Less common diseases include *iron deficiency* (PUD), *warm AIHA, Felty's syndrome* (splenomegaly, *neutropenia* due to antineutrophil antibodies and hypersplenism).]

Table continued on following page

Table 4–6. AUTOIMMUNE DISEASES (ADs) *Continued*

Most Common...	Answer and Explanation
cause of sero-negative RA in children	*juvenile RA*
type of juvenile RA presenting like an infectious disease	*Still's disease (20%)* [It presents with spiking fever, generalized lymphadenopathy, hepato-splenomegaly, joint disease, rash, and neu-trophilic leukocytosis.]
type of juvenile RA with disabling arthritis	*polyarticular type of juvenile RA (40%)*
type of juvenile RA with blindness	*pauciarticular type of juvenile RA (40%)* [Uveal tract inflammation is commonly noted.]
presentation of SLE	*arthritis* and *arthralgia* (95%)
cutaneous lesions in SLE	**butterfly rash**, *alopecia* [Skin disease is due to deposition of anti-DNA antibodies along the basement membrane in normal and involved skin (only involved skin in discoid lupus).]
cardiovascular finding in SLE	*fibrinous pericarditis with effusion* [*Libman-Sacks endocarditis* may also occur.]
pulmonary findings in SLE	*pleuritis with pleural effusion* [It may also produce *interstitial fibrosis.*]
hematologic disease in SLE	*warm AIHA* [Other autoimmune diseases include *thrombocytopenia, neutropenia,* and *lymphopenia.*]
coagulation disorder in SLE	*antiphospholipid syndrome due to the presence of lupus anticoagulant and/or anticardiolipin antibodies* [Antibodies are produced against phospholipids and produce thrombosis rather than anticoagulation. They produce recurrent spontaneous abortions owing to thrombosis of the placental bed.]
renal disease associated with SLE	*diffuse proliferative GN* [It presents slightly more commonly as a nephrotic than a nephritic syndrome. It is a common cause of death.]

Table 4–6. AUTOIMMUNE DISEASES (ADs) *Continued*

Most Common...	Answer and Explanation
lab abnormality in SLE	*positive serum ANA (99%)*
confirmatory tests for SLE	**anti–double-stranded DNA** and *anti-Sm*
COD in SLE	*infection secondary to corticosteroid and immunosuppressive therapy*
findings in drug-induced SLE that differ from those in sporadic SLE	*low incidence of renal and CNS involvement, absence of anti–double-stranded DNA and anti-Sm antibodies, normal complement levels, elevated antihistone and single-stranded-DNA antibodies, reversible disease with discontinuation of the drug*
drug resulting in SLE	*procainamide* [Hydralazine is also a common offender.]
cause of PSS and CREST syndrome	**small vessel vasculitis** followed by *excessive deposition of normal collagen in interstitial tissue*
initial sign of PSS and CREST syndrome	*Raynaud's phenomenon* [color changes in the digits from digital vasospasm/fibrosis]
skin findings in PSS	*symmetric swelling of the fingers, hands, and face* [Additional findings include telangiectasias over the face, fingers, and lips.]
GI tract findings in PSS	*dysphagia for solids and liquids due to a motor disorder of the distal esophagus* (smooth muscle is replaced by collagen) *with lack of peristalsis and relaxation of the LES* [Other: wide-mouthed diverticula in the small intestine.]
kidney findings in PSS	*vasculitis* (hyperplastic arteriolosclerosis), *immune complex GN, malignant hypertension, acute* and *chronic renal failure* (common cause of death)
lab findings in PSS	**positive serum ANA** (70–90%), anti-Scl antibodies (70%)
COD in PSS	*respiratory failure secondary to interstitial fibrosis and restrictive lung disease*

Table continued on following page

Table 4-6. AUTOIMMUNE DISEASES (ADs) *Continued*

Most Common...	Answer and Explanation
S/S of PM/DM	*purple-red discoloration and puffiness of the eyelids* (heliotrope eyelids), *muscle weakness and atrophy, increased incidence of lung cancer, dysphagia for solids/liquids, shiny patches* (Gottron's patches) *over the PIP joints*
lab findings in DM and PM	*increased serum CK* [Other test abnormalities include a *positive anti-JO-1 antibody*].
confirmatory test in DM and PM	*muscle biopsy demonstrating a lymphocytic infiltrate*
lab abnormality in MCTD	*anti-RNP antibodies* (95%)
S/S of Sjögren's syndrome	*RA, dry eyes* (keratoconjunctivitis sicca), *and a dry mouth* (xerostomia) *due to autoimmune destruction of lacrimal and minor salivary glands*, and *increased incidence of malignant lymphoma*
lab findings in Sjögren's syndrome	*positive serum ANA* (50–80%), *positive anti-SS-A* (70–80%), *positive anti-SS-B* (50–70%), *positive RF* (75–90%)
confirmatory test for Sjögren's syndrome	*lip biopsy demonstrating autoimmune destruction of the minor salivary glands*

Question: Which AD is most often associated with syndromes involving the hematologic system, lungs, and the minor salivary glands?
- (A) SLE
- (B) RA
- (C) PSS
- (D) MCTD
- (E) CREST syndrome

Answer: (B): RA is associated with Felty's syndrome (splenomegaly + neutropenia), Caplan's syndrome (RA + pneumoconiosis), and Sjögren's syndrome (RA + dry eyes and dry mouth). None of the other ADs listed have this many syndromes associated with them.

AD = autoimmune disease, AIHA = autoimmune hemolytic anemia, ANA = antinuclear antibodies, anti-Scl = anti-scleroderma, anti-Sm = anti-Smith, CK = creatine kinase, CNS = central nervous system, COD = cause of death, CREST = **c**alcinosis, **R**aynaud's phenomenon, **e**sophageal motility disorders, **s**clerodactyly, and **t**elangiectasia, DM = dermatomyositis, GI = gastrointestinal, GN = glomerulonephritis, HLA = human leukocyte antigen, Ig = immunoglobulin, LE = lupus erythematosus, LES = lower esophageal sphincter, MCP = metacarpophalangeal, MCTD = mixed connective tissue disease, PF = pleural fluid, PIP = proximal interphalangeal joint, PM = polymyositis, PSS = progressive systemic sclerosis, PUD = peptic ulcer disease, RA = rheumatoid arthritis, RF = rheumatoid factor, RNP = ribonucleoprotein, Scl = scleroderma, SLE = systemic lupus erythematosus, S/S = signs and symptoms, SS-A/SS-B = Sjögren's syndrome.

CHAPTER

FLUIDS AND HEMODYNAMICS

CONTENTS

Table 5–1. EDEMA AND HYPEREMIA

Most Common...	Answer and Explanation
sites for edema [fluid accumulation]	*interstitial space* [part of the ECF compartment] and *body fluid cavities*
Starling's force keeping fluid within blood vessels	*plasma oncotic pressure* [Oncotic pressure is synonymous with the plasma albumin concentration.]
Starling's force pushing fluid out of blood vessels	*plasma hydrostatic pressure*
types of edema fluid	*transudates, exudates, lymphedema*
type of edema fluid associated with an alteration in Starling's forces	*transudate* [It is a low protein (<3.0 g/dL) fluid with a scanty number of cells.]
Starling's force alterations producing transudates	*increased hydrostatic pressure* and/or a *decreased oncotic pressure*
sign of an alteration in Starling's forces	*pitting edema* and *body effusions (ascites, pleural effusion)* [Transudates settle to the most dependent portion of the body (e.g., the feet in a person who is standing).]

Table continued on following page

Table 5-1. EDEMA AND HYPEREMIA *Continued*

Most Common...	Answer and Explanation
form of edema secondary to an increase in hydrostatic pressure	*pulmonary edema in LHF* [When the left heart fails, the increase in LVEDP is transmitted back into the left atrium, pulmonary veins and out into the alveoli once hydrostatic pressure is greater than pulmonary capillary oncotic pressure.]
cause of pitting edema from a decrease in oncotic pressure	*alcoholic cirrhosis* [Albumin is synthesized in the liver. Other causes include *malabsorption*, *malnutrition* (kwashiorkor), and *nephrotic syndrome*.]
cause of ascites [edema in the peritoneal cavity]	*alcoholic cirrhosis* [It is due to increased hydrostatic pressure (portal vein hypertension), decreased oncotic pressure (decreased albumin synthesis), and secondary aldosteronism (decreased metabolism; activation of the RAA system).]
cause of a hydrothorax and hydropericardium [transudate in the pleural/pericardial cavity]	*CHF*
term for generalized edema	*anasarca*
cause of an exudate	*acute inflammation with increased vessel permeability* [Exudates are high protein (>3 g/dL) fluids with an increase in cells, usually neutrophils.]
hemothorax/peritoneum/pericardium [blood in the pleural/peritoneal/pericardial cavities]	*trauma to the chest wall, traumatic rupture of the spleen or liver, penetrating thoracic injury*, respectively
lymphedema in the United States	*radiation post-mastectomy for breast cancer*

Table 5–1. EDEMA AND HYPEREMIA *Continued*

Most Common...	Answer and Explanation
cause of active hyperemia (congestion) [increased arterial/ arteriolar blood flow]	*acute inflammation* (histamine-induced vaso-dilatation)
cause of CPC in the liver [local or systemic reduction in venous blood flow]	*RHF* [Congestion of blood in the THV of the liver produces the classic nutmeg liver, which may eventuate in fibrosis (cardiac cirrhosis).]
cause of CPC in the lungs	*LHF* [Hemorrhage into the alveoli leads to hemosiderin and fibrosis in the lung parenchyma (called brown induration of the lungs).]
cause of rust-colored sputum	*alveolar macrophages with phagocytosed hemosiderin in patients with CPC of the lungs in chronic heart failure* [They are called heart failure cells.]

Question: Which of the following represent an exudate rather than a transudate? **SELECT 3 answers**
  (A) Effusion in the pleural cavity in CHF
  (B) Swelling of the legs in pregnancy
  (C) Peritoneal effusion in alcoholic cirrhosis
  (D) Pericardial effusion in SLE
  (E) Pitting edema in the nephrotic syndrome
  (F) Swelling after a bee sting
  (G) Synovial fluid in RA

Answers: (D), (F), (G): A pericardial effusion in SLE is most likely due to acute fibrinous pericarditis with an increase in vessel permeability. Swelling of tissue in a bee sting is an exudate from increased vessel permeability. RA is an inflammatory joint disease. Choices A and B are transudates due to an increase in hydrostatic pressure. Choice C is a transudate due to an increase in hydrostatic pressure and decrease in oncotic pressure. Choice E is due to a decrease in oncotic pressure.

CHF = congestive heart failure, CPC = chronic passive congestion, ECF = extracellular fluid compartment, LHF = left heart failure, LVEDP = left ventricular end-diastolic pressure, RA = rheumatoid arthritis, RAA = renin-angiotensin-aldosterone, RHF = right heart failure, SLE = systemic lupus erythematosus, THV = terminal hepatic venule.

Table 5–2. VOLUME AND ELECTROLYTE DISORDERS

Most Common...	Answer and Explanation
sites for total body water (TBW) and total body sodium (TBNa$^+$)	*TBW is distributed in both the ECF and ICF compartments; TBNa$^+$ is distributed in the ECF compartment* (plasma in the vascular compartment and interstitial fluid)
lab test evaluating plasma solute concentration	*plasma osmolality (POsm in mOsm/kg)*
formula for calculating POsm	*POsm = (2) Na$^+$ + serum glucose/18 + serum blood urea nitrogen (BUN)/2.8 = 275–295 mOsm/kg*
cause of a decreased POsm	*hyponatremia*
cause of an increased POsm	*hyperglycemia*
solute controlling water movements between the ECF and ICF compartments	*sodium via osmosis, where water moves from a point of low to high concentration*
pathologic causes of water movement between the ECF and ICF	*hyponatremia and hyperglycemia* [Only Na$^+$ and glucose establish osmotic gradients between the ECF and ICF, since both are limited to the ECF compartment. Urea, a permeant solute, equalizes itself between the two compartments without establishing a gradient.]
measure of the tonicity of fluid [fluid osmolality responsible for water movements between the ECF and ICF]	*effective osmolality (EOsm)* [A normal EOsm represents an isotonic state and no gradient for water movements. A low EOsm indicates a hypotonic state, in which fluid moves from the ECF into the ICF compartment (ICF expansion). A high EOsm represents a hypertonic state (e.g., hypernatremia or hyperglycemia; not an increase in BUN), in which water moves out of the ICF into the ECF (ICF contraction).]
effect of hyperglycemia on the serum Na$^+$ concentration	*dilutional hyponatremia, as the osmotic gradient favors water movement out of the ICF into the ECF compartment*

Table 5–2. VOLUME AND ELECTROLYTE DISORDERS
Continued

Most Common...	Answer and Explanation
factors controlling plasma volume	**kidney reabsorption of salt and water** [Additional factors include *thirst* (function of POsm [decreased inhibits, increased stimulates] and *AT II* [decreased inhibits, increased stimulates]), *low and high pressure baroreceptors, RAA system, ADH.*]
factors activating the RAA system	**a decrease in renal blood flow** and *increase in catecholamines* (activation of baroreceptors from decreased cardiac output) [They both stimulate the JG apparatus (modified smooth muscle cell in the afferent arteriole) to release renin (an enzyme) → renin cleaves angiotensinogen into AT I → ACE in the lungs converts AT I into AT II (stimulates thirst, increases TPR) → AT II stimulates release of AT III and aldosterone (increases Na⁺ reabsorption).]
clinical term that reflects volume status	*effective arterial blood volume (EABV)* [It represents the total circulating volume of blood that is necessary to stimulate volume receptors.]
cause of a decrease in EABV and increase in ECF	*Starling's force abnormality* [Normally, EABV and ECF volume status parallel each other (e.g., decreased EABV, decreased ECF volume). However, if hydrostatic pressure is increased or oncotic pressure decreased, fluid moves out of the vascular compartment into the ISF, which increases the ECF volume. In either condition, the venous return to the right side of the heart is decreased, hence decreasing EABV.]
sites of the low- and high-pressure baroreceptors	low-pressure types: *left atrium* and *major intrathoracic veins.* high-pressure types: *aortic arch* and *carotid sinus* [These are innervated by cranial nerves IX and X.]
effect on the kidneys of a decreased EABV	*they reabsorb a slightly hypotonic solution (more water than salt) back into the ECF* [In addition, stimulation of the baroreceptor reflex increases catecholamine release, leading to venoconstriction, increased cardiac output, increased TPR, and stimulation of the

Table continued on following page

Table 5–2. VOLUME AND ELECTROLYTE DISORDERS
Continued

Most Common...	Answer and Explanation
Continued	RAA system. (AT II stimulates thirst, increases TPR, and stimulates aldosterone release, and aldosterone increases Na^+ reabsorption.) *Neural reflexes in the left atrium stimulate ADH release* (reabsorbs free water). The *decrease in renal blood flow further activates the RAA system.* There is also a *decrease in peritubular hydrostatic pressure (P_H) and increase in peritubular oncotic pressure (P_o),* leading to increased proximal tubule reabsorption of salt and water in isosmotic proportions.]
effect on the kidneys of an increased EABV	*there is no activation of the baroreceptor reflex, no release of ADH, no activation of the RAA system, and $P_H > P_o$* [no proximal tubule reabsorption of salt and water]
functions of ANP	*ANP is released with distention of the left atrium and suppresses all of the baroreceptor events listed above, vasodilates peripheral vessels, and directly inhibits Na^+ reabsorption in the kidneys*
functions of prostaglandin E_2	*inhibits ADH, blocks Na^+ reabsorption in the kidneys, and is an intrarenal vasodilator*
nephron site for Na^+ reabsorption	*the proximal tubules* [They reabsorb 60–80% of the filtered Na^+. In addition, they reabsorb K^+, urea, phosphate, bicarbonate (major site of reclamation), glucose, and amino acids. They are the principal site for generation of NH_3 used in the excretion of excess acid. P_o must be greater than P_H to reabsorb these solutes.]
nephron site with the highest UOsm	*thin descending limb* [This segment increases water reabsorption without Na^+, hence the UOsm may increase to a maximum of 1200 mOsm/kg.]
nephron site for the generation of free water	*the thick ascending limb (TAL) in the medullary segment which contains the Na^+-K^+-$2Cl^-$ cotransport pump* [Water that must accompany solute for excretion (20 mL of water per mOsm of solute) is called obligated

Table 5–2. VOLUME AND ELECTROLYTE DISORDERS
Continued

Most Common...	Answer and Explanation
Continued	water. In the TAL segment, Na^+, K^+, Cl^- reabsorbed without water produce free water (20 mL per mOsm of solute), which is what the kidneys either reabsorb when concentrating urine (ADH function) or excrete in diluting urine. Fluid in the tubular lumen of the TAL is very hypotonic, since the amount of free water is greater than obligated water.]
pump blocked by loop diuretics	Na^+-K^+-$2Cl^-$ cotransport pump in the TAL segment [Calcium is also lost by blocking this pump, hence the role of loop diuretics in treating hypercalcemia.]
nephron site and pump blocked by thiazide diuretics	*cortical segment of the TAL, which houses a pump that reabsorbs Na^+ and Cl^- ions* [Since calcium uses the same channel as Na^+ for PTH-enhanced absorption, thiazides enhance calcium reabsorption by blocking Na^+ reabsorption (useful in treating calcium stone formers).]
nephron site of the macula densa	*cortical segment of the TAL* [The macula densa is a modified chemoreceptor that senses volume and Na^+ alterations. A low volume or decreased Na^+ in the urine prompts stimulation of the JG apparatus and vice versa.]
nephron sites where the aldosterone-enhanced ATPase pumps for Na^+ reabsorption are located	*distal convoluted tubules (DCTs) and collecting tubules* [Aldosterone increases Na^+ reabsorption in exchange for either K^+ or H^+ ions. Na^+ ions are reabsorbed without water (generates free water).]
cause of hypokalemia in patients taking either a loop or thiazide diuretic	*increased delivery of unreabsorbed Na^+ to the aldosterone-enhanced Na^+ pumps in the DCT and collecting tubules leads to a greater exchange of Na^+ for K^+ with subsequent development of hypokalemia* (hence the need for K^+ supplements)
acid-base/electrolyte abnormalities in patients taking either a loop or thiazide diuretic	*metabolic alkalosis, hyponatremia, hypokalemia* [Once K^+ is depleted (*hypokalemia*), Na^+ ions primarily exchange with H^+, which reclaim HCO_3^- by combining with HCO_3^- ions in the urine to form carbonic acid, which

Table continued on following page

Table 5–2. VOLUME AND ELECTROLYTE DISORDERS
Continued

Most Common...	Answer and Explanation
Continued	dissociates into CO_2 + H_2O. CO_2 diffuses back into the tubular cell and combines with water to form carbonic acid. The latter dissociates into H^+ and HCO_3^- ions, which are reabsorbed into the blood (*metabolic alkalosis*). H^+ ions are used to reclaim more HCO_3^-. Loss of unreabsorbed Na^+ in the urine in hypertonic proportions (more Na^+ than H_2O) results in *hyponatremia*.]
acid-base/electrolyte abnormalities associated with aldosterone blockers	*metabolic acidosis, hyponatremia, hyperkalemia* [Aldosterone blockers (e.g., spironolactone) block the DCT and collecting duct Na^+ reabsorption pump, resulting in hyponatremia, retention of K^+ (potential for hyperkalemia), and retention of H^+ ions (potential for metabolic acidosis). Similar events occur in hypoaldosteronemia (e.g., Addison's disease).]
variable affecting K^+ loss in the DCT and collecting tubule	*increased distal delivery of Na^+ from more proximally acting diuretics* [Other variables include the *presence of aldosterone* (increased exchange of Na^+ for K^+) and *alkalosis* (H^+ ions enter the ECF [mechanism to combat alkalosis] from the renal tubules in exchange for K^+, which causes Na^+ to primarily exchange with K^+ ions, leading to hypokalemia).]
nephron sites for dilution and concentration of urine	*late distal and collecting ducts* [Dilution and concentration of urine depend on the absence or presence of ADH, respectively (see below).]
nephron site for secretion of H^+ ions	*collecting ducts where the aldosterone-enhanced H^+/K^+ ATPase pumps are located* [The H^+ ions secreted combine with HPO_4^- to form NaH_2PO_4 [titratable acid] or with NH_3 to form NH_4Cl.]
nephron site for regeneration of bicarbonate	*collecting ducts where the aldosterone-enhanced H^+/K^+ ATPase pumps are located* [CO_2 from the blood (not the urine) enters the collecting tubule, combines with H_2O to form

Table 5–2. VOLUME AND ELECTROLYTE DISORDERS
Continued

Most Common...	Answer and Explanation
Continued	H_2CO_3. The latter dissociates into H^+ and HCO_3^-. HCO_3^- (newly synthesized, not reclaimed from the urine) is reabsorbed and the H^+ ions are exchanged with K^+ in the pump.]
nephron sites for excretion of free water (dilution of urine)	*late distal and collecting tubules* [In the absence of ADH, hypotonic fluid containing obligated and free water is excreted. This is called a positive free water clearance ($+CH_2O$; see below) and is marked by a low UOsm. The amount of free water lost reflects the amount of water produced in the TAL segment that is necessary to bring the POsm back into the normal range.]
nephron sites for reabsorption of free water (concentration of urine)	*late distal and collecting tubules* [In the presence of ADH, free water is reabsorbed, hence raising the UOsm. This is called a negative free water clearance ($-CH_2O$; see below). The amount of free water reabsorbed reflects the amount of water generated in the TAL segment that must be added to plasma to bring the POsm back into the normal range.]
formula used to calculate CH_2O (free water clearance)	$CH_2O = V - COsm$, *where V = volume of urine in mL and COsm (osmolar clearance) equals the obligated water that must be excreted with solute* [$COsm = UOsm \times V/POsm$. If the CH_2O is positive, dilution is occurring (ADH is absent), and conversely, if it is negative, concentration is occurring (ADH is present).]
determinant of the serum Na^+ concentration	*total body osmolality, which equals $TBNa^+/TBW$* (TBK$^+$ has been left out of the numerator) [Serum Na^+ reflects the ratio of TBNa$^+$ to TBW, hence changes in either TBNa$^+$ or TBW produce changes in the serum Na^+ (= TBNa$^+$/TBW).]
patient alteration reflecting volume loss or gain	*daily weight*

Table continued on following page

Table 5–2. VOLUME AND ELECTROLYTE DISORDERS
Continued

Most Common...	Answer and Explanation
signs correlating with decreased TBNa$^+$	*dry mucous membranes, hypotension, reduced skin turgor (tenting of the skin),* and *weight loss* [A decreased TBNa$^+$ correlates with volume depletion. Skin turgor (sense of skin fullness) and dry mucous membranes reflect volume alterations in the ISF compartment, while hypotension parallels changes in plasma volume.]
signs correlating with increased TBNa$^+$	*pitting edema and ascites* [Since TBNa$^+$ is limited to the ECF compartment and the ISF compartment is two-thirds larger than the plasma volume, most of the increase in Na$^+$ is in the ISF, which produces pitting edema. An increase in TBW alone does not produce pitting edema, since most of the water is redirected into the ICF compartment by osmosis.]
electrolyte disturbance in the general population	*hyponatremia*
cause of a normal serum Na$^+$ and volume depletion (↓ TBNa$^+$)	*an isotonic loss of fluid,* which is most commonly due to adult secretory diarrhea (serum *Na$^+$ = ↓ TBNa$^+$/ ↓ TBW)* [An equal loss of Na$^+$ and water does not alter the serum Na$^+$; however, the loss of TBNa$^+$ produces volume depletion without any changes in the ICF compartment in the absence of a gradient for osmosis. If the patient had access to water, the TBW could increase and potentially result in hyponatremia.]
cause of a normal serum Na$^+$ and pitting edema (↑ TBNa$^+$)	*an isotonic gain of fluid most commonly due to excessive infusion of isotonic saline (serum Na$^+$ = ↑ TBNa$^+$/ ↑ TBW)* [The ECF compartment is expanded but the ICF compartment is normal (no gradient for osmosis).]
cause of hyponatremia [serum Na$^+$ <135 mEq/L] and volume depletion (↓ TBNa$^+$)	*a hypertonic loss of fluid,* most commonly secondary to diuretics (↓ serum Na$^+$ = ↓ ↓ TBNa$^+$/ ↓ TBW) [A proportionately greater loss of salt than water produces hyponatremia.]

Table 5-2. VOLUME AND ELECTROLYTE DISORDERS
Continued

Most Common...	Answer and Explanation
cause of hyponatremia and pitting edema ($\uparrow$ TBNa$^+$)	*a hypotonic gain of more water than salt, most commonly secondary to CHF ($\downarrow$ serum Na$^+$ = $\uparrow$ TBNa$^+$/$\uparrow$$\uparrow$ TBW)* [A greater gain in water than in salt produces not only hyponatremia but also pitting edema, owing to the increase in TBNa$^+$, which accumulates primarily in the ISF compartment. The increased TBW is distributed into the ICF compartment and to a lesser extent into the ECF compartment owing to osmosis. Other causes of this pitting edema/hyponatremia scenario are *cirrhosis, malabsorption, malnutrition,* and the *nephrotic syndrome.* All of these disorders are associated with hypoalbuminemia and a decrease in EABV due to decreased venous return to the heart as fluid is redirected into the ISF compartment by the reduced oncotic pressure. In CHF, the alteration that distributes fluid into the ISF is an increase in hydrostatic pressure.]
nonpharmacologic treatment of the pitting edema states	*restriction of both water and salt*
cause of hyponatremia and a normal physical exam (normal TBNa$^+$)	*hypotonic gain of pure water, which is most commonly due to SiADH ($\downarrow$ serum Na$^+$ = TBNa$^+$/$\uparrow$$\uparrow$ TBW)* [SiADH is most often associated with a small cell carcinoma of the lung. Other causes include *chlorpropamide, CNS disease,* and *TB.* The increased TBW is mainly redirected into the ICF compartment by osmosis; however, the ECF compartment is also volume overloaded (no pitting edema, since the TBNa$^+$ is normal). This causes an increased EABV, which suppresses the RAA system and reduces the proximal reabsorption of Na$^+$ ($P_H > P_o$ in the peritubular capillaries). However, ADH is not suppressed, hence urine concentration is still occurring ($-CH_2O$). A random urine Na$^+$ is increased (>40 mEq/L), owing to loss of Na$^+$ reabsorption in the proximal tubule.]

Table continued on following page

Table 5-2. VOLUME AND ELECTROLYTE DISORDERS
Continued

Most Common...	Answer and Explanation
nonpharmacologic treatment of SiADH	*restrict water but not salt*
cause of hypernatremia [serum Na^+ >145 mEq/L] with volume depletion ($\downarrow$ TBNa$^+$)	*hypotonic loss of more water than salt, which is most often osmotic diuresis secondary to* **DKA**, *sweating, baby diarrhea ($\uparrow$ serum Na^+ = $\downarrow$ TBNa$^+$/ $\downarrow$ $\downarrow$ TBW)* [If a patient had access to water, the increase in TBW could lead to a normal or low serum Na^+ concentration. Both the ECF and ICF compartments are volume depleted owing to an osmotic gradient favoring movement of water into the ECF, which is then lost in urine, sweat, or diarrheal fluid, respectively.]
cause of hypernatremia with pitting edema ($\uparrow$ TBNa$^+$)	*hypertonic gain of more salt than water most often secondary to excessive NaHCO$_3$ infusions or Na$^+$ salt antibiotics (e.g., carbenicillin; $\uparrow$ serum Na^+ = $\uparrow$ $\uparrow$ TBNa$^+$/ $\uparrow$ TBW)* [In this case, the ECF compartment is volume overloaded and the ICF compartment is volume depleted owing to osmosis.]
cause of hypernatremia with a normal physical exam (normal TBNa$^+$)	*hypotonic loss of pure water, which may be due to insensible water loss (fever, evaporation of water over mucous membranes) or diabetes insipidus ($\uparrow$ serum Na^+ = TBNa$^+$/ $\downarrow$ $\downarrow$ TBW)* [A loss of pure water without salt and signs of volume depletion is called dehydration. In this case, both the ECF and ICF compartments are contracted.]
cause of hyponatremia	*diuretics* [Hyponatremia always involves a defect in the generation or excretion of free water, which leads to a dysfunctional dilution process. The block in Na^+ reabsorption in either the Na^+-K^+-$2Cl^-$ cotransport pump by loop diuretics or the Na^+-Cl^- pump in the cortical segment by thiazides decreases formation of free water, which is essential for the dilution process.]
cause of hypernatremia	*insensible water loss due to fever* [Hypernatremia always involves a problem with access to water (e.g., infants, the elderly). In the

Table 5–2. VOLUME AND ELECTROLYTE DISORDERS
Continued

Most Common...	Answer and Explanation
Continued	above examples, access to water could potentially change a hypernatremia into a ratio favoring normo- or hyponatremia.]
CNS effect if hyponatremia is corrected too rapidly with saline	*central pontine myelinolysis* [Isotonic saline is "hypertonic" compared with the hypotonic state in the CNS; hence, rapid movement of water out of the brain cells results in demyelination. This more commonly occurs in alcoholics.]
compartment site for K^+ storage	*ICF compartment* [K^+ is important in neuromuscular transmission and in intracellular regulation of protein and glycogen synthesis.]
causes of hypokalemia [serum K^+ <3.5 mEq/L]	*renal loss* [Renal loss may be due to *diuretics*, primary aldosteronism, osmotic diuresis (e.g., glucosuria), type I and type II RTA). Other causes include *GI loss* (vomiting, diarrhea), *decreased intake* (poor diet), *transcellular shift* (see below).]
factors promoting movement of K^+ into cells (transcellular shift into the ICF) leading to hypokalemia	**insulin**, *epinephrine, alkalosis* (H^+ moves out of cells while K^+ moves in to maintain electroneutrality), β_2-*agonists* (e.g., albuterol)
factors promoting movement of K^+ out of cells into the ECF compartment leading to hyperkalemia	*insulin deficiency, inorganic metabolic acidoses* (e.g., renal failure, not ketoacidosis or lactic acidosis, which are due to organic acids), β-*antagonists* (e.g., propranolol), *digitalis toxicity* (inhibits the Na^+/K^+ ATPase pump), *succinylcholine* (muscle relaxant), *tissue breakdown* (e.g., rhabdomyolysis)
S/S of hypokalemia	**muscle weakness**, *constipation, paralytic ileus* (absent bowel peristalsis)
ECG findings in hypokalemia	*U waves* (positive wave after the T wave)
nonpathologic cause of hyperkalemia	*pseudohyperkalemia secondary to iatrogenic hemolysis of RBCs*

Table continued on following page

Table 5–2. VOLUME AND ELECTROLYTE DISORDERS
Continued

Most Common...	Answer and Explanation
pathophysiologic causes of hyperkalemia	**decreased renal excretion** (e.g., renal failure, aldosterone deficiency [e.g., Addison's]), *transcellular shift* (see above)
S/S of hyperkalemia	**weakness from problems in neuromuscular conduction,** *cardiac arrhythmias* (e.g., ventricular arrhythmias, heart stops in diastole)
early ECG findings in hyperkalemia	*peaked narrow T waves*

Question: Which of the following would most likely result in a decrease in POsm, mental status abnormalities, and a normal physical exam?
  (A) SiADH
  (B) Right-sided heart failure
  (C) Insensible water loss
  (D) Diuretic therapy
  (E) Overzealous infusion of isotonic saline

Answer: (A): In SiADH, there is hypotonia of pure water without salt, hence the physical exam is normal (normal TBNa$^+$) and the patient has hyponatremia ($\uparrow$ POsm). Choice B produces hyponatremia, but pitting edema is present. Choice C produces hypernatremia ($\downarrow$ POsm) and a normal physical exam, owing to a loss of pure water. Choice D results in hyponatremia, but skin turgor is poor ($\uparrow$ TBNa$^+$). Choice E does not alter the serum Na$^+$, and the patient has signs of pitting edema ($\downarrow$ TBNa$^+$).

ACE = angiotensin-converting enzyme, ADH = antidiuretic hormone, AT I = angiotensin I, AT II = angiotensin II, AT III = angiotensin III, ANP = atrial natriuretic peptide, ATP = adenosine triphosphate, BUN = blood urea nitrogen, CNS = central nervous system, DCT = distal convoluted tubule, DKA = diabetic ketoacidosis, EABV = effective arterial blood volume, ECF = extracellular fluid, ECG = electrocardiogram, EOsm = effective osmolality, GI = gastrointestinal, ICF = intracellular fluid, ISF = interstitial fluid, JG = juxtaglomerular, P$_H$ = peritubular hydrostatic pressure, P$_O$ = peritubular oncotic pressure, POsm = plasma osmolality, PTH = parathormone, RAA = renin-angiotensin-aldosterone, RBC = red blood cell, RTA = renal tubular acidosis, SiADH = syndrome of inappropriate ADH, S/S = signs and symptoms, TAL = thick ascending limb, TB = tuberculosis, TBK$^+$ = total body potassium, TBNa$^+$ = total body sodium, TBW = total body water, TPR = total peripheral resistance, UOsm = urine osmolality.

Table 5–3. SHOCK

Most Common...	Answer and Explanation
types of shock	**hypovolemic,** *cardiogenic, septic, neurogenic*
pathophysiologic effect of shock	*tissue hypoxia*
cause of hypo-volemic shock	*hemorrhage*
cause of cardiogenic shock	*acute myocardial infarction*
cause of septic shock	*gram-negative septicemia due to Escherichia coli*
cause of neurogenic shock	*fainting*
S/S of hypovolemic and cardiogenic shock	**sinus tachycardia**; *cold, clammy skin (vaso-constriction of vessels); hypotension; positive tilt test* [increase in pulse and decrease in blood pressure when moving from a supine to upright position]
S/S of endotoxic shock	*sinus tachycardia, variable blood pressure, warm skin* [Endotoxins activate the alternative complement pathway, causing the release of anaphylatoxins (C3a and C5a), leading to arteriolar vasodilatation (warm skin). Damaged endothelial cells release nitric oxide (vasodilator). Vasodilatation increases venous return of blood to the heart, hence increasing cardiac output (high output failure).]
complications in endotoxic shock	**ischemic acute tubular necrosis,** *ARDS, multiorgan failure, DIC, heart failure*
WBC effect of endotoxic shock	*absolute neutropenia due to increased adhesion molecule synthesis*
effect of acute blood loss on the Hb and Hct	*no effect* [An equal loss of plasma and RBCs does not alter the Hb and Hct. Fluid entry into the vascular compartment occurs before the replacement of RBCs by the marrow, hence the RBC deficit is uncovered in a few hours to a few days.]

Table continued on following page

Table 5–3. SHOCK *Continued*

Most Common...	Answer and Explanation
effect of acute blood loss when crystalloids are infused	*drop in Hb and Hct* [Crystalloid solutions like isotonic saline and Ringer's lactate remain in the ECF compartment, hence uncovering the RBC deficit by acting like "plasma."]
effect of hypovolemic and cardiogenic shock on the mixed venous oxygen content [MVOC = O_2 content in blood in right side of the heart]	*decreased MVOC due to reduction in cardiac output allows tissue cells to extract more O_2 from blood*
effect of endotoxic shock on the MVOC	*increased MVOC due to rapid flow of blood through the microcirculation from massive vasodilatation of the arterioles* (peripheral resistance vessels)
effect of hypovolemic shock on the PCWP versus cardiogenic shock [PCWP is a Swan-Ganz measurement reflecting LVEDP]	*the PCWP in hypovolemic shock is decreased (reduced volume of blood in the left ventricle) and increased in cardiogenic shock (volume of blood increases in the failed left ventricle)*
organ adversely affected in shock	*renal medulla of the kidney* [Since only 10% of the blood distributed to the kidneys is directed into the medulla, hypovolemia increases the chances of ischemic ATN.]
lab findings in hypovolemic shock	*increased anion gap metabolic acidosis due to anaerobic glycolysis and build-up of lactate, hyperglycemia* [release of cortisol, glucagon, and catecholamines increases glycogenolysis], and *elevated WBC count* [cortisol and catecholamines decrease adhesion molecule synthesis, which releases the WBC marginating pool into the circulating pool]
type of shock with the highest mortality	*endotoxic shock (20–80%)*

Table 5–3. SHOCK *Continued*

Question: Which of the following is more likely to occur in endotoxic than in hypovolemic shock?
(A) Tissue hypoxia
(B) Metabolic acidosis
(C) Sinus tachycardia
(D) Warm skin
(E) Low MVOC

Answer: (D): Warm skin is more likely to occur in endotoxic shock owing to arteriolar vasodilation from histamine and nitric oxide. Both types of shock have metabolic acidosis, sinus tachycardia, and tissue hypoxia. Hypovolemic shock has a decreased MVOC, while endotoxic shock has an increased MVOC.

ARDS = adult respiratory distress syndrome, ATN = acute tubular necrosis, DIC = disseminated intravascular coagulation, ECF = extracellular fluid, Hb = hemoglobin, Hct = hematocrit, LVEDP = left ventricular end-diastolic pressure, MVOC = mixed venous oxygen content, PCWP = pulmonary capillary wedge pressure, RBC = red blood cell, S/S = signs and symptoms, WBC = white blood cell.

Table 5–4. ACID-BASE DISORDERS

Most Common...	Answer and Explanation
acid-base disorder	*respiratory acidosis* (decreased arterial pH due to an increase in $PaCO_2$) [*Respiratory alkalosis* (increased arterial pH due to a decrease in $PaCO_2$), *metabolic acidosis* (decreased arterial pH due to a decrease in HCO_3^-), and *metabolic alkalosis* (increased arterial pH due to an increase in HCO_3^-) are the other acid-base disorders.]
renal response for respiratory acidosis [pH <7.35 and $PaCO_2$ >44 mm Hg (33–44 mm Hg)]	*reclaim/regenerate HCO_3^- producing metabolic alkalosis as compensation* [It requires 4–5 days for the kidneys to fully reclaim/regenerate bicarbonate as compensation for respiratory acidosis. Compensation brings pH back toward normal range (7.35–7.45). *Full compensation* is when pH is brought back into the normal range (extremely rare); *partial compensation*, when both compensation and pH are outside the normal range; and *no compensation* (uncompensated), when compensation has not extended beyond its normal range. Compensation moves in the same

Table continued on following page

Table 5–4. ACID-BASE DISORDERS *Continued*

Most Common...	Answer and Explanation
Continued	direction as the primary disease to try to bring the ratio of HCO_3^- to $PaCO_2$ back close to the normal of 20:1.]
renal response for respiratory alkalosis [pH >7.45 and $PaCO_2$ <33 mm Hg (33–44 mm Hg)]	*loss of HCO_3^- in urine, producing metabolic acidosis as compensation*
pulmonary response for metabolic acidosis [pH <7.35 and HCO_3^- <22 mEq/L (22–28 mEq/L)]	*blow off CO_2 (hyperventilation), producing respiratory alkalosis as compensation* [It requires 12–24 hours for the lungs to reach a steady state of compensation in primary metabolic disorders.]
pulmonary response for metabolic alkalosis [pH >7.45 and HCO_3^- >28 mEq/L (22–28 mEq/L)]	*retain CO_2 (hypoventilation), producing respiratory acidosis as compensation*
acid-base disorder producing tissue hypoxia	*metabolic alkalosis* [Respiratory acidosis is compensation for metabolic alkalosis. An increase in alveolar PCO_2 is always accompanied by a corresponding decrease in alveolar PO_2 and PaO_2. Alkalosis left-shifts the ODC (decreases release of O_2 from Hb). The combination of hypoxemia and a left-shifted ODC produces tissue hypoxia, which often precipitates ventricular arrhythmias.]
acid-base disorder producing a PaO_2 >100 mm Hg	*respiratory alkalosis* [As alveolar PCO_2 decreases from hyperventilation (blowing off CO_2), alveolar PO_2 has a corresponding increase, hence increasing the PaO_2.]
stimulus for central chemoreceptors in the medulla	*H^+ ions derived from CO_2 entering the CSF and combining with H_2O to form H_2CO_3, which dissociates into H^+ ions and HCO_3^- anions* [An increase in H^+ ions secondary to an increase in $PaCO_2$ (more CO_2 enters the

Table 5–4. ACID-BASE DISORDERS *Continued*

Most Common...	Answer and Explanation
Continued	CSF) stimulates respirations (blows off CO_2), while a decrease in H^+ ions due to a decrease in $PaCO_2$ reduces respirations (retains CO_2).]
stimuli for the peripheral chemoreceptors [carotid bodies and aortic bodies]	*hypoxemia, increase in $PaCO_2$, increase in H^+ ions* [The carotid bodies are the most important of the two receptors. Unlike central receptors, the peripheral receptors are responsive to hypoxemia.]
causes of acute respiratory acidosis [$PaCO_2$ >44 mm Hg, HCO_3^- ≤30 mEq/L]	*depression of the medullary respiratory center* (e.g., barbiturates) [Other causes include: *upper airway obstruction* (e.g., cafe coronary [food caught in the upper airway]), *chest bellows* [diaphragm, intercostal muscles] *dysfunction* (e.g., paralysis of muscles of respiration), *primary lung disease* (e.g., acute exacerbation of COPD).]
cause of chronic respiratory acidosis [$PaCO_2$ >44 mm Hg, HCO_3^- >30 mEq/L]	*primary lung disease* (e.g., **COPD**)
S/S in respiratory acidosis	**somnolence**, *increased intracranial pressure* [increased $PaCO_2$ vasodilates cerebral vessels and increases vessel permeability], *secondary polycythemia* [hypoxemic stimulus for erythropoietin release]
electrolyte abnormalities in respiratory acidosis	*HCO_3^- moves out of cells as compensation and Cl^- ions move into the cells (hypochloremia) to maintain electroneutrality* [This exchange increases the serum HCO_3^- concentration ~3–4 mEq/L (up to 30 mEq/L) without involving the kidneys.]
causes of acute respiratory alkalosis [$PaCO_2$ <33 mm Hg, HCO_3^- ≥18 mEq/L]	**CNS respiratory medullary center stimulation** (e.g., **anxiety**, endotoxemia [endotoxin effect], salicylates), *primary lung disease* (e.g., initial phase of bronchial asthma, pulmonary embolus)
causes of chronic respiratory alkalosis [$PaCO_2$ <33 mm Hg, HCO_3^- ≥12 but <18 mEq/L]	**CNS respiratory medullary center stimulation** (e.g., **cirrhosis** [toxic products], *residence at high altitude, pregnancy* [progesterone effect]), *primary lung disease* (e.g., restrictive lung diseases [e.g., sarcoidosis])

Table continued on following page

Table 5–4. ACID-BASE DISORDERS *Continued*

Most Common...	Answer and Explanation
S/S of respiratory alkalosis	**light-headedness**, *tetany* (alkalosis increases negative charges on albumin, hence more ionized calcium binds to albumin, resulting in lower ionized calcium levels), *circumoral and digital paresthesias* [numbness]
electrolyte abnormalities in respiratory alkalosis	*HCO_3^- moves into the cells as compensation and Cl^- ions move out of the cells (hyperchloremia) to maintain electroneutrality*
causes of metabolic alkalosis [pH >7.45 and HCO_3^- >28 mEq/L]	**diuretics**, *vomiting*, *primary mineralocorticoid excess states* (e.g., primary aldosteronism [Conn's syndrome]) [To maintain the increase in plasma HCO_3^- concentration, the kidneys must reclaim/regenerate HCO_3^-. Volume depletion is the primary mechanism for maintaining the high HCO_3^- in metabolic alkalosis produced by diuretics and vomiting. Volume depletion leads to secondary aldosteronism and increased distal exchange of Na^+ ions with H^+ ions, which reclaims HCO_3^-. In addition, volume depletion causes the proximal renal tubules to increase Na^+ reabsorption in exchange for H^+ ions, the latter reclaiming more HCO_3^-. In primary aldosteronism, increased exchange of Na^+ for K^+ in the distal tubules/collecting ducts leads to hypokalemia, leaving H^+ as the primary cation for Na^+ exchange, which, in turn, increases HCO_3^- reclamation (see Table 5–2). Finally, the aldosterone-enhanced H^+/K^+ pump increases regeneration of HCO_3^-.]
causes of the saline-responsive types of metabolic alkalosis	**diuretics**, *vomiting* [Replacing volume with isotonic saline reverses the condition, since the stimulus to reclaim HCO_3^- has been removed.]
causes of saline-resistant types of metabolic alkalosis	*primary aldosteronism* (Conn's syndrome) [Since the problem in mineralocorticoid excess is not volume depletion (see above), replacing saline does not correct the alkalosis.]
cause of primary aldosteronism	*benign adenoma in the adrenal cortex autonomously secreting excess aldosterone*

Table 5–4. ACID-BASE DISORDERS *Continued*

Most Common...	Answer and Explanation
symptom of primary aldosteronism	*muscle weakness* from severe hypokalemia due to increased exchange of K$^+$ for Na$^+$ [Other S/S include: *diastolic hypertension* (increased plasma volume, chronic retention of Na$^+$), *absence of pitting edema* (increased plasma volume increases the EABV, which increases P_H in the proximal tubule, causing enough loss of Na$^+$ in the urine to offset the gain of Na$^+$ distally caused by aldosterone).]
lab finding in primary aldosteronism	*hypokalemia* due to increased distal exchange of K$^+$ for Na$^+$ [Other findings include *increased urinary loss of K$^+$* (excellent screening test), *metabolic alkalosis* (increased distal exchange of Na$^+$ with H$^+$ when K$^+$ is depleted reclaims HCO$_3^-$), *low plasma renin activity* (increased plasma volume suppresses renin release).]
types of metabolic acidosis [pH <7.35 and HCO$_3^-$ <22 mEq/L]	**increased anion gap** and *normal anion gap metabolic acidosis*
formula used to distinguish increased from normal anion gap (AG) metabolic acidosis	*AG = serum Na$^+$ − (serum Cl$^-$ + serum HCO$_3^-$)* [Using normal values: AG = 140 − (104 + 24) = 12 mEq/L +/− 4. The 12 mEq/L represents anions that are unaccounted for by the formula. An increase in unmeasured anions (e.g., AcAc, β-OHB, lactate, salicylate, formate [metabolic product of methyl alcohol], oxalate [metabolic product of ethylene glycol], phosphate, and sulfates [renal failure]) increases the AG. Buffering of excess H$^+$ ions lowers the HCO$_3^-$ concentration. Every H$^+$ buffered leaves the corresponding anion of the acid behind, hence balancing the loss of HCO$_3^-$ depleted in the buffering process.]
mechanism for ketoacidosis in uncontrolled DM	*increased β-oxidation of fatty acids leading to increased production of acetyl CoA, which is converted into acetone, AcAc, and β-OHB*
type of ketoacidosis in alcoholics	β-OHB acidosis [In alcohol metabolism, increased acetyl CoA results in increased ketogenesis in the liver. Increased NADH favors conversion of AcAc into β-OHB. β-OHB is

Table continued on following page

Table 5–4. ACID-BASE DISORDERS *Continued*

Most Common...	Answer and Explanation
Continued	not detected by standard tests for ketones using the nitroprusside reaction, which only detects acetone and AcAc.]
clinical and lab findings in methyl alcohol poisoning	*blindness due to conversion of methyl alcohol (alcohol in shellac, Sterno, deicing solutions) to formaldehyde and then formic acid (increased AG metabolic acidosis), which attacks the optic nerve* [It is treated with infusion of ethyl alcohol, since both alcohols compete for alcohol dehydrogenase in their metabolism; hence, methyl alcohol is left unmetabolized and is removed by dialysis
clinical and lab findings in ethylene glycol (antifreeze) poisoning	*renal failure secondary to conversion of ethylene glycol into oxalic acid (increased AG metabolic acidosis), which binds with calcium to form crystals (easily identified in the urine) that block the renal tubules* [It is also treated with infusion of ethyl alcohol, which competes with ethylene glycol for metabolism.]
mechanism for increased AG metabolic acidosis in renal failure	*inability to excrete all of the daily load of H^+ (1 mEq per kg of body weight)*
cause of lactic acidosis	*tissue hypoxia, most often secondary to shock* [It may also occur with *severe hypoxemia* (<35 mm Hg), *CHF, CO poisoning, cyanide poisoning.* Some cases are *not associated with tissue hypoxia* (e.g., cirrhosis [cannot metabolize lactate]).]
causes of a normal AG metabolic acidosis	**loss of HCO_3^- in the GI tract** (e.g., **diarrhea**) or *GU tract* (e.g., RTA) [For example, if 10 mEq/L of HCO_3^- are lost in the stool, the serum HCO_3^- concentration is now 14 mEq/L (24 − 10). The loss in anions is counterbalanced by an equal gain in Cl^- ions to maintain electroneutrality; hence, the serum Cl^- concentration is now 114 mEq/L (104 + 10). The AG = 140 − (114 + 14) = 12 mEq/L.]

Table 5–4. ACID-BASE DISORDERS *Continued*

Most Common...	Answer and Explanation
type of RTA	*type I distal RTA, which is most commonly due to a defective aldosterone-enhanced H^+/K^+ ATPase pump in the collecting tubule* (see Table 5–2) [Protons are retained and combine with Cl^- to form HCl, K^+ is lost in the urine (hypokalemia), and the urine pH consistently remains >5.5 (less titratable acid and loss of NH_4Cl).]
mechanism for proximal RTA (type II RTA)	*decreased proximal tubule renal threshold for HCO_3^- reclamation* [If the threshold is lowered to 15 mEq/L, then the serum HCO_3^- concentration eventually becomes 15 mEq/L. The acidosis begins with HCO_3^- loss in the urine (urine pH >5.5), since the filtered HCO_3^- is not all reabsorbed. However, as the serum HCO_3^- approaches renal threshold, reabsorption matches the amount filtered and the urine pH becomes acid again (urine pH <5.5).]
causes of proximal RTA	**nephrotoxic agents** (e.g., heavy metals, aminoglycosides), *carbonic anhydrase inhibitors* (block HCO_3^- reclamation) [A genetic disease called *Fanconi's syndrome* produces proximal RTA and loss of glucose, urea, uric acid, phosphate, and amino acids.]
S/S in metabolic acidosis	*hyperventilation* (Kussmaul's breathing [rapid, deep breathing]; compensation is respiratory alkalosis) [Other S/S include *decreased myocardial contractility, osteoporosis* (bone buffers excess H^+), *warm shock, abdominal pain, vomiting.*]
lab finding in metabolic acidosis	*acidemia, respiratory alkalosis* (compensation), *low HCO_3^-* (primary abnormality) [Other findings: *hyperkalemia* (inorganic type of metabolic acidosis; not diarrhea or type I or II RTA [hypokalemia]), *hyperglycemia* (acidosis inhibits glycolysis), *hyperuricemia* (acids compete with uric acid for excretion in the kidneys).]
components of an ABG that are directly measured	*pH, $PaCO_2$, PO_2* [SaO_2, O_2 content, HCO_3^-, base excess/deficit are calculated.]

Table continued on following page

Table 5–4. ACID-BASE DISORDERS *Continued*

Most Common...	Answer and Explanation
noninvasive method for measuring SaO_2	*pulse oximeter* [It measures the differential absorption of two wavelengths of light (for oxyHb and deoxyHb) in pulsatile fashion, which reflects the SaO_2. It is dependent on the rate of blood flow (e.g., vasoconstriction alters the readings), position of the ODC, and type of Hb present (e.g., it cannot detect CO or metHb).]
term applied when two or more ABG disorders occur simultaneously	*mixed ABG disorders* [They are called simple disorders if only one is present.]
method of detection of a mixed ABG disorder	*careful history and physical exam* (e.g., knowing what to expect) [Other clues include a *normal pH in the presence of grossly abnormal $PaCO_2$ or HCO_3^-* (acidosis/alkalosis together; full compensation is extremely rare; hence a normal pH represents a mixed disorder), *markedly increased arterial pH* (two alkaloses together), *markedly decreased arterial pH* (two acidoses together).]
mixed disorder expected in a cardiorespiratory arrest	*primary metabolic acidosis (increased AG type from lactic acidosis) + primary respiratory acidosis (hypoventilation)* [This produces a very low pH.]
mixed disorder expected in salicylate intoxication	*primary metabolic acidosis* (salicylic acid + lactic acidosis) + *primary respiratory alkalosis* (salicylates overstimulate the respiratory center) [The pH is normal rather than decreased owing to the presence of a primary (not compensatory) respiratory alkalosis.]
method of interpreting simple ABGs	although various ratios are available for calculating the expected compensation, the following represents the easiest method to begin interpreting ABGs: *step 1:* define the $PaCO_2$—if <33 mm Hg = respiratory alkalosis; if >44 mm Hg = respiratory acidosis *step 2:* define the HCO_3^-—if <22 mEq/L = metabolic acidosis; if >28 mEq/L = metabolic alkalosis

Table 5-4. ACID-BASE DISORDERS *Continued*

Most Common...	Answer and Explanation
Continued	*step 3:* define the pH—if <7.35 = acidosis; if >7.45 = alkalosis *step 4:* the pH defines what is the primary disorder versus the compensation; e.g., $PaCO_2$ = 60 mm Hg [respiratory acidosis], HCO_3^- = 31 mEq/L [metabolic alkalosis], pH = 7.33 [acidemia], the primary disease is respiratory acidosis and partial compensation is metabolic alkalosis

Question: The patient is a 42-year-old woman with chronic headaches who presents with an altered sensorium and ecchymoses. pH = 7.37 (7.35–7.45), $PaCO_2$ = 20 mm Hg (33–44 mm Hg), serum HCO_3^- = 11 mEq/11 (22–28 mEq/L), serum Na^+ 140 mEq/L (136–145), serum K^+ 3.8 mEq/L (3.5–5.0), serum Cl^- 106 mEq/L (95–105), HCO_3^- 12 mEq/L (22–28). You suspect the patient has which of the following?

(A) Simple metabolic acidosis
(B) Simple respiratory alkalosis
(C) Mixed metabolic acidosis and respiratory alkalosis
(D) Mixed metabolic acidosis and metabolic alkalosis
(E) Mixed metabolic alkalosis and respiratory alkalosis

Answer: (C): pH = 7.37 (normal), $PaCO_2$ = 20 mm Hg (respiratory alkalosis), HCO_3^- = 11 mEq/L (metabolic acidosis), serum Na^+ = 140 mEq/L (normal), serum K^+ = 3.8 mEq/L (normal), serum Cl^- = 106 mEq/L (increased), HCO_3^- = 12 mEq/L (low; metabolic acidosis), calculated AG = 140 − (106 + 11) = 23 mEq/L, which is increased. The normal pH represents a mixed disorder, since full compensation rarely occurs. Therefore, primary metabolic acidosis (increased AG type) and primary respiratory alkalosis are present. (Note: the pH would have been <7.35 in the presence of a primary metabolic acidosis with compensated respiratory alkalosis.) Diagnosis: mixed primary metabolic acidosis + respiratory alkalosis. With the history of headaches, salicylate intoxication is the most likely cause.

AcAc = acetoacetic acid, ABG = arterial blood gas, AG = anion gap, ATP = adenosine triphosphate, β-OHB = β-hydroxybutyric acid, CHF = congestive heart failure, COPD = chronic obstructive pulmonary disease, CSF = cerebral spinal fluid, DM = diabetes mellitus, EABV = effective arterial blood volume, GI = gastrointestinal, GU = genitourinary, Hb = hemoglobin, metHb = methemoglobin (iron +3), NADH = nicotinamide adenine dinucleotide, ODC = oxygen dissociation curve, O_2 content = 1.34 (Hb) × O_2 saturation + PaO_2, $PaCO_2$ = partial pressure of CO_2 in arterial blood, PaO_2 = partial pressure of O_2 in arterial blood, PCO_2 = partial pressure of CO_2, P_H = peritubular hydrostatic pressure, PO_2 = partial pressure of O_2, PRA = plasma renin activity, RTA = renal tubular acidosis, SaO_2 = oxygen saturation, S/S = signs and symptoms.

Table 5–5. HEMOSTASIS SYSTEM AND LABORATORY TESTING

Most Common...	Answer and Explanation
components of the hemostasis system	*blood vessels, platelets, coagulation system, fibrinolytic system*
endothelial cell–derived anticoagulants	*tissue plasminogen activator* (tPA) [activates plasminogen to form plasmin], *heparin-like products* [enhance AT III activity], *prostacyclin* (PGI$_2$) [prevents platelet aggregation and vasodilates; endothelial cell prostacyclin synthetase converts PGH$_2$ into PGI$_2$]
liver-derived anticoagulants	*ATIII* [inhibits coagulation factors that are serine proteases (e.g., thrombin, factor X)] *proteins C and S* [enhance fibrinolytic activity, inactivate factors V and VIII]
endothelial cell–derived procoagulants [enhance vessel thrombosis]	*von Willebrand's factor VIII* (VIII:vWF; platelet adhesion factor; also synthesized by megakaryocytes), *VIII:Ag* (VIII antigen, carrier protein for VIII:vWF), *tissue thromboplastin* (activates factor VII in the extrinsic coagulation system)
platelet-derived procoagulants	*thromboxane A$_2$* (TXA$_2$) [platelet aggregator and vasoconstrictor; thromboxane synthetase converts PGH$_2$ into TXA$_2$], *VIII:vWF* [synthesized by megakaryocytes and stored in α granules within platelets; circulates as multimers], *ADP* [platelet aggregator located in dense bodies]
liver-derived procoagulants	*all the coagulation factors except VIII:vWF, VIII:Ag*
site of platelet production	*bone marrow by cytoplasmic fragmentation of megakaryocytes to produce 1000–3000 platelets per megakaryocyte* [They live ~10 days and ~one third are stored in the spleen.]
platelet enzyme blocked by aspirin and NSAIDs	*platelet cyclooxygenase* [converts arachidonic acid into PGG$_2$, which is converted into PGH$_2$, and by thromboxane synthetase into TXA$_2$] [Endothelial cell cyclooxygenase is not as affected by these drugs.]

Table 5–5. HEMOSTASIS SYSTEM AND LABORATORY
TESTING *Continued*

Most Common...	Answer and Explanation
binding agent for the vitamin K–dependent factors [factors II (prothrombin), VII, IX, and X, and proteins C and S]	*calcium binds the vitamin K–dependent factors to platelet factor 3 (PF3), which is the phospholipid substrate upon which coagulation occurs*
sequence of reactions used by the extrinsic coagulation system to generate thrombin	*it contains factor VII, which is activated by tissue thromboplastin* [Activated factor VII activates factor X in the final common pathway (see below), which produces thrombin to convert fibrinogen into fibrin.]
sequence of reactions used by the intrinsic coagulation system to generate thrombin	*it contains factor XII (Hageman's factor; activated by exposed subendothelial collagen and kallikrein), factor XI, factor IX, and factor VIII:C* [Factor XII, factor XI, HMWK, and prekallikrein are called contact factors. Activated XIIa activates prekallikrein to produce kallikrein, which activates HMWK to produce bradykinin.]
sequence of reactions used by the final common pathway to generate thrombin	*both coagulation systems activate the final common pathway, which includes factor X, factor V, factor II (prothrombin; converted into thrombin) and factor I (fibrinogen)* [Thrombin acts on fibrinogen to form fibrin monomer + fibrinopeptides A and B. Fibrin monomers then form fibrin aggregates, which form soluble fibrin (urea soluble), which is converted to insoluble fibrin with cross-links to form a stable clot (urea insoluble) by factor XIII.]
site for synthesis of the vitamin K–dependent factors	*the liver, which produces nonfunctional precursors that become functional (able to bind with calcium) when vitamin K_1 γ-carboxylates their terminal glutamic acid residues*
coagulation factors consumed in forming a fibrin clot	*factors I (fibrinogen), II (prothrombin), V, and VIII* [These factors are absent in serum.]

Table continued on following page

Table 5–5. HEMOSTASIS SYSTEM AND LABORATORY
TESTING *Continued*

Most Common...	Answer and Explanation
activators of plasminogen in the fibrinolytic pathway	**tPA,** *factor XII, streptokinase, urokinase* [tPA, streptokinase, and urokinase are used clinically in activating the system to dissolve clots.]
substrates degraded by plasmin	*circulating fibrinogen, clot-associated fibrinogen, and clot-associated fibrin monomers to form degradation products X, Y, D, and E as well as D-dimers* (cross-linked fragments; indicates factor XIII activity) *in clot-associated fibrin monomers*
vessel response in small vessel injury	*vasoconstriction* [reduces blood flow to facilitate platelet adhesion]
platelet response in small vessel injury	*platelet adhesion to exposed VIII:vWF via their GPIb receptors* [This is followed by the platelet release reaction of ADP (begins platelet aggregation) → platelet synthesis of TXA$_2$ (further enhances platelet aggregation and vasoconstriction) → platelet aggregation in the vessel lumen with fibrinogen cross-links between subjacent GPIIb/IIIa platelet fibrinogen receptors and cross-links with circulating VIII:vWF and subjacent platelet GPIb receptors for VIII:vWF to form a primary (temporary) hemostatic plug → cessation of bleeding. The above events are evaluated by the bleeding time (see below).]
coagulation system response in small vessel injury	*release of tissue thromboplastin (activates the extrinsic pathway) and activation of factor XII in the intrinsic system* [Both systems generate thrombin, which converts platelet-associated fibrinogen into fibrin with the formation of a stable clot.]
fibrinolytic system response in small vessel injury	*plasminogen is activated by tPA and activated factor XII* [This results in the release of plasmin, which dissolves the stable clot and re-establishes blood flow.]
test to evaluate platelets	*platelet count (150,000–400,000 cells/μL)* [10–15 platelets per oil powered field in a peripheral smear is ~ equivalent to a normal platelet count.]

Table 5–5. HEMOSTASIS SYSTEM AND LABORATORY
TESTING *Continued*

Most Common...	Answer and Explanation
platelet function test	*bleeding time (BT; normally <10 minutes)* [It evaluates vessel and platelet function up to the formation of a primary hemostatic plug. It does not evaluate the coagulation system.]
cause of a prolonged BT	*patient on aspirin or NSAIDs* [Other causes include *thrombocytopenia (<90,000 cells/µL), VWD, vascular disease* (e.g., scurvy).]
test to measure VIII:vWF	*ristocetin cofactor assay (single best test for VWD)* [Ristocetin normally aggregates platelets containing the GPIb receptor or VIII:vWF. If either component is missing, platelets cannot aggregate, which is the basis of the test. Agar gel electrophoresis is useful for identifying circulating vWF multimers (polymers of increasing molecular weight and size).]
coagulation system tests	*prothrombin time* (PT) and *activated partial thromboplastin time* (aPTT)
extrinsic coagulation system test	*PT* [It measures the extrinsic system down to the formation of a fibrin clot: VII → X → V → II → I → clot (normally 11–15 seconds). Protein-lipid tissue factor is added to the plasma to replace PF3, hence eliminating the role of platelets. The PT is prolonged if the above factors are <40% of normal. It is not sensitive for factor I or factor XIII deficiencies.]
use of the PT	*follow patients on coumarin* [Other uses: evaluating the severity of liver disease, detecting factor VII, X, V, and II deficiencies.]
use of the International Normalized Ratio (INR) for reporting the PT	*to follow coumarin anticoagulation* [The INR standardizes the PT regardless of the protein-lipid tissue reagents used in test kits anywhere in the world. INR = (patient PT/control PT) × International Sensitivity Index (value assigned to the particular type of protein-lipid tissue factor used in the test kit).]

Table continued on following page

Table 5–5. HEMOSTASIS SYSTEM AND LABORATORY TESTING *Continued*

Most Common...	Answer and Explanation
intrinsic coagulation system test	*aPTT* [It evaluates the intrinsic system down to the formation of a clot: XII → XI → IX → VIII → X → V → II → I → clot (normal 25–35 seconds). Thromboplastin is added to the test system to replace PF3, hence eliminating the role of platelets. The aPTT is prolonged if the above factors (not sensitive to fibrinogen or factor XIII), HMWK, or prekallikrein is below 30–40% of normal.]
use of the aPTT	*follow patients on heparin anticoagulation* [Other uses: An aPTT >150 seconds is highly predictive of a contact factor deficiency (XII, XI, HMWK, prekallikrein). Less prolonged values are present in the other factor deficiencies.]
vitamin K–dependent factor not detected by the PT	*factor IX, which is in the intrinsic pathway*
test used to evaluate the final stage of clotting	*thrombin time (TT)* [It detects abnormalities in conversion of fibrinogen into a fibrin clot by adding thrombin to the test system.]
uses of the TT	*fibrinogen deficiency, dysfibrinogenemia* (structurally abnormal fibrinogen commonly seen in liver disease), *heparin therapy* (heparin via AT III inhibits thrombin added to the test system)
test used for detecting circulating anticoagulants [antibodies, inhibitors of coagulation factors]	*mixing studies* [It distinguishes coagulation factor deficiencies from decreased production versus deficiencies due to antibody destruction (called inhibitors/circulating anticoagulants). 0.5 mL of patient plasma and 0.5 mL of normal plasma are mixed together. Correction of the previously prolonged PT and/or aPTT implies a true factor deficiency (normal plasma added the missing factor), while lack of correction indicates destruction of the factor by an antibody in both the patient and normal plasma.]

Table 5–5. HEMOSTASIS SYSTEM AND LABORATORY
TESTING *Continued*

Most Common...	Answer and Explanation
fibrinolytic system tests	*fibrin(ogen) degradation (split) products (FDPs)* and *D-dimer assay* [FDPs include the X, Y, D, and E fragments of plasmin degradation of fibrinogen alone, clot-associated fibrinogen, or clot-associated fibrin. D-dimers are cross-linked FDPs indicating factor XIII activity in a clot-associated fibrin clot rather than plasmin activity on fibrinogen alone or clot-associated fibrinogen. A positive FDP assay with a negative D-dimer assay indicates primary fibrinolysis (see below), whereas positive results in both assays indicate intravascular clotting (e.g., DIC, see below).]

Question: Which of the following results is expected in a patient taking aspirin?
(A) Thrombocytopenia
(B) Prolonged aPTT
(C) Prolonged PT
(D) Prolonged TT
(E) Prolonged BT

Answer: (E): Only the BT is prolonged with aspirin usage, since it produces a qualitative rather than a quantitative platelet defect. None of the coagulation studies evaluate platelet function, hence they are all normal.

aPTT = activated partial thromboplastin time, ADP = adenosine diphosphate, AT III = antithrombin III, BT = bleeding time, DIC = disseminated intravascular coagulation, FDP = fibrinogen degradation product, HMWK = high molecular weight kininogen, INR = International Normalized Ratio, NSAIDs = nonsteroidal anti-inflammatory drugs, PF = platelet factor, PG = prostaglandin, PGI$_2$ = prostacyclin, PT = prothrombin time, tPA = tissue plasminogen activator, TT = thrombin time, TXA$_2$ = thromboxane A$_2$, VIII:Ag = factor VIII antigen, VIII:C = factor VIII coagulant, VIII:vWF = von Willebrand's factor, VWD = von Willebrand's disease.

Table 5–6. SELECTED VASCULAR AND PLATELET DISORDERS

Most Common...	Answer and Explanation
sign associated with platelet disorders	*epistaxis* [nosebleeds] [Other signs include *petechiae* [1–3 mm, red, nonblanching, non-palpable hemorrhages on the skin and mucous membranes], *ecchymoses* [purpuric lesions about the size of a quarter], *easy or spontaneous bruising, bleeding from superficial scratches* (no primary hemostatic plug).]
genetic vascular disorder	*hereditary hemorrhagic telangiectasia (Osler-Weber-Rendu disease)* [An AD disease, it presents as epistaxis and pinpoint, dilated vascular channels in the mouth (tongue, lips), GI tract (produces iron deficiency), and skin. Less common genetic diseases include *Marfan's syndrome* (AD defect in fibrillin) and *Ehlers-Danlos syndrome* (multifactorial; defect in collagen).]
vessel disease in the elderly	*senile purpura due to atrophy of the perivascular support leading to purpura (ecchymoses) on the extensor surfaces.*
nutritional vascular disease	*scurvy due to vitamin C deficiency* [It leaves collagen structurally weak owing to lack of hydroxylation of proline and lysine.]
metabolic vascular disease	*excess glucocorticoids* (e.g., **patient on steroids**, Cushing's syndrome)
infectious vascular diseases	**viral infections** (e.g., rubella, rubeola), *RMSF* (rickettsial vasculitis transmitted by a tick), *scarlet fever* (toxin-induced)
cause of thrombocytopenia	*increased destruction* (e.g., **immune**, consumed in platelet clots or fibrin clots) [Other causes: *decreased production* (e.g., bone marrow suppression, marrow infiltration [e.g., metastasis, leukemia], *abnormal sequestration* (e.g., splenomegaly).]
cause of thrombocytopenia in children	*idiopathic thrombocytopenic purpura (ITP)* [IgG antibodies develop against the platelet GPIIb/IIIa receptor (type II hypersensitivity). It presents with an abrupt onset of epistaxis and petechiae, usually following a URI.

Table 5–6. SELECTED VASCULAR AND PLATELET DISORDERS *Continued*

Most Common...	Answer and Explanation
Continued	Megakaryocytes are present in the marrow. Splenomegaly is not present. Recovery is the rule. Steroids are used in symptomatic cases.]
cause of thrombocytopenia in systemic immune diseases	*autoimmune thrombocytopenia, particularly in patients with SLE* [IgG antibody develops against platelets with extravascular removal by macrophages (type II hypersensitivity). Unlike ITP in children, it is more insidious, more likely to be chronic, less responsive to therapy, and more likely to exhibit splenomegaly.]
mechanism for drug-induced thrombocytopenia	*"innocent bystander" immune destruction* [Drug-antibody complexes deposit on the surface of platelets and activate complement with destruction of the platelet (type III hypersensitivity). Common drug offenders include quinidine, sulfa drugs, penicillin, heparin, and thiazides. Withdrawal of the drug reverses the condition.]
virus-associated immune thrombocytopenias	**HIV, CMV, EBV** [Thrombocytopenia is the most common coagulation abnormality in AIDS.]
cause of TTP	*small vessel damage by a circulating toxin* (unknown) *that causes platelets to form platelet thrombi on damaged endothelial cells throughout the body*
S/S of TTP	*fever, thrombocytopenia, microangiopathic hemolytic anemia with schistocytes* [fragmented RBCs], *neurologic abnormalities, and renal failure*
lab findings in TTP	*thrombocytopenia, prolonged BT, normal PT and aPTT* [It is not DIC, since there is no intravascular consumption of clotting factors.]
cause of HUS in children	*similar in pathogenesis to TTP; one cause is toxin-induced endothelial damage by Escherichia coli serotype O157:H7 obtained by eating undercooked hamburger meat* [Some drugs have been associated with HUS (e.g., mitomycin, cyclosporine, cisplatin). Plasmapheresis is life-saving.]

Table continued on following page

Table 5–6. SELECTED VASCULAR AND PLATELET DISORDERS *Continued*

Most Common...	Answer and Explanation
S/S of HUS	*similar to TTP* (see above) [The renal disease is worse in HUS than in TTP, whereas the CNS disease is worse in TTP than in HUS.]
lab findings in HUS	*similar to TTP* (see above)
cause of primary thrombocytosis [elevated platelet count]	*myeloproliferative disease (e.g., PRV, essential thrombocythemia)* [These disorders are associated with thrombosis and bleeding.]
cause of secondary thrombocytosis	*malignancy, due to IL-6 stimulation of platelet production* (35% as part of a paraneoplastic syndrome) [Other causes include *infection* (e.g., TB), *rebound after thrombocytopenia, chronic iron deficiency,* and *splenectomy.*]
acquired cause of a qualitative platelet defect with a normal platelet count	*patient taking aspirin or NSAIDs, which block platelet cyclooxygenase and prevent the synthesis of TXA₂ and the platelet release reaction*
genetic cause of a qualitative platelet defect	*VWD with absence of VIII:vWF, the platelet adhesion factor* [In addition, patients have low VIII:Ag and VIII:C.]
platelet abnormality in uremia	*guanidinosuccinic acid inhibits PF3 and also interferes with platelet adhesion and aggregation* [It is reversed with dialysis, desmopressin (ADH), and combined estrogen/progestin pills.]

Question: A 44-year-old woman presents with fever, epistaxis, petechiae, mental status abnormalities, oliguria, and a normocytic anemia with numerous schistocytes present in the peripheral smear. You would expect the laboratory studies to reveal which of the following? **SELECT 2 answers**
   (A) A prolonged PT
   (B) A prolonged aPTT
   (C) A prolonged BT
   (D) Thrombocytopenia
   (E) An abnormal ristocetin cofactor assay

Answer: (C) and (D): The patient has TTP with the formation of platelet thrombi (thrombocytopenia and prolonged BT) without consumption of coagulation factors (normal PT and aPTT) or abnormalities in platelet adhesion (normal ristocetin cofactor assay).

aPTT = activated partial thromboplastin time, AD = autosomal dominant, ADH = antidiuretic hormone, AIDS = acquired immunodeficiency
virus, BT = bleeding time, CMV = cytomegalovirus, CNS = central
nervous system, DIC = disseminated intravascular coagulation, EBV =
Epstein-Barr virus, GI = gastrointestinal, HIV = human immunodeficiency virus, HUS = hemolytic uremic syndrome, Ig = immunoglobulin,
IL = interleukin, ITP = idiopathic thrombocytopenic purpura, NSAID
= nonsteroidal anti-inflammatory drug, PF = platelet factor, PRV =
polycythemia rubra vera, PT = prothrombin time, RBC = red blood
cell, RMSF = Rocky Mountain spotted fever, SLE = systemic lupus
erythematosus, S/S = signs and symptoms, TB = tuberculosis, TTP =
thrombotic thrombocytopenic purpura, URI = upper respiratory infection, VIII:Ag = factor VIII antigen, VIII:C = factor VIII coagulant,
VIII:vWF = von Willebrand's factor, VWD = von Willebrand's disease.

Table 5–7. COAGULATION AND FIBRINOLYTIC DISORDERS

Most Common...	Answer and Explanation
signs of a coagulation disorder	*delayed bleeding* (e.g., after a molar dental extraction; a primary hemostatic plug is present but not a stable clot), *hemarthroses* (severe hemophilia A and B), *bleeding into spaces* (severe hemophilia A and B), *hematuria, GI bleeds*
cause of a coagulation deficiency	*defective production* (e.g., hereditary, **acquired** [e.g., **liver disease**, **vitamin K deficiency**]) [Other causes: *increased consumption* (e.g., **DIC**), *increased destruction* (e.g., circulating anticoagulants [antibodies, inhibitors]), *combinations of the above.*]
SXR hereditary coagulation disorder	*hemophilia A* [It is an SXR disorder with a deficiency of VIII:C (asymptomatic female carrier transmits the disease to 50% of her sons). Severe disease is a VIII:C concentration <1% of normal (never changes throughout life). Mild cases (VIII:C between 25 and 50%) are asymptomatic unless stressed by major surgery or trauma. *Hemophilia B* (factor IX deficiency) is the second most common cause of hemarthroses.]
method of detecting asymptomatic female carriers of hemophilia A or B	*DNA techniques with identification of the abnormal locus on the X chromosome* [A ratio of VIII:C to VIII:Ag <0.75 is also very suggestive of a hemophilia A carrier (VIII:Ag is normal in hemophilia A).]

Table continued on following page

Table 5–7. COAGULATION AND FIBRINOLYTIC
DISORDERS *Continued*

Most Common...	Answer and Explanation
treatment of severe hemophilia A	*recombinant factor VIII concentrates* [There is no risk of transmitting HIV. ~75% of hemophilia A patients treated with factor VIII concentrates (pooled VIII:C from multiple donors) before 1985 (before screening was available) became infected with HIV. Infusion of products containing VIII:C causes an immediate nonsustained increase in de novo synthesis of VIII:C but not in excess of the amount infused.]
hereditary coagulation disorder	*VWD* [Classic VWD is an AD disorder. Other VWD variants are uncommon.]
S/S of VWD	*patients present with signs of platelet and coagulation defects* (e.g., epistaxis, menorrhagia)
GI association with VWD	*angiodysplasia* [dilated vessels that bleed; second most common cause of a massive lower GI bleed]
lab findings in VWD	*low VIII:vWF, VIII:Ag, and VIII:C; low RCoFA; prolonged BT*
treatment for mild VWD	*cryoprecipitate* [concentrate of factor VIII molecules, fibrinogen, factor XIII] *used to be the gold standard*, but **DDAVP (desmopressin) is now the treatment of choice** (stimulates synthesis of all factor VIII conponents) [*Estrogen* is useful in women with menorrhagia, since it increases all factor VIII components. Infusion of products containing factor VIII causes a slow but sustained increase in de novo synthesized factor VIII that is in excess of the amount infused.]
circulating anticoagulant [inhibitor, antibody]	*antibodies against factor VIII* (most commonly in the treatment of hemophilia A) [The prolonged aPTT does not correct with the addition of normal plasma (mixing studies). Additional causes include the *postpartum state* and *chlorpromazine therapy.*]
circulating anticoagulant against platelet PF3	*lupus anticoagulant (LA)* [This prolongs the aPTT (90%) and less commonly the PT (20%). Addition of phospholipid to the test system corrects the aPTT.]

Table 5–7. COAGULATION AND FIBRINOLYTIC DISORDERS *Continued*

Most Common...	Answer and Explanation
circulating anticoagulant against cardiolipin	*anticardiolipin antibody (ACA)* [This produces a false positive syphilis serology.]
syndrome associated with LA and/or ACA	*antiphospholipid (APL) syndrome* [Both antibodies are present in 60% of cases (one antibody in 40%).]
coagulation abnormality associated with APLs	*arterial and venous thrombosis* [The antibodies react against phospholipids in endothelial cells, resulting in damage and thrombosis. Clinical disorders include *repeated spontaneous abortions* (placental bed thrombosis), *stroke, hepatic vein thrombosis* (Budd-Chiari syndrome), *thromboembolization.*]
fat soluble vitamin deficiency resulting in a coagulation disorder	*vitamin K deficiency* [Vitamin K_1 is the active vitamin, while vitamin K_2 is inactive and requires epoxide reductase to convert it back into its functional state. Colon bacteria synthesize vitamin K_2.]
cause of vitamin K deficiency in newborns	*lack of bacterial colonization of the bowel* [The lowest values are between days 2 to 5, hence the practice of intramuscular vitamin K shots in newborns to prevent *hemorrhagic disease of the newborn* (e.g., CNS hemorrhage, ecchymoses, hemorrhage). Breast milk has no vitamin K.]
adult cause of vitamin K deficiency	*coumarin anticoagulation* [Coumarin derivatives inactivate epoxide reductase; therefore, vitamin K–dependent factors are nonfunctional. Less common causes include *malabsorption* and the use of *broad-spectrum antibiotics* (e.g., third-generation cephalosporins, neomycin; the latter drug is commonly used in liver failure to destroy colonic bacteria and production of ammonia).]
reason why heparin and coumarin anticoagulation are started simultaneously in the treatment of venous thrombosis	*heparin immediately anticoagulates the patient, while coumarin requires 4–5 days for full anticoagulation owing to the different half-lives of vitamin K–dependent factors that have already been γ-carboxylated* [Protein C and factor VII have the shortest half-lives (4–6 hours) and factor II the longest (72 hours).]

Table continued on following page

Table 5–7. COAGULATION AND FIBRINOLYTIC
DISORDERS *Continued*

Most Common...	Answer and Explanation
treatment of life-threatening hemorrhage in a patient on coumarin	*infusion of fresh frozen plasma (FFP)* [It contains functional coagulation factors. Oral or intramuscular vitamin K is provided in less serious bleeds.]
cause of DIC	*septicemia* [Other causes include *obstetrical problems* (e.g., amniotic fluid embolism), *massive trauma, disseminated cancer* (e.g., acute progranulocytic leukemia). It is a thrombohemorrhagic disorder with intravascular clotting and consumption of clotting factors with secondary fibrinolysis.]
factors consumed in DIC	*fibrinogen, factors II, V, VIII, and platelets* [In addition, *AT III* is used up in neutralizing serine proteases.]
S/S of DIC	*oozing of blood from wounds and venipuncture sites* [Other S/S include *hypovolemic shock* (activation of the complement system by plasmin with the release of anaphylatoxins), *widespread ecchymoses* (platelet dysfunction from FDPs, thrombocytopenia), *widespread organ dysfunction* (e.g., renal failure).]
lab findings in DIC	*presence of FDPs and D-dimers (best overall tests)* [Other findings include *prolonged aPTT and PT* (due to consumption of coagulation factors), *thrombocytopenia* (consumed in clots), *normocytic anemia with schistocytes* (fragmented RBCs from intravascular hemolysis), *decreased fibrinogen* (consumed in clots and destroyed by plasmin), *decreased AT III* (used up in neutralizing serine proteases).]
treatment of DIC	*treat the underlying cause of DIC* [Stopgaps to keep the patient hemostatically stable include infusion of *packed RBCs, FFP, platelet concentrates*, and *cryoprecipitate* (contains fibrinogen and factor VIII). *Subcutaneous heparin* attacks the thrombosis part of the syndrome by inactivating thrombin.]

Table 5–7. COAGULATION AND FIBRINOLYTIC DISORDERS *Continued*

Most Common...	Answer and Explanation
pathologic cause of multiple factor deficiencies	*severe liver disease* [Less common causes include *DIC* and *vitamin K deficiency.* Most coagulation factors are synthesized in the liver, hence severe liver disease produces multiple deficiencies.]
cause of secondary fibrinolysis	*DIC* [Activation of factor XII leads to concomitant activation of plasminogen.]
causes of primary fibrinolysis	*radical prostatectomy* (release of urokinase), *metastatic prostate cancer, open heart surgery* [Serious bleeding is likely to occur once α_2-plasmin inhibitor is used up in neutralizing excess plasmin.]
lab findings in primary fibrinolysis	**increased FDPs and normal D-dimers**, *decreased fibrinogen, prolonged aPTT and PT* [coagulation factors are degraded by plasmin; FDPs interfere with clotting], *normal platelet count*

Question: Which of the following represents hemophilia A rather than classic VWD?
  (A) Normal BT
  (B) Prolonged aPTT
  (C) Normal PT
  (D) Low VIII:C
  (E) Low VIII:Ag

Answer: (A): Hemophilia A has a normal BT (no platelet adhesion defect; VWD is missing VIII:vWF), prolonged aPTT (also in VWD), normal PT (also in VWD), low VIII:C (also in VWD), normal VIII:Ag (low in VWD).

ACA = anticardiolipin antibody, AD = autosomal dominant, APL = anti-phospholipid, aPTT = activated partial thromboplastin time, AT III = antithrombin III, BT = bleeding time, CNS = central nervous system, DIC = disseminated intravascular coagulation, FDPs = fibrin(ogen) degradation products, FFP = fresh frozen plasma, GI = gastrointestinal, LA = lupus anticoagulant, PT = prothrombin time, RBC = red blood cell, RCoFA = ristocetin cofactor assay, S/S = signs and symptoms, SXR = sex-linked recessive, VIII:Ag = factor VIII antigen, VIII:C = factor VIII coagulant, VWD = von Willebrand's disease, VIII:vWF = von Willebrand's factor.

Table 5–8. THROMBOEMBOLIC DISORDERS

Most Common...	Answer and Explanation
blood components in a pale thrombus	*primarily platelets and small amounts of fibrin* [They develop in areas of rapid arterial blood flow where there is endothelial damage (e.g., TTP, components in cigarette smoke) or turbulence (e.g., **atherosclerotic plaque**, branching points in arteries).]
blood components in a red thrombus	*coagulation factors* (fibrinogen, factors V, VIII, and II), *fibrin, platelets, entrapped RBCs* [They develop in areas of stasis (e.g., venous system) or in hypercoagulable states (e.g., AT III deficiency). They contain *lines of Zahn*, representing alternating pale (platelets) and red (RBCs) areas.]
risk factors for venous thrombosis	**stasis** (e.g., **postoperative state**), *CHF* (decreased venous return to the heart), *obesity, oral contraceptives* (decreased AT III levels), *smoking*
risk factors for arterial thrombosis	**age** (>45 years in a man, >55 in a woman), *LDL >160 mg/dL, HDL <35 mg/dL, diabetes mellitus, hypertension, smoking, family history of premature CAD/stroke, increased plasma homocysteine levels* (damage to vessel endothelium)
cause of a mural thrombus [thrombus that is adherent to the endothelial surface of the atrium or ventricle]	*acute myocardial infarction* [These are mixed pale and red clots, since there is an element of stasis (red clot) and endothelial injury (pale clot). Other causes include *ventricular aneurysm* and *left atrial dilatation* (e.g., mitral stenosis).]
site for venous thrombosis	*deep saphenous veins in the calf* [These red clots propagate toward the heart. Once they reach the femoral and iliac veins, the chance of breaking off and embolizing to the lungs is increased.]
complication of venous thrombosis	*thromboembolization with or without pulmonary infarction* [The most common site for thromboembolization is the femoral veins in the thigh.]
complication of arterial thrombosis	*infarction*

Table 5–8. THROMBOEMBOLIC DISORDERS *Continued*

Most Common...	Answer and Explanation
treatment for venous thrombosis	*heparin and coumarin anticoagulants* [Heparin enhances AT III activity with subsequent neutralization of serine proteases (particularly thrombin and factor X), whereas coumarin blocks vitamin K_1 production; therefore, factors II, VII, IX, and X are nonfunctional. Heparin does not dissolve clots.]
treatment of arterial thrombosis	*low-dose aspirin* [It blocks platelet cyclooxygenase, thereby preventing synthesis of TXA_2 and the release reaction for platelet aggregation. *Fibrinolytic agents* (e.g., tPA, streptokinase) are used to dissolve large clots (e.g., coronary artery thrombosis).]
treatment of venous thrombosis in pregnancy	*heparin* [Coumarin derivatives are teratogenic.]
complication of anticoagulant therapy	*bleeding*
treatment of heparin overcoagulation and bleeding	*protamine sulfate*
acquired causes of a hypercoagulable state	*cancer* (patients commonly have an increase in fibrinogen, factor V, and factor VIII), *oral contraceptives*
hereditary cause of a hypercoagulable state	**factor V Leiden deficiency** (resistant to protein C degradation) [Deficiencies of protein C/S, AT III are less common.]
clues favoring hereditary hyper-coagulable state	**recurrent deep venous thrombosis (DVT) with or without pulmonary embolus (PE),** *family history of the above, DVT or PE at an early age, unusual sites for venous thrombosis* (e.g., axilla, dural sinuses)
cause of hemor-rhagic skin necrosis in a patient placed on coumarin	*heterozygote carrier with protein C deficiency* [These patients have 30–60% protein C levels. When placed on coumarin, they become "homozygous," since the protein C they do have is now nonfunctional.

Table continued on following page

Table 5–8. THROMBOEMBOLIC DISORDERS *Continued*

Most Common...	Answer and Explanation
Continued	Since the half-life of the protein is only 4–6 hours, thrombosis occurs before patients become fully anticoagulated. Thrombosis mainly occurs in the vessels of the skin. It may also occur with *protein S deficiency.*]
origin of emboli to the lungs in the venous system [an embolus is a mass (gas, liquid, solid) transmitted in the blood from one site to another site]	*femoral veins in the upper thigh* (propagation from thrombus in the deep saphenous veins of the lower leg)
origin of emboli in the arterial system	*clots dislodged from the left side of the heart* (e.g., mural thrombus, vegetations on the aortic or mitral valve)
cause of paradoxical embolization	*thromboembolism from the venous system through a patent foramen ovale into the systemic circulation*
cause of fat embolization	*fractures of the long bones or pelvis* [Fat enters the microcirculation to produce, within 24–72 hours, signs of CNS dysfunction, respiratory failure (hypoxemia, dyspnea), and thrombocytopenia (platelets stick to the fat globules in the circulation; petechiae develop in the upper half of the body). Mortality is <10%.]
cause of death in amniotic fluid embolization	*DIC* [Amniotic fluid embolism usually accompanies a difficult delivery. Amniotic fluid is rich in thromboplastin, thereby initiating DIC. Lanugo hair and fetal squamous cells are noted in the lungs of women who die (>80% mortality) of complications related to the disease.]
cause of right-sided air embolization	*surgery in the head and neck area* or *catheter insertion into the jugular or subclavian vein* [Air is sucked into the venous system owing to the negative intrathoracic pressure. It froths up the blood in the pulmonary artery, restricting blood flow. It is treated with 100% oxygen while the patient is head down with feet up in a left lateral decubitus position.]

Table 5–8. THROMBOEMBOLIC DISORDERS *Continued*

Most Common...	Answer and Explanation
cause of decompression sickness (caisson disease)	*deep-sea diving* [rapid ascension to the surface releases nitrogen gas into the blood vessels of muscles and joints (bends)] [Atmospheric pressure increases by 1 atmosphere for every 33 feet of descent. Nitrogen gas is dissolved in tissue as one descends in the water. Treatment is the administration of O_2 in a hyperbaric chamber.]

Question: Which of the following will **MOST LIKELY** result in a bleeding diathesis?
  (A) Presence of LA
  (B) Protein C deficiency
  (C) Polycythemia
  (D) Oral contraceptives
  (E) Malabsorption

Answer: (E): Malabsorption results in vitamin K deficiency, which, in turn, would lead to an anticoagulated state. LA is a misnomer, since Protein C deficiency (leaves factors V and VIII activated and the fibrinolytic system activity reduced), polycythemia (increased RBCs produce hyperviscosity), and oral contraceptives (decreases AT III levels) all predispose to hypercoagulability.

AD = autosomal dominant, AT III = antithrombin III, CAD = coronary artery disease, CHF = congestive heart failure, CNS = central nervous system, DIC = disseminated intravascular coagulation, DVT = deep venous thrombosis, HDL = high density lipoproteins, LA = lupus anticoagulant, LDL = low density lipoproteins, PE = pulmonary embolus, RBC = red blood cell, TTP = thrombotic thrombocytopenic purpura, TXA_2 = thromboxane A_2, tPA = tissue plasminogen activator.

CHAPTER

NUTRITION

CONTENTS

Table 6–1. NUTRITION IN DISEASE, NUTRITIONAL ASSESSMENT, EATING DISORDERS, AND PROTEIN ENERGY MALNUTRITION

Most Common...	Answer and Explanation
nutritionally related causes of death	**heart disease,** *cancer, stroke* (These 3 account for two thirds of all deaths in the United States.) [Dietary factors (e.g., low fiber/high saturated fat) are the second most common (smoking is first) contributors to increased morbidity and mortality in the United States.]
test to evaluate total body fat composition	*caliper skinfold measurements at multiple sites*
test to evaluate immune competence	*cutaneous hypersensitivity reactions to common antigens* [Lack of response indicates anergy and poor cellular immunity. *A total lymphocyte count* is also used.]
tests to evaluate lean body mass	*urinary measurement of creatinine* (metabolic product of creatine in muscle) *and 3-methylhistidine* (component of actin and myosin)
tests to evaluate visceral protein mass	**retinol-binding protein** (1 day half-life; best test), *prealbumin* (half-life, 2–3 days), *transferrin* (half-life, 8–10 days), *albumin* (half-life, 18–20 days) [The shorter the protein half-life, the better the correlation with protein mass.]

Table continued on following page

105

Table 6–1. NUTRITION IN DISEASE, NUTRITIONAL ASSESSMENT, EATING DISORDERS, AND PROTEIN ENERGY MALNUTRITION *Continued*

Most Common...	Answer and Explanation
eating disorder with distortion of body image	*anorexia nervosa* [A distorted body image most clearly separates it from the weight loss syndrome (e.g., exercise enthusiasts) and bulimia.]
S/S in anorexia nervosa	**secondary amenorrhea** [body weight below 15% of normal decreases GnRH, and decreases FSH and LH, which decreases estrogen], *osteoporosis* [lack of estrogen], *cardiovascular abnormalities* (heart failure, ventricular arrhythmias) [Stress hormones are increased (ACTH, cortisol, GH).]
COD in anorexia nervosa	*ventricular arrhythmias*
S/S of bulimia nervosa	*an eating disorder associated with self-induced vomiting; S/S include bruising of the knuckles, acid injury to the enamel* [Boerhaave's and Mallory-Weiss syndromes may also occur (distal esophagus/stomach rupture or tear, respectively).]
acid-base disorder in bulimia nervosa	*hypochloremic hypokalemic metabolic alkalosis* (from vomiting)
definition of obesity	*body mass index (BMI) >30 kg/m²* (weight in kilograms divided by height in meters squared) [A BMI of 27.5–30 kg/m² is mild obesity, 31–40 kg/m² moderate obesity, and >40 kg/m² morbid obesity. Body fat >20% above the ideal weight is also used as a definition of obesity].
ethnic groups predisposed to obesity	**Native Americans,** *African Americans, Hispanics, white Americans*
cause of obesity	*genetic factors (50–75%)* [Energy intake is greater than energy expenditure at rest and with exercise, owing to alterations in the hypothalamic feeding and satiety center. The obesity gene codes for a protein called leptin, which normally controls appetite. Inactivation of the gene leads to obesity. Hyperplasia of adipose cells occurs in children and hypertrophy in adults.]

Table 6–1. NUTRITION IN DISEASE, NUTRITIONAL ASSESSMENT, EATING DISORDERS, AND PROTEIN ENERGY MALNUTRITION *Continued*

Most Common...	Answer and Explanation
medical complication in obesity	*hypertension* (? hyperinsulinemia with increased renal sodium reabsorption) [Other complications include *LVH, thromboembolism, CAD* (a waist-to-hip ratio >1:1 is the greatest risk), *stroke, sleep apnea, gallstones, cancer* (colorectal, breast, endometrial, ovarian), *osteoarthritis, type II DM, lipid abnormalities* (increased LDL and TG, decreased HDL).]
COD in calorie-restricted diets	*ventricular arrhythmias*
effect of PEM on nitrogen balance	*negative nitrogen balance* (intake [protein intake 24 hrs/6.25] − excretion [urine urea nitrogen 24 hrs + 4/total urine volume in liters]) *owing to inadequate protein intake, nutrient losses, increased nutrient requirements* [Normal people should have a value approaching zero.]
examples of PEM	*kwashiorkor, marasmus,* or combinations of the two
S/S of marasmus	*muscle wasting and loss of subcutaneous fat leading to "broomstick extremities" (due to a total reduction in caloric intake)*
S/S in kwashiorkor	*pitting edema (hypoalbuminemia, due to an inadequate intake of protein* [normal total caloric intake]), *hepatomegaly with fatty change* (VLDL cannot be excreted from hepatocytes due to decreased apolipoprotein synthesis in the liver) [Other findings: flaky paint dermatitis, diarrhea, anemia, decreased immune response, reddish hair (flag sign), and apathy.]

Table continued on following page

Table 6–1. NUTRITION IN DISEASE, NUTRITIONAL ASSESSMENT, EATING DISORDERS, AND PROTEIN ENERGY MALNUTRITION *Continued*

Question: Which of the following is more commonly associated with kwashiorkor than with marasmus?
(A) Broomstick extremities
(B) Hypoalbuminemia
(C) Severe muscle wasting
(D) Decreased caloric intake
(E) Growth failure

Answer: (B): Owing to decreased protein intake, serum albumin is decreased. Choices (A), (C), and (D) are present in marasmus. Both conditions have growth failure.

ACTH = adrenocorticotropic hormone, BMI = body mass index, CAD = coronary artery disease, COD = cause of death, DM = diabetes mellitus, FSH = follicle stimulating hormone, GnRH = gonadotropin releasing hormone, GH = growth hormone, HDL = high-density lipoprotein, LDL = low-density lipoprotein, LH = luteinizing hormone, LVH = left ventricular hypertrophy, PEM = protein-energy malnutrition, S/S = signs and symptoms, TG = triglyceride, VLDL = very low density lipoprotein.

Table 6–2. VITAMIN DISORDERS

Most Common...	Answer and Explanation
vitamins associated with toxicity	*fat-soluble vitamins A, D, E, and K* [Fat-soluble vitamins are stored in fat, whereas water-soluble vitamins, when in excess, are excreted in urine.]
vitamins that serve as cofactors in biochemical reactions	*water-soluble vitamins*
vitamin deficiencies producing growth retardation in children	*vitamins A, D* (rickets), *and C* (scurvy)
vitamin toxicity producing increased intracranial pressure and hypercalcemia in children	*vitamin A toxicity* [Increased intracranial pressure causes papilledema, bulging fontanelles, and convulsions. Vitamin A (retinoic acid) enhances the activity of vitamin D in reabsorbing calcium and phosphorus in the small bowel.]

Table 6–2. VITAMIN DISORDERS *Continued*

Most Common...	Answer and Explanation
vitamin deficiencies with hair abnormalities	*deficiencies of vitamin A, vitamin C, and biotin* [Vitamin A deficiency causes follicular hyperkeratosis; vitamin C deficiency, perifollicular hemorrhages; and biotin deficiency, patchy areas of baldness.]
vitamin toxicities producing hypercalcemia	*vitamins A and D* [Vitamin A enhances the action of vitamin D, which reabsorbs calcium and phosphorus from the small bowel.]
vitamin deficiencies with eye abnormalities	*vitamin A deficiency* (leads to squamous metaplasia of the conjunctiva, keratomalacia [corneal softening leading to blindness], and nyctalopia [loss of night vision]) and *riboflavin deficiency* (corneal neovascularization)
vitamin deficiencies with glossitis	*deficiencies of niacin, riboflavin* (magenta tongue), *pyridoxine, vitamin C, B₁₂, and folate*
vitamin deficiency with skin hyperpigmentation and dementia	*niacin deficiency* (pellagra) [Niacin is involved in the synthesis of nicotinamide adenine dinucleotide (NAD$^+$) and nicotinamide adenine dinucleotide phosphate (NADP$^+$), which are cofactors in oxidation/reduction reactions.]
vitamin deficiencies with a hemorrhagic diathesis	*vitamin C* (scurvy) and *vitamin K deficiency* [Scurvy, owing to defective collagen synthesis, produces ecchymoses and hemarthroses. Vitamin K deficiency in newborns is called hemorrhagic disease of the newborn. See Chapter 5.]
vitamin deficiency producing tetany	*vitamin D deficiency,* which causes hypocalcemia and tetany [Decreased ionized calcium causes neuromuscular hyperexcitability.]
vitamin deficiencies producing paresthesias and decreased position and vibratory sensation	*deficiencies of thiamine* (common in alcoholics) *and vitamin B₁₂* (subacute combined degeneration involving the dorsal columns and the lateral corticospinal tract)
vitamin deficiency producing cerebellar disease and spinocerebellar ataxia	*vitamin E deficiency* [Deficiency is most commonly associated with chronic malabsorption in patients with cystic fibrosis.]

Table continued on following page

Table 6–2. VITAMIN DISORDERS *Continued*

Most Common...	Answer and Explanation
vitamin deficiencies producing anemia	*deficiencies of vitamin E* (hemolytic anemia in newborns), *vitamin C* (produces iron and folate deficiencies), *pyridoxine* (sideroblastic anemia; defect in heme synthesis), B_{12} (macrocytic anemia), and *folate* (macrocytic anemia)
vitamin deficiency producing ophthalmoplegia, nystagmus, ataxia, confusion, and memory deficits	*thiamine deficiency* [Confusion, ataxia, nystagmus, and ophthalmoplegia characterize Wernicke's encephalopathy, and confabulation with antegrade and retrograde memory deficits is Korsakoff's psychosis. Thiamine deficiency is most commonly due to alcoholism.]
vitamin deficiency associated with poor wound healing	*vitamin C deficiency* (scurvy) [Vitamin C is responsible for hydroxylation of proline and lysine in collagen. These are the sites of cross-bridging of collagen fibrils for increased tensile strength.]
vitamin deficiency producing high output failure and congestive cardiomyopathy	*thiamine deficiency* [Thiamine is a cofactor for pyruvate dehydrogenase, which converts pyruvate into acetyl CoA, the latter combining with OAA to form citrate. Deficiency leads to ATP depletion, which reduces contractility in the heart, and to volume overload with dilatation (congestive cardiomyopathy). Thiamine deficiency also causes peripheral vasodilatation of arterioles, which increases the return of blood to the heart, causing high output failure.]
vitamin deficiency due to eating raw eggs	*biotin deficiency* [Avidin in raw eggs binds biotin. Biotin is the cofactor for pyruvate carboxylase, which converts pyruvate to OAA.]
vitamin deficiencies producing diarrhea	*deficiencies of niacin, B_{12}, and folate* [Niacin deficiency (pellagra) is characterized by diarrhea, dermatitis (hyperpigmentation), and dementia. Folate and B_{12} deficiency lead to a reduction in DNA synthesis. In the intestinal cells, this causes malabsorption.]
vitamin deficiency secondary to tryptophan deficiency	*niacin deficiency* [Tryptophan, an essential amino acid, can be converted into niacin. Deficiency may occur with corn-based diets (corn lacks tryptophan), carcinoid syndrome (tryptophan also forms serotonin), and Hartnup's disease (defect in the uptake of neutral amino acids in the intestine and kidneys).]

Table 6–2. VITAMIN DISORDERS *Continued*

Most Common...	Answer and Explanation
vitamin deficiencies produced by drinking goat's milk	*folate* and *pyridoxine deficiency*
vitamin deficiency producing bleeding gums	*vitamin C deficiency* [There is also a loss of teeth.]
vitamin deficiency causing a prolonged PT	*vitamin K deficiency* [Vitamin K γ-carboxylates glutamate residues in coagulation factors II (prothrombin), VII, IX, X, and proteins C and S. The PT evaluates the following factors: VII → X → V → II → I (fibrinogen) → clot.]
vitamin deficiency causing atrophic gastritis and achlorhydria	B_{12} *deficiency* (specifically PA) [In PA, autoantibodies destroy parietal cells, which synthesize acid and intrinsic factor.]
antioxidant vitamins	*vitamins E* (inhibits lipid peroxidation in the cell membrane) and *C* (FR scavenger; reducing agent)
vitamin whose function is to prevent squamous metaplasia	*vitamin A* [Metaplasia of corneal epithelium produces Bitot's spot (focal area of squamous metaplasia) and keratomalacia (softening of the cornea), the latter leading to blindness. Other sites for metaplasia include the bronchi (chronic bronchitis, pneumonia), hair follicles (follicular hyperkeratosis), bladder (stones).]
endocrine disorder producing β-carotenemia	*primary hypothyroidism* [Thyroid hormone enhances conversion in the small intestinal cells of β-carotenes into retinoic acid. Deficiency leads to a buildup of the former compound, resulting in yellow skin (not conjunctiva). Unlike retinoic acid, β-carotenes are not toxic in high doses.]
source of vitamin D	*sunlight* [Skin-derived 7-dehydrocholesterol after UVB exposure is converted into cholecalciferol (vitamin D_3).]
sites involved in vitamin D synthesis	*skin, small intestine, liver* (first hydroxylation to 25-(OH)-D_3 cholecalciferol [calcidiol]), *kidneys* (second hydroxylation to 1,25(OH)$_2$-D_3 cholecalciferol [calcitriol])

Table continued on following page

Table 6–2. **VITAMIN DISORDERS** *Continued*

Most Common...	Answer and Explanation
stimuli for synthesis of 1α-hydroxylase	**PTH,** *hypophosphatemia* [It is synthesized in the proximal tubules. Calcitriol and hyperphosphatemia inhibit the enzyme.]
functions of vitamin D	*reabsorb calcium and phosphorus* from the small intestine to establish a solubility product ($Ca^{++} \times PO_4^{--}$) to *mineralize bone and cartilage*
clinical differences between vitamin D deficiency in children and in adults	*craniotabes* (increased recoil of the skull; first sign of rickets), *rachitic rosary* (increased osteoid in the epiphyses of the ribs) [Vitamin D deficiency in children is called rickets and in adults, osteomalacia. Both have a reduction in bone mineralization causing softening of bone and an excess of osteoid leading to bowing of the legs.]
radiologic findings in vitamin D deficiency	**osteopenia** (rarefied bone) and *pseudofractures* (Looser's lines, Milkman's fractures), representing linear lines in the metaphysis where blood vessels push aside the soft osteoid
cause of vitamin D deficiency	*chronic renal disease,* owing to reduced second hydroxylation of vitamin D
lab test used to assess vitamin D status	*calcidiol* (owing to its longer circulating half-life [3 weeks] than calcitriol [4–6 hours])
lab findings in vitamin D deficiency in chronic renal disease	**hypocalcemia,** *normal to high serum phosphorus* [kidneys are the main excretory route; may be normal owing to phosphaturic effect of increased PTH], *high alkaline phosphatase* [response to reduced bone mineralization], *increased PTH* [stimulus of hypocalcemia; secondary hyperparathyroidism], *normal calcidiol, decreased calcitriol*
lab findings in vitamin D deficiency secondary to malabsorption	*same as above except for a decreased serum phosphorus and decreased calcidiol*
cause of type I vitamin D–dependent rickets	*decreased 1α-hydroxylase* [There is a decrease in serum calcium, phosphorus, and calcitriol. PTH is increased and calcidiol normal.]

Table 6–2. VITAMIN DISORDERS *Continued*

Most Common...	Answer and Explanation
cause of type II vitamin D–dependent rickets	*absent receptors for vitamin D* [Serum calcium and phosphorus are both decreased. PTH is increased, calcidiol is normal, and calcitriol is increased (key distinction from type I).]
vitamin deficiency producing the brown bowel syndrome	*vitamin E deficiency* [The brown bowel is due to a buildup of lipofuscin and is most commonly seen in cystic fibrosis.]
cause of pyridoxine deficiency	*isoniazid* [Pyridoxine is involved in heme synthesis, synthesis of neurotransmitters, transamination reactions (e.g., conversion of alanine into pyruvate).]
supplements required in pregnancy	*folate* and *iron* [Folate stores last ~3–4 months. Women have ~400 mg of iron stores and normally lose 500 mg per pregnancy.]
vitamin deficiency produced by methotrexate, phenytoin, and BCPs	*folate deficiency* [With methotrexate there is a block in dihydrofolate reductase, which converts DHF into THF. Phenytoin blocks intestinal conjugase, which converts polyglutamates (form of folate in food) into monoglutamates. BCPs block the uptake of monoglutamates in the jejunum.]

Question: Which of the following is an abnormality associated with a fat-soluble vitamin rather than a water-soluble vitamin deficiency?

    (A) Wernicke's encephalopathy
    (B) Dementia
    (C) Hypocalcemia
    (D) Hyperpigmentation
    (E) Sideroblastic anemia

Answer: (C): Hypocalcemia is seen in vitamin D deficiency. Choices (B) and (D) are present in niacin deficiency. Choice (A) is a feature of thiamine deficiency. Choice (E) is characteristic of pyridoxine deficiency.

ATP = adenosine triphosphate, BCP = birth control pills, DHF = dihydrofolate, FR = free radical, OAA = oxaloacetic acid, PA = pernicious anemia, PT = prothrombin time, PTH = parathormone, THF = tetrahydrofolate, UVB = ultraviolet light B.

Table 6–3. TRACE ELEMENT DISORDERS, DIETARY FIBER, NUTRITION AND CANCER, NUTRITIONAL CHANGES WITH AGING, SPECIAL DIETS

Most Common...	Answer and Explanation
cause of trace element deficiencies	*total parenteral nutrition*
trace element deficiency associated with anemia	*copper deficiency* [Copper is a cofactor for ferroxidase, which converts iron to $+3$. This enables iron to bind to transferrin. Hence, copper deficiency produces a microcytic anemia, since iron cannot be delivered to normoblasts in the bone marrow.]
trace element deficiency associated with poor wound healing and dysgeusia [lack of taste sense]	*zinc deficiency* [Deficiency is common in diabetics and alcoholics. Growth retardation, hypogonadism, and dry, scaly skin around the eyes and mouth also occur.]
trace element deficiency associated with dissecting aortic aneurysms	*copper deficiency* [Copper is a cofactor for lysyl oxidase, which forms cross-links in collagen and elastic tissue, hence deficiency leaves the aorta, an elastic artery, structurally weakened.]
trace element deficiency associated with dental caries	*fluoride deficiency*
cause of mottling of the teeth and calcifications of ligaments and tendons	*excess fluoride*
trace element that is an antioxidant	*selenium* [Selenium is a cofactor in glutathione peroxidase, which forms GSH. GSH neutralizes peroxide in the cytosol.]
insoluble fibers	*wheat bran, wheat germ* [Insoluble fiber is nonfermentable. It is composed of lignin, hemicellulose, and cellulose.]
soluble fibers	*oat brain, fruits, psyllium seeds* [Soluble fiber is fermentable. It is composed of pectins, gums, mucilages, and hemicellulose.]

Table 6–3. TRACE ELEMENT DISORDERS, DIETARY FIBER, NUTRITION AND CANCER, NUTRITIONAL CHANGES WITH AGING, SPECIAL DIETS *Continued*

Most Common...	Answer and Explanation
fiber type that has a hypoglycemic and hypocholesterolemic effect	*soluble fiber*
effects of fiber on stool	*fiber decreases stool transit time, increases stool bulk, decreases stool pH, decreases the amount of estrogen reabsorbed, and decreases the effect of lithocholic acid* (secondary bile acid associated with colorectal cancer) *on the bowel mucosa by decreasing stool transit time and absorbing it into the fiber*
cancers whose incidence is decreased by a high fiber diet	*colorectal, endometrial, ovarian, breast*
group of vegetables linked to a reduction in cancer	*cruciferous vegetables* (e.g., broccoli, cauliflower) [They contain high amounts of β-carotenoids, vitamin C, and vitamin E.]
food contaminant that increases the risk for hepatocellular carcinoma	*aflatoxins* [This mold is a cocarcinogen with hepatitis B in producing hepatocellular carcinoma.]
S/S of essential fatty acid deficiency	*dry skin, thrombocytopenia, hair loss, impaired wound healing* [Linoleic and linolenic acid are the essential fatty acids. They supply double bonds in fatty acid synthesis. Linoleic acid is also utilized in the synthesis of arachidonic acid.]
effects of a high saturated fat diet [saturated fat + ω-6 polyunsaturated lipids]	*enhance atherosclerosis, carcinogenic* [They enhance uptake of estrogen in the bowel, hence predisposing to cancers of the breast, endometrium, and ovary. They are converted into secondary bile acids (e.g., lithocholic acid), which increase the risk for colorectal cancer. Ideally, saturated fat should account for <7% of the fat intake and total fat intake <25% of the total calories.]

Table continued on following page

Table 6–3. TRACE ELEMENT DISORDERS, DIETARY FIBER, NUTRITION AND CANCER, NUTRITIONAL CHANGES WITH AGING, SPECIAL DIETS *Continued*

Most Common...	Answer and Explanation
nutritional changes associated with aging	*decrease in body weight, lean body mass* (relative increase in fat), *energy requirements*
dietary inadequacies associated with aging	*pyridoxine, vitamin D, folate, calcium, and zinc* [Iron is not recommended as a supplement, owing to generation of FRs and formation of oxidized LDL.]
recommendations for the prevention of osteoporosis in postmenopausal women	*estrogen, calcium* (1000–1500 mg daily), *vitamin D* (400–800 IU daily), *exercise*
indications for a low sodium diet	*essential hypertension, CHF, chronic renal disease, cirrhosis*
indications for a low protein diet	*chronic renal disease* (low protein diet decreases the urea load on the kidneys) and *cirrhosis* (low protein diet decreases the formation of ammonia by urease-producing bacteria in the bowel).
problem associated with a pure vegan diet	B_{12} *deficiency* (B_{12} is only in animal products)

Question: Which of the following is **NOT** considered a preventive measure for osteoporosis in postmenopausal women?
- (A) Swimming
- (B) Estrogen
- (C) Calcium
- (D) Vitamin D
- (E) Walking

Answer: (A): Swimming does not place enough stress on the bones (similar to the effect of gravity). All the other choices are recommended.

CHF = congestive heart failure, FRs = free radicals, GSH = glutathione, LDL = low-density lipoprotein, S/S = signs and symptoms.

CHAPTER

GENETICS

CONTENTS

Table 7–1. DIAGNOSTIC TECHNIQUES, MUTATIONS, CHROMOSOME DISORDERS

Most Common...	Answer and Explanation
genetic disorders in blacks	**sickle cell trait/disease,** α- *and* β-*thalassemia, G6PD deficiency*
genetic disorders in Jews	**Tay-Sachs disease,** *Gaucher's disease, factor XII deficiency*
genetic disorder in Northern Europeans	*cystic fibrosis*
types of prenatal tests	**amniocentesis** (16 weeks), *chorionic villus biopsy* (9–12 weeks), *fetal blood sampling, fetal biopsy, ultrasonography*
routine maternal screening tests for genetic disorders	**AFP,** β-*hCG, unconjugated estriol* [A low AFP and unconjugated estriol + a high β-hCG occurs in Down syndrome in 60% of cases.]
screening test abnormality in open neural tube defects	*increased AFP* [AFP is fetal albumin. It must be correlated with gestational age.]
DNA technique used to locate gene abnormalities	*nucleic acid probes* [Probes contain specific amino acid sequences of portions of DNA. They are spliced into DNA strands and are allowed to hybridize with a corresponding segment of DNA from a patient sample.]

Table continued on following page

Table 7–1. DIAGNOSTIC TECHNIQUES, MUTATIONS, CHROMOSOME DISORDERS *Continued*

Most Common...	Answer and Explanation
gene technique used when the exact site of an abnormal gene is unknown	*restriction fragment length polymorphism (RFLP)* [Abnormal genetic sites must be linked to a harmless marker gene on the same chromosome. DNA fragments on the abnormal chromosome (DNA is cleaved by restriction endonucleases) are compared from both normal family members and those with the disease, and variations in fragment lengths that separate the two are studied. Future children in that family can then be studied and compared with normal and affected family members.]
cause of a genomic mutation [abnormal number of chromosomes]	*nondisjunction* [In nondisjunction, there is a failure of one set of homologous chromosomes to separate during the first phase of meiosis. Hence, the gamete contains either 22 or 24 chromosomes (normal haploid number is 23).]
cause of a chromosome mutation	*translocations* [A translocation is where one part of a chromosome is transferred to a nonhomologous chromosome. It is a balanced translocation if the translocated fragment is still functional. A robertsonian translocation is a type of balanced translocation in which there is a reciprocal translocation between the same two acrocentric chromosomes (e.g., chromosome 21) with the formation of one long chromosome (patient has 45 chromosomes but is normal, since both translocated fragments work).]
causes of gene mutations (mendelian disorders)	*deletions or insertions of nucleotide bases resulting in an altered code for the gene product*
technique used to identify translocations, deletions, and other rearrangements	*chromosome analysis using banding and/or high-resolution techniques* [The Y chromosome has a strong fluorescence under UV light when stained with quinacrine.]
genetic cause of mental retardation	*Down syndrome*

Table 7–1. DIAGNOSTIC TECHNIQUES, MUTATIONS, CHROMOSOME DISORDERS *Continued*

Most Common...	Answer and Explanation
cause of Down syndrome	*nondisjunction resulting in trisomy 21* (extra chromosome is of maternal origin) [Increasing maternal age increases the risk for nondisjunction.]
COD in childhood in Down syndrome	*endocardial cushion defects* (combined ASD and VSD)
factor affecting longevity in older patients with Down syndrome	*Alzheimer's disease* [Chromosome 21 codes for β-amyloid protein, which is converted into amyloid, which is toxic to neurons.]
GI abnormalities in Down syndrome	*duodenal atresia* (vomiting of bile-stained material at birth; double bubble sign on a flat plate of the abdomen) and *Hirschsprung's disease* (absent ganglion cells in the rectum; failure to pass meconium)
hematologic problem in Down syndrome	*acute myelogenous leukemia* (<3 years of age) and *acute lymphoblastic leukemia* (>3 years of age)
risk factor for having a child with Down syndrome	*maternal age* [Any woman >35 years of age is at increased risk.]
genetic cause of primary amenorrhea [no menses by 16 years of age]	*Turner's syndrome* [Owing to the absence of oocytes by 2 years of age, these patients have decreased estradiol levels, hence they lack secondary sex characteristics and do not menstruate.]
cause of Turner's syndrome	*nondisjunction leading to a 45 XO genotype* (~50–60%) [Mosaics may also occur (XO/XY; XO/XX). Since one of the two X chromosomes is randomly inactivated to become a nuclear appendage called a Barr body, Turner's syndrome patients do not have any Barr bodies (a normal woman has one Barr body).]
study used to identify Barr bodies	*smear of the buccal mucosa squamous cells and identification of nuclear appendages representing Barr bodies*
newborn presentation of Turner's syndrome	**lymphedema of the hands and feet,** *cystic hygroma* (dilated lymphatic channels) in the neck, *preductal coarctation of the aorta*

Table continued on following page

Table 7–1. DIAGNOSTIC TECHNIQUES, MUTATIONS, CHROMOSOME DISORDERS *Continued*

Most Common...	Answer and Explanation
ovarian tumor associated with Turner's syndrome	*dysgerminoma* (germ cell tumor) [Presence of a Y chromosome confers an increased risk for ovarian cancer.]
lab findings in Turner's syndrome	*decreased estradiol, increased FSH and LH levels* [Decreased estradiol results in an increase in gonadotropins owing to a negative feedback relationship.]
cause of Klinefelter's syndrome	*nondisjunction resulting in an XXY genotype* [In contrast to a normal male, there is one Barr body.]
testicular findings in Klinefelter's syndrome	*atrophy with fibrosis of the seminiferous tubules and hyperplasia of Leydig cells*
cause of hyperestrinism in Klinefelter's syndrome	*aromatization of testosterone into estradiol in the Leydig cells* [Sertoli cells in the seminiferous tubules normally synthesize inhibin, an inhibitor of FSH. Absence of inhibin increases FSH, which increases the synthesis of aromatase in Leydig cells. Patients have female secondary sex characteristics (e.g., gynecomastia).]
lab findings in Klinefelter's syndrome	*decreased testosterone, azoospermia* (no sperm), *increased FSH, LH, and estradiol*
S/S of the cri-du-chat syndrome	*mental retardation, cat-like cry, and a VSD (due to a partial deletion of chromosome 5)*
microdeletion syndromes	*Prader-Willi and Angelman's syndromes* [Both have a microdeletion at the same location on chromosome 15, but in the former syndrome, chromosome 15 is of paternal origin, and in the latter syndrome, it is of maternal origin. This is an example of genomic imprinting.]

Genetics **121**

Table 7–1. DIAGNOSTIC TECHNIQUES, MUTATIONS, CHROMOSOME DISORDERS *Continued*

Question: Which of the following is common to Down syndrome, Turner's syndrome, and Klinefelter's syndrome?
(A) Cardiac defects
(B) Nondisjunction
(C) Hematologic abnormalities
(D) Mental retardation
(E) Abnormal number of Barr bodies

Answer: (B): All of them have abnormalities in chromosome number (nondisjunction is the most common cause). Only Down syndrome and Turner's have cardiac abnormalities. Only Down syndrome patients have hematologic problems. Only Turner's and Klinefelter's patients have abnormal Barr body counts. Only Down syndrome patients have mental retardation. Both Klinefelter's and Turner's patients have learning disabilities but not mental retardation.

AFP = alpha-fetoprotein, ASD = atrial septal defect, β-hCG = human chorionic gonadotropin, COD = cause of death, FSH = follicle-stimulating hormone, GI = gastrointestinal, G6PD = glucose 6-phosphate dehydrogenase, LH = luteinizing hormone, S/S = signs and symptoms, UV = ultraviolet, VSD = ventricular septal defect.

Table 7–2. MENDELIAN DISORDERS, MULTIFACTORIAL INHERITANCE, MITOCHONDRIAL DNA DISORDERS

Most Common...	Answer and Explanation
Mendelian disorder	*autosomal dominant* (AD) [Dominant means that the gene is strong enough to express itself in a heterozygous state (one normal allele and one abnormal allele; an allele is an alternative form of the same gene). Homozygous AD diseases are rare. 50% of siblings are affected and 50% are normal when one of the parents is normal and the other has an AD disease.]

male with disease
($\underline{a}$ = abnormal gene,
A = normal gene)

	A	$\underline{a}$
normal female A	AA	A$\underline{a}$
A	AA	A$\underline{a}$

Table continued on following page

Table 7–2. MENDELIAN DISORDERS, MULTIFACTORIAL INHERITANCE, MITOCHONDRIAL DNA DISORDERS
Continued

Most Common...	Answer and Explanation
characteristics of AR diseases	*recessive indicates a weak gene that must be present in a homozygous state* (both alleles are abnormal) *for it to express itself; heterozygotes are asymptomatic carriers* [Both parents must be carriers of the abnormal gene to transmit the disease to their children. Two asymptomatic carriers have a 25% chance of having a child with the disease, a 50% chance of a child who is an asymptomatic carrier, and a 25% chance of a normal child.
characteristics of SXR disorders	*an affected male transmits the disease to all of his daughters, who are asymptomatic carriers, and to none of his sons. An asymptomatic carrier female transmits the disease to 50% of her sons and 50% of her daughters, the latter representing asymptomatic carriers*
characteristics of SXD disorders	*the percentages of children with the abnormal gene are the same as with SXR; however, the gene is dominant, so both males and females are symptomatic* [An affected woman transmits symptomatic disease to 50% of her daughters and 50% of her sons and an affected man transmits disease to all of his daughters and none of his sons.]

For the AR diseases row, the Punnett square reads:

		asymptomatic male carrier	
		A	a
asymptomatic female carrier	A	AA	Aa
	a	Aa	aa has disease

For the SXR disorders row:

		asymptomatic male		
		X	Y	XX = asymptomatic
normal female	X	XX	XY	matic
	X	XX	XY	female carrier

		normal male		
		X	Y	
asymptomatic female carrier	X	XX	XY	50% of males
	X	XX	XY	with disease

Table 7–2. MENDELIAN DISORDERS, MULTIFACTORIAL INHERITANCE, MITOCHONDRIAL DNA DISORDERS
Continued

Most Common...	Answer and Explanation
Mendelian disorder exhibiting penetrance	AD [Penetrance is where a person with the abnormal gene may or may not express the disease. If two children are A$\overline{\text{a}}$ but only one of the two expresses the disease, there is 50% penetrance (100% penetrance if both express the disease). The asymptomatic person can still transmit the disease to his or her children.]
Mendelian disorder exhibiting variable expressivity	AD [Variable expressivity is where there can be varying degrees of expression of the disease. Unlike with penetrance, the patient does manifest the disease to some minor or major extent.]
Mendelian disorder in which the disease may occur later in life	AD [Examples of this phenomenon are Huntington's chorea, adult polycystic kidney disease, and familial polyposis. Chorea, renal cysts, and polyps, respectively, are not present at birth.]
AD disease	*von Willebrand's disease* (1 in 125)
AR disease	*hemochromatosis* (1 in 100)
SXR disease	*fragile X syndrome* (1 in 1000)
genetic disease in blacks	*sickle cell disease* (1 in 625)
Mendelian disorder associated with enzyme deficiencies	AR [A few SXR diseases have enzyme deficiencies (e.g., G6PD deficiency, Lesch-Nyhan syndrome), and rarely, AD diseases (e.g., AIP, C1 esterase inhibitor deficiency).]
Mendelian disorder associated with structural defects in proteins and receptors	AD [For example, congenital spherocytosis has a defect in spectrin in the RBC membrane. Familial hypercholesterolemia has a defect in the LDL receptor.]

Table continued on following page

Table 7–2. MENDELIAN DISORDERS, MULTIFACTORIAL INHERITANCE, MITOCHONDRIAL DNA DISORDERS
Continued

Most Common...	Answer and Explanation
skin lesions associated with neurofibromatosis	*AD disease with cafe au lait spots; pigmented, pedunculated neurofibromas;* and *plexiform neurofibromas* [Cafe au lait spots are coffee-colored flat lesions whose long axes parallel an underlying cutaneous nerve. Pedunculated neurofibromas are benign tumors that involve all elements of the peripheral nerve. Plexiform neurofibromas lead to grotesque overgrowth of soft tissue (e.g., "elephant man").]
tumors associated with neurofibromatosis	**acoustic neuromas** (benign tumor arising from Schwann cells involving the eighth cranial nerve), *meningiomas, optic nerve gliomas, pheochromocytomas* (produces hypertension), and *Lisch nodules* on the iris (really hamartomas, not true neoplasms)
defect in Marfan's syndrome (AD)	*defect in fibrillin,* a component of elastin in elastic tissue
skeletal defects in Marfan's syndrome	*eunuchoid proportions* (lower body length greater than upper body length; arm span greater than height), *arachnodactyly* (spider hands)
cardiovascular abnormalities in Marfan's syndrome	*dissecting aortic aneurysm* (most common cause of death), *mitral valve prolapse* (common cause of sudden death)
eye defect in Marfan's syndrome	*dislocated lens* [The suspensory ligament is defective.]
enzyme deficiency in PKU (AR)	*phenylalanine hydroxylase deficiency,* which catalyzes the conversion of phenylalanine into tyrosine [Phenylalanine is increased and tyrosine is decreased. A blood sample must be taken a few days after birth and not on cord blood, since the baby must be exposed to phenylalanine in breast milk.]
S/S in PKU	**mental retardation,** *projectile vomiting* (resembles congenital pyloric stenosis), *hypopigmentation* (decreased tyrosine = decrease in melanin synthesis)

Table 7–2. MENDELIAN DISORDERS, MULTIFACTORIAL
INHERITANCE, MITOCHONDRIAL DNA DISORDERS
Continued

Most Common...	Answer and Explanation
buildup products in PKU	**phenylalanine,** *phenylpyruvic acid, phenyl-lactic acid,* and *phenylacetic acid* [The last three compounds are minor pathway products derived from phenylalanine. They impart a mousy odor to sweat.]
treatment for PKU	*phenylalanine-free diet*
enzyme deficiency in galactosemia (AR)	*GALT, which converts galactose 1-PO$_4$ into glucose 1-PO$_4$, the latter converted into glucose 6-PO$_4$* (fuel for gluconeogenesis)
S/S of galactosemia	*toxic effects on multiple organs and osmotic damage to the lens and peripheral nerves* [An increase in galactose 1-PO$_4$ is toxic to neurons (mental retardation), hepatocytes (liver failure), and the kidneys (aminoaciduria). Galactose is converted into galactitol, an alcohol sugar, which produces osmotic damage to the lens (cataracts) and peripheral nerve (peripheral neuropathy).]
lab findings in galactosemia	*galactosuria, hypoglycemia* [Galactose spills into the urine, producing a positive test result for reducing substances. The decrease in glucose 6-PO$_4$ causes fasting hypoglycemia.]
treatment for galactosemia	*lactose-free diet* [Lactose is glucose + galactose.]
enzyme deficiency in essential fructosuria (AR)	*fructokinase, which catalyzes the reaction that converts fructose into fructose 1-PO$_4$* [Unlike hereditary fructose intolerance, it is a benign disease with an excess of fructose in the urine.]
enzyme deficiency in hereditary fructose intolerance (AR)	*aldolase B* [Aldolase B catalyzes the reaction that converts fructose 1-PO$_4$ into glyceraldehyde and DHAP, which are three carbon intermediates in the glycolytic cycle.]
S/S of hereditary fructose intolerance	*a buildup of fructose 1-PO$_4$, which is toxic to neurons* (mental retardation) and *hepatocytes* (liver failure)

Table continued on following page

Table 7–2. MENDELIAN DISORDERS, MULTIFACTORIAL
INHERITANCE, MITOCHONDRIAL DNA DISORDERS
Continued

Most Common...	Answer and Explanation
lab findings in hereditary fructose intolerance	*fructosuria, hypophosphatemia, hypoglycemia* [Fructose spills into the urine, producing a positive test result for reducing substances. Phosphorylation of fructose intracellularly depletes PO_4 stores (hypophosphatemia). The decrease in three carbon intermediates reduces substrates for gluconeogenesis (fasting hypoglycemia).]
enzyme deficiency in homocystinuria (AR)	*cystathione synthetase, which converts homocysteine into cystathione*
S/S of homocystinuria	*homocysteine is increased, leading to vessel damage and thrombosis* [Other features resemble Marfan's syndrome (dislocated lens, arachnodactyly). Two diseases that are dissimilar to each other in pathogenesis but similar in clinical findings are an example of genetic heterogeneity.]
enzyme deficiency in alkaptonuria (AR)	*homogentisate oxidase, which converts homogentisate into maleylacetoacetate* [Homogentisic acid is increased.]
S/S of alkaptonuria	*homogentisic acid* (oxidized into a black pigment) *binds to collagen* (severe joint disease, intervertebral disc disease) *and produces black urine on exposure to light*
enzyme deficiency in von Gierke's disease (AR)	*it is a glycogen storage disease caused by a deficiency of the gluconeogenic enzyme glucose 6-phosphatase, which catalyzes the conversion of glucose 6-PO_4 into glucose*
signs of von Gierke's disease	*hepatorenomegaly due to glycogen excess with liver and renal failure* (gluconeogenic enzymes are in these organs) [Glucose 6-PO_4 is the substrate for producing glycogen (glucose 6-PO_4 → glucose 1-PO_4 → UDP-glucose → glycogen), hence its increase leads to an excess production of normal glycogen in organs containing the missing gluconeogenic hormones.]

Table 7–2. MENDELIAN DISORDERS, MULTIFACTORIAL
INHERITANCE, MITOCHONDRIAL DNA DISORDERS
Continued

Most Common...	Answer and Explanation
lab findings in von Gierke's disease	**hypoglycemia,** *lactic acidosis, hyperuricemia* [Glucose cannot be synthesized in the fasting state (hypoglycemia) and there is an increase in anaerobic metabolism (lactic acidosis). Glucagon, cortisol, or fructose challenges do not increase glucose because of the enzyme block. Glycogen accumulation in the kidneys interferes with uric acid excretion.]
enzyme deficiency in Pompe's disease (AR)	*it is the only glycogenosis that is a lysosomal storage disease, since it is deficient in the lysosomal enzyme acid maltase, which is necessary to degrade glycogen* [Normal glycogen accumulates in the heart, leading to a restrictive cardiomyopathy at an early age.]
enzyme deficiency in McArdle's disease (AR)	*it is a glycogenosis due to a deficiency of muscle phosphorylase, hence muscle glycogen cannot be catabolized into glucose for energy*
S/S of McArdle's disease	*patients fatigue easily and rhabdomyolysis (muscle necrosis) may occur* [Lactic acid does not accumulate after exercise, since anaerobic glycolysis cannot occur without glucose.]
types of glycogenoses associated with an accumulation of abnormal glycogen	*brancher and debrancher enzyme deficiency types of glycogenoses.* [Von Gierke's disease, Pompe's disease, and McArdle's disease all have an accumulation of normal glycogen.]
enzyme deficiency in Tay-Sachs disease (AR)	*it is a sphingolipidosis* (lysosomal storage disease) *due to a deficiency of hexosaminidase leading to an accumulation of GM2 gangliosides in lysosomes* (forms whorled configurations on EM) [It is associated with a cherry red spot in the macula and severe mental retardation.]
enzyme deficiency in Niemann-Pick disease (AR)	*it is a sphingolipidosis (lysosomal storage disease) with a deficiency of sphingomyelinase leading to an accumulation of sphingomyelin* (forms zebra bodies on EM) [Macrophages have a bubbly cytoplasm. Patients are mentally retarded and have hepatosplenomegaly.]

Table continued on following page

Table 7–2. MENDELIAN DISORDERS, MULTIFACTORIAL INHERITANCE, MITOCHONDRIAL DNA DISORDERS
Continued

Most Common...	Answer and Explanation
enzyme deficiency in Gaucher's disease (AR)	*it is a sphingolipidosis* (lysosomal storage disease) *due to a deficiency of* β-*glucocerebrosidase leading to an accumulation of glucocerebroside* [Macrophages have a fibrillar-appearing cytoplasm. Hepatosplenomegaly is prominent.]
enzyme deficiency in metachromatic leukodystrophy (AR)	*it is a sphingolipidosis* (lysosomal storage disease) *due to a deficiency of arylsulfatase A with an accumulation of sulfatides* [An abnormal myelin is produced.]
enzyme deficiency in Krabbe's disease (AR)	*it is a sphingolipidosis* (lysosomal storage disease) *due to a deficiency of galactosylceramidase and an accumulation of galactocerebroside* [In the CNS, the galactocerebroside is phagocytosed by histiocytes producing multinucleated giant cells called globoid bodies.]
lysosomal storage diseases that are SXR	*Fabry's disease* and *Hunter's syndrome* [The former is due to a deficiency of α-galactocerebrosidase A with an accumulation of ceramide trihexoside and the latter a deficiency of L-iduronosulfate sulfatase and an accumulation of dermatan and heparan sulfate.]
mucopolysaccharidosis	*Hurler's syndrome* (AR), *which is due to a deficiency of* α-1-iduronidase *and an accumulation of dermatan sulfate and heparan sulfate* [Patients have severe mental retardation, coarse facial features, premature CAD, and abnormal circulating lymphocytes with vacuoles.]
enzyme deficiency in Lesch-Nyhan syndrome (SXR)	*it is due to a deficiency of HGPRT, an inhibitor of PRPP, hence purine metabolism is left unchecked and uric acid is increased* [Patients have mental retardation, hyperuricemia, and self-mutilation.]
cause of fragile X syndrome (SXR)	*associated with triplet repeats of three nucleotides (CGG)* [It is the second most common genetic cause of mental retardation and most common cause of retardation in males. Patients have macroorchidism appearing at puberty and an increased incidence of MVP. A special chromosome study must be performed to identify the fragile X chromosome.]

Table 7–2. MENDELIAN DISORDERS, MULTIFACTORIAL INHERITANCE, MITOCHONDRIAL DNA DISORDERS
Continued

Most Common...	Answer and Explanation
inheritance pattern for diseases like hypertension, gout, and CAD	*multifactorial (polygenic) inheritance, which refers to multiple small mutations plus environmental factors* [Other examples include type II DM, cleft lip/palate, congenital pyloric stenosis, hair/eye/skin color, open neural tube defects, and congenital heart disease.]
pattern of inheritance in mitochondrial DNA disorders	*maternal inheritance* [Mitochondrial DNA codes for enzymes involved in oxidative phosphorylation; affected females transmit the disease to all of their children, while affected men do not transmit the disease to any of their children (mitochondrial DNA is in the tail of the sperm, which is lost with fertilization).]

Question: Which of the following is common to all four of the mendelian inheritance disorders?
(A) Females express the disease
(B) Late manifestations
(C) Penetrance
(D) Variable expressivity
(E) Males express the disease

Answer: (E): All four types can have symptomatic males. SXR diseases do not usually have symptomatic females. Only AD diseases have penetrance, variable expressivity, and late manifestations.

AD = autosomal dominant, AIP = acute intermittent porphyria, AR = autosomal recessive, CAD = coronary artery disease, CNS = central nervous system, DM = diabetes mellitus, DHAP = dihydroxyacetone phosphate, EM = electron microscopy, GALT = galactose-1-phosphate uridyl transferase, G6PD = glucose-6-phosphate dehydrogenase, HGPRT = hypoxanthine-guanine-phosphoribosyl-transferase, LDL = low-density lipoprotein, MVP = mitral valve prolapse, PKU = phenylketonuria, PRPP = 5-phospho-α-D-ribosyl-1-pyrophosphate, RBC = red blood cell, S/S = signs and symptoms, SXD = sex-linked dominant, SXR = sex-linked recessive, UDP = uridine diphosphate.

Table 7–3. SEX DIFFERENTIATION DISORDERS, DEVELOPMENTAL DISORDERS

Most Common...	Answer and Explanation
determinant of genetic sex	*presence or absence of the Y chromosome* [Presence of the Y chromosome causes development of a testis from germinal tissue. Mullerian inhibitory factor prevents mullerian structures from developing. Absence of the Y chromosome results in formation of ovaries and inhibition of wolffian structures.]
functions of fetal testosterone	*development of the epididymis, seminal vesicles,* and *vas deferens*
functions of fetal dihydrotestosterone	*development of the prostate and external male genitalia by fusion of the labia to form the scrotum and extension of the clitoris to form a penis*
function of 5-α-reductase	*converts testosterone into DHT*
cause of male pseudohermaphroditism	*testicular feminization* (SXR) [A male pseudohermaphrodite is a genotypic male who has the phenotypic appearance of a female.]
cause of testicular feminization	*deficiency of androgen receptors* [Neither testosterone nor DHT can develop male accessory structures, and the external genitalia remain female. Testicles are located in the inguinal canal. Absence of androgen receptors leaves estrogen unopposed, hence secondary female characteristics are present. The vagina is partially developed and ends in a blind pouch (the vagina normally develops from the urogenital sinus and mullerian epithelium).]
lab findings in testicular feminization	*normal testosterone, increased LH* (testosterone does not inhibit LH)
cause of female pseudohermaphroditism	*adrenogenital syndrome* (AR) [A female pseudohermaphrodite is a genotypic female with a male phenotype. Adrenogenital syndrome involves enzyme deficiencies in steroid synthesis.]

Table 7–3. SEX DIFFERENTIATION DISORDERS, DEVELOPMENTAL DISORDERS *Continued*

Most Common...	Answer and Explanation
enzyme deficiency in adrenogenital syndrome	*21-hydroxylase (OHase) deficiency* [Normally, the enzyme converts 17-OH-progesterone into 11-deoxycortisol. 11-OHase converts 11-deoxycortisol into cortisol. The latter two compounds and their metabolites are measured as 17-OHCS. Proximal to these reactions, 17-OHase converts pregnenolone into DHEA and progesterone into androstenedione, which are weak androgens that are measured as 17-KS. Androstenedione is converted (oxidoreductase reaction) into testosterone. 21-OHase also converts progesterone into 11-deoxycorticosterone, which is further converted by 11-OHase into corticosterone. 18-OHase in the zona glomerulosa (only location) converts corticosterone into aldosterone, the most powerful mineralocorticoid.]
S/S of 21-OHase deficiency	*weakness and hypovolemia* (loss of the weak mineralocorticoids causes the renal loss of sodium), *female pseudohermaphroditism* (accumulation of 17-KS proximal to the block converts female to male genitalia), *males develop precocious puberty* (increased 17-KS), *diffuse hyperpigmentation* (low cortisol increases ACTH)
lab findings in 21-OHase deficiency	*hyponatremia and hyperkalemia, increased 17-KS, decreased 17-OHCS* (11-deoxycortisol and cortisol are distal to the block), *hypocortisolism, increased ACTH, increased urine sodium*
S/S of 11-OHase deficiency	*salt retention with hypertension* (increased 11-deoxycorticosterone proximal to the block), *female pseudohermaphroditism* (accumulation of 17-KS proximal to the block), *precocious puberty in males, diffuse hyperpigmentation*
lab findings in 11-OHase deficiency	*increased 17-KS, increased 17-OHCS* (increase in 11-deoxycortisol proximal to the block), *hypocortisolism, increased ACTH*
S/S of 17-OHase deficiency	*retention of salt with hypertension* (the entire mineralocorticoid pathway is left open), *male pseudohermaphroditism* (decreased 17-KS) but *females look female, diffuse hyperpigmentation*

Table continued on following page

Table 7–3. SEX DIFFERENTIATION DISORDERS, DEVELOPMENTAL DISORDERS *Continued*

Most Common...	Answer and Explanation
lab findings in 17-OHase deficiency	*decreased 17-KS and 17-OHCS, hypocortisolism, increased ACTH*
cause of malformations [defect in morphogenesis]	*unknown* (40–60%) [Known causes include genetic factors, exposure to teratogens, and maternal factors. Deformations are mechanical defects inflicted on the fetus after organ development has occurred.]
malformation	*hypospadias*, where the urethra opens on the undersurface of the penis [Club feet and congenital heart disease are also common malformations.]
period for development of open neural tube defects	*23rd to 28th days of gestation*, which is when the tube normally closes [Low maternal folate levels increase the risk for open neural tube defects.]
cause of macrosomia in newborns	*maternal DM* [Hyperglycemia in the mother increases insulin in the fetus. Insulin increases fat deposition and muscle mass.]
causes of open neural tube defects	**folate deficiency,** *maternal DM, valproic acid*
cause of vaginal adenosis and clear cell carcinoma of the vagina	*history of maternal exposure to DES* [DES inhibits mullerian differentiation, hence all mullerian structures are negatively affected (e.g., tube abnormalities, uterine abnormalities, cervical incompetence).]
fetal site of involvement in maternal cocaine abuse	*CNS* (infarcts, intraventricular hemorrhage)
S/S of the fetal alcohol syndrome	**mental retardation** [Other findings include *IUGR, ASD* (least common defect), *maxillary hypoplasia*.]
teratogenic effects of isotretinoin	*craniofacial defects* (e.g., cleft palate), *cardiac defects, CNS malformations* (e.g., hydrocephalus) [A pregnancy test is always ordered when placing a female on isotretinoin for acne. Patients must use contraception while taking the medication.]

Table 7–3. SEX DIFFERENTATION DISORDERS, DEVELOPMENTAL DISORDERS *Continued*

Most Common...	Answer and Explanation
teratogens/ developmental disorders associated with cardiac defects	*maternal DM* (transposition of the great vessels), *rubella* (PDA), *fetal alcohol syndrome* (ASD), *isotretinoin, lithium* (Ebstein's anomaly involving the tricuspid valve), *phenytoin, maternal SLE* (complete heart block from maternal passage of anti-Rh_0 [SS-A] antibodies)
teratogenic effects of smoking	*low birth weight* [There is also a danger of SIDS.]
teratogenic effects of thalidomide	*amelia* [absent limbs] or *phocomelia* [*partial development of limbs*]
anticoagulant used in pregnancy	*heparin* (no teratogenic effects) [Warfarin is contraindicated (CNS defects, nasal hypoplasia).]
congenital infection	*CMV* [Most cases are asymptomatic.]
types of vertical transmission [mother to fetus]	**transplacental,** *passage through the birth canal, breast feeding*
congenital infections transmitted transplacentally	**CMV,** *toxoplasmosis, syphilis* (only after the 5th month), *rubella, varicella-zoster, HIV*
congenital infections transmitted at delivery through the vaginal tract	*herpes simplex* (endocervical lesions), *Chlamydia trachomatis* (endocervical secretions), *HBV* (blood)
congenital infection associated with cardiac defects	*rubella* (PDA) [Nerve deafness is the most common malformation and PDA the least common. Cataracts and mental retardation also occur.]
congenital infections associated with deafness	**rubella** (most common manifestation), *late syphilis*
congenital infections associated with CNS calcifications	**CMV,** *toxoplasmosis, herpes simplex*
congenital infection diagnosed by urine culture and cytology	*CMV* [CMV produces basophilic intranuclear inclusions. Urine culture is the gold standard for diagnosis. Ganciclovir and foscarnet have been used in therapy.]

Table continued on following page

Table 7–3. SEX DIFFERENTIATION DISORDERS, DEVELOPMENTAL DISORDERS *Continued*

Most Common...	Answer and Explanation
congenital infection transmitted by maternal exposure to cat litter or undercooked meat	*toxoplasmosis* [The later toxoplasmosis is contracted in pregnancy, the greater the chance of infection and the greater the severity of infection.]
congenital infections associated with eye abnormalities	**CMV** (chorioretinitis), *rubella* (cataracts), *toxoplasmosis* (chorioretinitis), *herpes simplex* (keratoconjunctivitis), *late syphilis* (interstitial keratitis)
early S/S for congenital syphilis	*mucocutaneous lesions, pneumonitis* (pneumonia alba), *snuffles* (persistent rhinitis), *hepatomegaly, anemia, generalized lymphadenopathy, osteochondritis*
late S/S in congenital syphilis	*teeth abnormalities* (Hutchinson's pegged teeth in the upper central incisors, mulberry molars), *interstitial keratitis* (potential for blindness), *sensorineural deafness*
target sites for congenital varicella/zoster infections	**CNS** (cortical atrophy of the brain), *limbs* (hypoplasia), and *skin* (vesicular lesions)
method of delivery in women with active *Herpes genitalis*	*Cesarean section* to avoid newborn contamination while passing through the infected vaginal tract
cause of stillbirths [delivery of a dead child]	**unknown** [Known causes include problems with the *placenta* (e.g., abruption), *umbilical cord* (e.g., strangulation), *ascending infection* (e.g., group B *Streptococcus*).]
cause of spontaneous abortions [pregnancy that terminates before the fetus can remain alive outside the uterus; ~22 weeks]	**fetal karyotype disorder** (~50%), usually trisomy 16 [Other causes include *maternal factors* (e.g., infection), *placental factors* (e.g., infarction), and *fetal factors* (e.g., congenital infection).]

Table 7–3. SEX DIFFERENTIATION DISORDERS, DEVELOPMENTAL DISORDERS *Continued*

Most Common...	Answer and Explanation
nomenclature for expressing newborn maturity	*appropriate for gestational age* (AGA), *small for gestational age* (SGA), *large for gestational age* (LGA) [Birth weight and gestational age are used to establish the above designations. *Term newborns* are those born between 38 and 42 weeks, *preterm newborns* <38 weeks, and *postterm newborns* >42 weeks.]
cause of SGA newborns	**maternal factors** (e.g., smoker, alcohol exposure) [Other causes involve *fetal* (e.g., chromosome disorder) or *placental abnormalities* (e.g., infection).]
components of the Apgar score	*Apgar scores are obtained at 1 and 5 minutes and include respiratory effort, heart rate, muscle tone, color, and response to a catheter in the nose*
cause of death in newborns [birth to 1 month of age]	**congenital malformations** and *RDS*
cause of death in infants [1 month to 1 year of age]	*SIDS*
cause of SIDS	*unknown* [Potential contributing factors include parental smoking, defects in fatty acid metabolism, sleeping prone, neural development delay, respiratory center abnormality.]
cause for the decrease in deaths due to SIDS over the last few years	*sleeping supine* [Some newborns when sleeping prone do not have CNS mechanisms to move their head when rebreathing their own CO_2.]
time frame for death due to SIDS	*at night, between 2 and 3 months of age* [It is rare in infants <1 month or >9 months of age.]
autopsy findings in SIDS cases	*abnormalities in the heart* (conduction defects, RVH), *lungs* (petechiae on the pleura, spotty inflammatory changes), and *CNS* (astrocyte proliferation)

Table continued on following page

Table 7–3. SEX DIFFERENTIATION DISORDERS, DEVELOPMENTAL DISORDERS *Continued*

Most Common...	Answer and Explanation
age-dependent [inevitable with age] findings in the lungs	*obstructive-type pattern* (so-called senile emphysema) *with decreased elasticity* (reduced recoil on expiration), *FEV_{1sec}, and FVC, and increased TLC, RV*
age-dependent change in the aorta	*loss of elasticity* [This predisposes to systolic hypertension (systolic pressure >160 mm Hg).]
age-dependent type of arthritis	*osteoarthritis*
age-dependent disorders involving the eyes	*cataracts, arcus senilis*
age-dependent disorders involving the ears	*presbycusis* (sensorineural hearing loss) and *otosclerosis* (fusion of the ear ossicles producing conductive hearing loss)
age-dependent changes in the immune system	*decreased CD_8 T suppressor cells leading to an increase in CD_4 T helper cells and an increase in autoantibody formation*
age-dependent changes in the skin	*loss of skin elasticity* (increased cross-bridging of collagen), *increased body fat, increased vessel instability* (senile purpura)
age-dependent disorders involving the reproductive tract in men	*prostate hyperplasia* and *prostate cancer, decreased testosterone*
age-dependent changes in the reproductive tract in women	*breast and vulvar atrophy, decreased estrogen, increased gonadotropins* (FSH and LH, owing to a decrease in estrogen and progesterone, respectively)
age-dependent changes in the endocrine system	*increased glucose intolerance* (increase in body fat, decrease in insulin receptor synthesis)
age-dependent changes in the renal system	*decreased GFR with concomitant reduction in the creatinine clearance*

Table 7–3. SEX DIFFERENTIATION DISORDERS, DEVELOPMENTAL DISORDERS *Continued*

Most Common...	Answer and Explanation
age-related [more common but not inevitable with aging] disorders involving in the cardiovascular system	**CAD,** *temporal arteritis, aortic stenosis*
age-related disorders involving the musculoskeletal system	**osteoporosis,** *Paget's disease of bone*
age-related disorders involving the respiratory system	**pneumonia** (usually *Streptococcus pneumoniae*) and *primary lung cancer*
age-related disorders involving the CNS	**Alzheimer's disease,** *Parkinson's disease, strokes, subdural hematomas*
age-related disorders involving the immune system	**monoclonal gammopathies of undetermined significance,** *multiple myeloma*
age-related disorders involving the skin	**basal cell carcinoma,** *squamous cell carcinoma, malignant melanoma,* all of which have a relation to UV light
age-related disorders involving the reproductive tract	women: cancers of the **breast,** *endometrium, ovary* men: *malignant lymphoma of testicle*
age-related disorders involving the kidneys	*renovascular hypertension secondary to atherosclerosis, renal adenocarcinoma*
age-related disorder involving the endocrine system	*type II DM*

Table continued on following page

Table 7–3. SEX DIFFERENTIATION DISORDERS, DEVELOPMENTAL DISORDERS *Continued*

Question: Which of the following congenital infections are transmitted most commonly during vaginal delivery? **SELECT 3**
  (A) HBV
  (B) CMV
  (C) Rubella
  (D) Syphilis
  (E) Toxoplasmosis
  (F) Herpes simplex virus
  (G) *Chlamydia trachomatis*

Answers: (A), (F), (G): HBV is primarily transmitted by contamination with infected blood during delivery. Both herpes simplex and *Chlamydia trachomatis* infections are incurred while passing through the cervix. All the other choices are primarily transplacentally transmitted.

ACTH = adrenocorticotropic hormone, AR = autosomal recessive, ASD = atrial septal defect, CAD = coronary artery disease, CMV = cytomegalovirus, CNS = central nervous system, DES = diethylstilbestrol, DHEA = dehydroepiandrosterone, DHT = dihydrotestosterone, DM = diabetes mellitus, FEV_{1sec} = forced expiratory volume in 1 second, FSH = follicle-stimulating hormone, FVC = forced vital capacity, GFR = glomerular filtration rate, HBV = hepatitis B virus, HIV = human immunodeficiency virus, IUGR = intrauterine growth retardation, 17-KS = 17-ketosteroid, LH = luteinizing hormone, OHase = hydroxylase, 17-OHCS = 17-hydroxycorticosteroid, PDA = patent ductus arteriosus, RDS = respiratory distress syndrome, RV = residual volume, RVH = right ventricular hypertrophy, SIDS = sudden infant death syndrome, SLE = systemic lupus erythematosus, S/S = signs and symptoms, SXR = sex-linked recessive, TLC = total lung capacity, UV = ultraviolet.

CHAPTER

ENVIRONMENTAL PATHOLOGY

CONTENTS

Table 8–1. Mechanical injuries.
Table 8–2. Chemical and drug injuries.

Table 8–1. MECHANICAL INJURIES

Most Common...	Answer and Explanation
cause of a pathologic fracture [fracture due to an abnormality in bone]	**metastasis to bone** [Other causes include *osteoporosis* (vertebral fracture most common), *cysts, Paget's disease of bone, osteogenesis imperfecta.*]
fracture in newborns	*clavicular fracture,* which frequently occurs with breech deliveries or delivery of LGA infants.
age bracket for greenstick fractures	*children* [A greenstick fracture is a break in the cortex on the convex side of the shaft and an intact concave side.]
complication of a supracondylar fracture in children	*Volkmann's ischemic contracture* [Supracondylar fractures are unstable and compress the brachial artery and median nerve, the former rendering the forearm compartment subject to ischemic damage.]
postmenopausal fracture associated with osteoporosis	*vertebral fracture* [Colles' fractures are the second most common fracture.]
fracture associated with ecchymoses of the mastoid	*basilar skull fracture* (petrous portion of the temporal bone) [Otorrhea (CSF fluid leaking out of the ear) may also occur.]
fracture associated with rhinorrhea [CSF leaking from the nose]	*orbital fractures* [Rhinorrhea occurs after a fracture of the cribriform plate. Orbital fractures also produce raccoon eyes (periorbital hemorrhage) and ophthalmoplegia (eye muscle entrapment).]
cause of a contusion [blood in tissue]	*blunt force injury to the skin*

Table 8–1. MECHANICAL INJURIES *Continued*

Most Common...	Answer and Explanation
cause of an abrasion [superficial excoriation of the epidermis]	*direct or tangential blow to the skin*
cause of a laceration [tear of skin with bridging by vessels, nerves, and connective tissue]	*blunt force injury that overstretches the skin*
cause of an incision [skin wound with sharp margins]	*surgery*
gunshot wound associated with fouling [deposition of gas and soot in the wound]	*contact wound,* where the muzzle is held against the body surface
gunshot wound associated with powder tattooing [stippling of gunpowder in the skin]	*intermediate wound* (1.5–3 feet away from the body surface) [Distant wounds do not have powder tattooing.]
feature distinguishing an exit from an entrance gunshot wound	*exit wounds are larger and more irregular than entrance wounds*
sign of manual strangulation and shake injuries in babies	*petechial hemorrhages in the conjunctiva and retinal hemorrhages, respectively*
cause of rigor mortis [postmortem hardening of muscles]	*breakdown of ATP in tissue and accumulation of lactic acid with denaturation of muscle proteins*
term applied to postmortem body cooling	*algor mortis* [The body cools ~1.5°F/hour.]

Table 8–1. MECHANICAL INJURIES *Continued*

Most Common...	Answer and Explanation
term applied to fixed dependent purplish discoloration after death	*livor mortis* [Blood leaking out of blood vessels is fixed after 12 hours.]
cause of accidental death from 1 to 24 years of age	*MVAs, most often associated with drunk driving* [In white males, it is also the most common cause of death between 25 and 44 years of age. AIDS is the most common cause of death in black males and in women between 25 and 44 years.]
site and type of aortic injury in car accidents	*tear in the aorta just below the ligamentum arteriosum*
site of drowning in children	*home swimming pools* [Drowning is the third most common cause of death in children from 1–14 years of age.]
type of drowning	*wet drowning* (90%), where there is an initial laryngospasm on contact with water followed by relaxation and aspiration of water into the lungs [Dry drowning has intense laryngospasm.]
injury associated with drowning	*asphyxia* [Both fresh and salt water in the lungs destroy surfactant, leading to massive atelectasis and intrapulmonary shunting of blood (severe hypoxemia, respiratory and metabolic acidosis).]
effect of salt water on plasma volume and sodium concentration	*hypernatremia and volume depletion*, since salt water draws fluid into the lungs from the pulmonary capillaries [Theoretically, death should be faster in salt water than in fresh water.]
effect of fresh water on plasma volume and serum sodium	*volume overload and hyponatremia*, since water moves into the pulmonary capillaries by osmosis [RBC hemolysis is more likely to occur.]
distinction between a first- and a second-degree burn	*second-degree burns have blisters, whereas first-degree burns only have reddening of the epidermis* [Both burns should heal without scarring.]

Table continued on following page

Table 8–1. MECHANICAL INJURIES *Continued*

Most Common...	Answer and Explanation
distinction between a second- and a third-degree burn	*absence of pain and the presence of scarring are more likely to occur with third-degree burns*
sites for re-epithelialization of burn wounds	*skin along the edges of the wound and residual adnexal epithelium*
COD in burns	**infection associated with** *Pseudomonas aeruginosa* [*ARDS, severe volume depletion*, and *multiorgan failure* also commonly occur.]
GI abnormality associated with burns	*Curling's stress ulcers in the stomach*
COD in a fire	*smoke inhalation*
poisonings in a house fire	*CO and cyanide poisoning* (originates from polyurethane in upholstery and other items)
distinctions between heat cramps and heat exhaustion	*heat exhaustion is associated with fever and significant signs of volume depletion; heat cramps lack the above*
distinction between heat exhaustion and heat stroke	*fever in heat exhaustion ranges from 37.5°C–39°C (101.2°F), while fever in heat stroke is ≥41°C (108.5°F).* [In heat stroke, patients frequently do not sweat.]
treatment for malignant hyperthermia (AD disease)	*dantrolene* [Malignant hyperthermia is precipitated in surgery when patients receive halothane or muscle relaxants. There is a defect in calcium release channels in the muscle sarcoplasmic reticulum.]
vessel changes in frostbite	*initial vasoconstriction is followed by vasodilatation, vessel thrombosis, nerve injury, and death of tissue* [Direct injury is due to ice crystallization in tissue.]
core body temperature defining hypothermia	<35°C (95°F) [Cold temperatures uncouple oxidative phosphorylation with eventual progression into circulatory failure.]
types of electrical current	*alternating and direct current*, the former primarily used in the United States

Table 8–1. MECHANICAL INJURIES *Continued*

Most Common...	Answer and Explanation
type of current involved in electrocutions	*AC* [AC produces tonic contractions of the hand and inability to release the object transmitting the current.]
variable responsible for electrocution	*current is more important than voltage in electrocutions* [Ohm's law states that I (current) = E (volts)/R (resistance). As R decreases (e.g., wet skin), I increases.]
COD in electrocution	*cardiorespiratory arrest*
types of ionizing radiation	*gamma rays, x-rays, particulate radiation* (alpha particles and beta particles) [The shorter the wavelength of the radiation, the greater the penetration (gamma rays have the greatest penetration and alpha particles and beta particles the least penetration).]
cell site for radiation injury	**DNA** (most susceptible), *RNA, and proteins* [Radiation produces FRs by hydrolysis of water in tissue, which damage the above structures. The G2 and mitosis phase of the cell cycle are most susceptible, while the G1 and S phase are least sensitive.]
tissue types susceptible to radiation	**lymphocytes** (hematopoietic cells are most sensitive to radiation), *germinal cells, skin, GI epithelium* [Bone, mature cartilage, muscle, and peripheral nerves are least sensitive to radiation.]
initial lab finding in total body irradiation	*lymphopenia*
portion of UV light with the greatest mutagenic effect	*UVB* [UVA is black light and UVC is germicidal. UVB produces an increase in thymidine dimers in DNA.]
skin cancer associated with UVB light	*basal cell carcinoma*
injury associated with laser radiation	*third-degree burn*
injuries associated with infrared light	*burns* and *cataracts*

Table continued on following page

Table 8–1. MECHANICAL INJURIES Continued

Most Common...	Answer and Explanation
injuries purported to be associated with microwaves	*cataracts, cancer, sterility*
type of acid-base disorders noted in high altitude	*respiratory alkalosis* [Hyperventilation lowers alveolar PCO_2, which raises both alveolar and arterial PO_2.]
type of high altitude sickness	*acute mountain sickness* associated with headache and fatigue [Hikers should increase fluids and take oxygen if available. High altitude pulmonary edema and cerebral edema are more serious conditions and require immediate descent.]

Question: Volume depletion is **LEAST LIKELY** associated with which of the following?
  (A) Third-degree burns
  (B) Heat cramps
  (C) High altitude climbing
  (D) Pelvic fractures
  (E) Salt water drowning

Answer: (B) Heat cramps are not associated with volume depletion or fever. All the other conditions listed have major problems with volume depletion.

AC = alternating current, AD = autosomal dominant, AIDS = acquired immunodeficiency syndrome, ARDS = adult respiratory distress syndrome, ATP = adenosine triphosphate, COD = cause of death, CSF = cerebrospinal fluid, FR = free radical, GI = gastrointestinal, LGA = large for gestational age, MVA = motor vehicle accident, PCO_2 = partial pressure of carbon dioxide, PO_2 = partial pressure of oxygen, RBC = red blood cell, UV = ultraviolet.

Table 8–2. CHEMICAL AND DRUG INJURIES

Most Common...	Answer and Explanation
age bracket associated with poisonings	*<5 years old*
infection associated with IV drug abuse	*skin abscesses*

Table 8–2. CHEMICAL AND DRUG INJURIES *Continued*

Most Common...	Answer and Explanation
systemic infection associated with IV drug abuse	**HBV** [Other common systemic infections are *HIV, infective endocarditis, brain abscesses,* and *tetanus.*]
serious pulmonary complication of IV heroin abuse	*noncardiogenic pulmonary edema*
treatment for heroin abuse	*naloxone*
COD due to a prescription drug in the United States	*tricyclic antidepressant overdose*
drug overdose associated with quinidine-like widening of the QRS	*tricyclic antidepressant overdose* [IV sodium bicarbonate is used in treatment.]
COD from an illicit drug in the United States	*cocaine overdose* [It blocks the uptake of neurotransmitters dopamine and norepinephrine by the presynaptic axon. It is a sympathomimetic drug (e.g., produces my**d**riasis; **d** = dilate). It predisposes to sudden death, ventricular arrhythmias, and myocarditis.]
metabolite measured to document marijuana use	*THC* [It has a high lipid solubility and remains measurable for more than a week.]
S/S of marijuana use	**delayed reaction time,** *inability to judge speed and distance, gynecomastia, lung disease*
beneficial effect of marijuana	*decreases nausea in cancer patients*
blood level for alcohol accepted in most states as legal drunkenness	*≥100 mg/dL*
blood alcohol level associated with death	*>500 mg/dL*

Table continued on following page

Table 8–2. CHEMICAL AND DRUG INJURIES *Continued*

Most Common...	Answer and Explanation
site of action of alcohol	*CNS,* where it exerts a depressant effect on the cerebral cortex, limbic system, cerebellum, and lower brain stem, in that order
sites for reabsorption of alcohol	**small intestine** (75%) and *stomach* (25%)
diseases with alcohol abuse as the primary cause	*thiamine deficiency* (Wernicke's encephalopathy and Korsakoff's psychosis), *folate deficiency, acquired sideroblastic anemia, Mallory-Weiss syndrome, Boerhaave's syndrome, cirrhosis* (esophageal varices indirectly via portal hypertension), *fatty change in the liver, chronic pancreatitis, acute pancreatitis* (shares the lead with biliary tract disease)
lab findings in alcohol abuse	*macrocytic anemia* (folate deficiency), *fasting hypoglycemia* and *lactic acidosis* [increased NADH in its metabolism converts pyruvate to lactate], *increased GGT* [synthesized by SER from alcohol induction of the system], *serum AST > ALT* [AST is primarily in hepatocyte mitochondria and alcohol is a mitochondrial poison], *hyperuricemia* [lactate and β-OHB compete with uric acid for renal excretion], β-*OHB ketoacidosis* [increased NADH converts AcAc into β-OHB], *hypertriglyceridemia* [increased NADH increases the synthesis of VLDL]
mechanism of injury of acetaminophen toxicity	*acetaminophen FR formation in the liver* [GSH is used up in neutralizing the FRs.]
target sites for acetaminophen toxicity	**liver** [hepatocellular necrosis] and *kidneys* [Along with aspirin, acetaminophen produces renal papillary necrosis.]
treatment of acetaminophen toxicity	*N-acetylcysteine,* which is a substrate for synthesis of GSH
alkylating agent associated with induction of second malignancies	*busulfan*

Table 8–2. CHEMICAL AND DRUG INJURIES *Continued*

Most Common...	Answer and Explanation
alkylating agent associated with bladder cancer and hemorrhagic cystitis	*cyclophosphamide* [It predisposes to transitional cell carcinoma of the bladder.]
drugs producing interstitial fibrosis in the lungs	*amiodarone, bleomycin, busulfan, nitrofurantoin, methysergide*
drug causing the gray baby syndrome	*chloramphenicol* [The gray baby syndrome is associated with hypothermia, bradycardia, cyanosis, and hypotension. Chloramphenicol also produces aplastic anemia.]
systems with clinical effects of excess unopposed estrogen	*hematologic:* venous thrombosis (DVT in the legs, pulmonary embolus); *cardiovascular:* AMI; *CNS:* stroke; *reproductive:* breast, endometrial, ovarian cancers, and gynecomastia in males; *hepatobiliary:* intrahepatic cholestasis, gallstones
systems with deleterious clinical effects of oral contraceptives	*hepatobiliary:* liver cell adenoma, hepatocellular carcinoma, gallstones; *reproductive:* possible connection with breast cancer in long-term users, cervical cancer
beneficial clinical effects of oral contraceptives	**contraception,** protective against *FCC, PID, ovarian cancer, endometrial cancer, acne, hirsutism, rheumatoid arthritis*
adverse effects of penicillin	**skin rash** (type I hypersensitivity), *acute interstitial nephritis* (type IV hypersensitivity), *hypersensitivity vasculitis* (type III hypersensitivity reaction), *hemolytic anemia* (type II hypersensitivity)
adverse effects of iron overdose	**gastritis,** *liver cell necrosis* leading to *liver failure* [Undigested pills can be seen on radiograph. It is treated with deferoxamine and sodium bicarbonate gastric lavage.]
adverse effects of salicylate intoxication	*gastritis, fulminant hepatitis, metabolic acidosis* (primarily in children), *mixed respiratory alkalosis and metabolic acidosis* (primarily in adults), *vertigo, tinnitus, hyperpyrexia* (uncouples oxidative phosphorylation) [Salicylates are in oil of wintergreen. The urine is alkalinized to increase excretion.]

Table continued on following page

Table 8–2. CHEMICAL AND DRUG INJURIES *Continued*

Most Common...	Answer and Explanation
intoxications seen in painters	*methylene chloride* (converted into CO), *lead poisoning*
intoxication seen in farmers	*organophosphate poisoning*
intoxication seen in dry cleaners	*Carbon tetrachloride toxicity* [It is converted into CCl_3 FRs, which produce hepatic necrosis.]
intoxication seen in automobile mechanics	*CO poisoning* [Lead poisoning is possible if batteries are being incinerated.]
chemical toxicities noted in the rubber/ chemical industry	*benzene* (aplastic anemia, acute leukemia), *aniline dyes* (bladder cancer)
clinical findings in isopropyl alcohol poisoning	coma [Unlike other alcohol poisonings, it does not produce an increased anion gap metabolic acidosis, since it is converted into acetone (fruity odor on the breath). The osmolal gap between the calculated and measured P_{osm} is >10 mOsm/kg.]
alcohol toxicity associated with blindness	*methyl alcohol poisoning* [It is converted into formic acid, which irritates the optic nerve. It produces an osmolal gap and increased anion gap metabolic acidosis.]
alcohol toxicity associated with renal failure	*ethylene glycol (antifreeze) poisoning* [It is converted into oxalic acid, which combines with calcium to form calcium oxalate crystals in the kidneys, leading to renal failure. It also produces an osmolal gap and an increased anion gap metabolic acidosis.]
treatment for ethylene glycol and methyl alcohol poisoning	*IV infusion of ethyl alcohol,* which competes with these other alcohols for alcohol dehydrogenase for metabolism
COD due to poisoning in the United States	*CO poisoning* [It blocks cytochrome oxidase, left-shifts the oxygen dissociation curve (less oxygen released), and decreases oxygen saturation (number of binding sites on Hb for carrying oxygen). The PaO_2 is normal.]
initial clinical finding in CO poisoning	*headache* [It produces a cherry red discoloration of skin. Concentrations >60% are lethal.]

Table 8–2. CHEMICAL AND DRUG INJURIES *Continued*

Most Common...	Answer and Explanation
source of CO poisoning	**automobile exhaust** [Other sources include *wood stoves, domestic and natural gases,* and *methylene chloride.*]
chronic effect of CO poisoning	*Parkinson's disease due to necrosis of the globus pallidus* [It also accelerates atherosclerosis.]
treatment of CO poisoning	*100% oxygen*
GI effect of ingested strong alkalis	*liquefactive necrosis of the esophageal epithelium with stricture formation*
GI effect of ingested strong acid	*coagulation necrosis of the epithelium*
toxicity associated with an almond smell to the breath	*cyanide poisoning* [It blocks cytochrome oxidase.]
treatment for cyanide poisoning	*nitrites* (amyl nitrite and sodium nitrite) are used first to create metHb, which competes with cytochrome oxidase for cyanide to form cyanmetHb. *Thiosulfate* is then added, which combines with cyanide in cyanmetHb to form harmless thiocyanate.
toxicity associated with 100% oxygen	**diffuse alveolar damage,** *bronchopulmonary dysplasia, retinopathy of prematurity* (in newborns) [These disorders are caused by superoxide FR formation.]
heavy metal associated with acute intoxication	*arsenic* [It is present in pet dips, pesticides, and Fowler's solution. It produces a garlic odor to the breath and affects the CNS (most common COD), skin (gray skin, skin squamous cancers), kidneys (ATN), lung (cancer), liver (angiosarcoma).]
heavy metal associated with chronic intoxication	*lead* [It denatures enzymes (ferrochelatase [sideroblastic anemia], ALA dehydrase [increases ALA], ribonuclease [coarse basophilic stippling]). It is treated with BAL and EDTA (some add penicillamine).]

Table continued on following page

Table 8–2. CHEMICAL AND DRUG INJURIES *Continued*

Most Common...	Answer and Explanation
target sites of lead poisoning in children	**CNS** (convulsions, demyelination), *hematopoietic system* (microcytic anemia), and *GI* (colic; densities are noted on plain radiographs of the abdomen)
target sites of lead poisoning in adults	*gingiva* (Pb line), *peripheral nerves* (e.g., wrist drop), *kidneys* (renal tubular acidosis, nephrotoxic ATN, interstitial nephritis), and *musculoskeletal system* (gout [Pb enhances the uptake of uric acid in the kidneys])
heavy metal identified on radiograph	*lead* [It deposits in the epiphyses and may be seen in the GI tract.]
lab findings in lead poisoning	**increased blood lead levels** (best screen); *microcytic, hypochromic anemia; coarse basophilic stippling* [ribonuclease is denatured, hence ribosomes remain in RBCs]; *increased FEP* [block in ferrochelatase increases FEP behind the block]; *increased serum iron, percent saturation,* and *ferritin; decreased TIBC; increased ALA* (due to block in ALA dehydrase)
heavy metal poisoning associated with eating contaminated fish	*mercury poisoning* [Treatment involves the use of dimercaprol (BAL) and penicillamine.]
cause of mushroom poisoning	*ingestion of mushrooms from the species* Amanita, *the toxin of which blocks RNA polymerase* [It targets the GI tract (vomiting, bloody diarrhea), liver (hepatic necrosis), and other sites.]
clinical findings in organophosphate poisoning	it irreversibly blocks acetylcholine esterase (decreases serum/RBC cholinesterase levels), *hence increasing acetylcholine at synapses and myoneural junctions. Initially, there is increased autonomic activity* (lacrimation, salivation, meiotic pupils) *and later nicotinic effects are noted* (muscle fasciculations and paralysis)

Table 8–2. CHEMICAL AND DRUG INJURIES *Continued*

Most Common...	Answer and Explanation
treatment of organophosphate poisoning	**atropine** and *pralidoxime*
toxicity resembling tetanus	*strychnine poisoning* [It is a powerful CNS stimulant and interferes with neurotransmission at spinal synapses of inhibitory neurons.]
poisons associated with garlic-smelling breath	*arsenic* and *yellow phosphorus poisoning*
overdose associated with frothing from the mouth	*heroin overdose leading to noncardiogenic pulmonary edema*
toxicity associated with an acneiform rash	*bromism*
antidote for benzodiazepine overdose	*flumazenil*
antidote for calcium channel blocker toxicity	*calcium*
antidote for digoxin toxicity	*digoxin-specific Fab (fragment antibodies)* [This will further falsely increase digoxin levels.]
antidote for anticholinergic overdoses	*physostigmine*
antidote for β-adrenergic drug toxicity	*glucagon*
antidote for narcotic overdoses	*naloxone*

Table continued on following page

Table 8–2. CHEMICAL AND DRUG INJURIES *Continued*

Most Common...	Answer and Explanation
cause of premature death in the United States	*cigarette smoking*
test used to indicate nicotine intake	*plasma or urine level of cotinine*
complication associated with smoking	*COPD* (chronic bronchitis and emphysema)
cancers for which smoking is the most common cause	**lung cancer** (squamous and small cell types), *oral squamous cancer, pancreatic adenocarcinoma, transitional cell carcinoma of the bladder, squamous carcinoma of the larynx*
cardiovascular effects of smoking	**AMI,** *sudden cardiac death, peripheral vascular disease*
GI effects of smoking	**GERD,** *delayed healing of peptic uclers*
S/S of a black widow spider bite (latrodectism)	*a sharp prick, usually felt after picking up wood from a wood pile; venom (a neurotoxin) causes muscle spasms in the thighs and abdomen* [An antivenin is available. Calcium gluconate helps reduce the muscle spasms.]
S/S of a brown recluse spider bite	*not as painful as the black widow bite; toxin is necrotoxic and produces an extensive necrotic lesion at the envenomation site; can produce ATN and a hemolytic anemia*
S/S associated with poisonous scorpion bites	*paresthesias at the envenomation site, hypertension, respiratory paralysis* (most common COD) [Only one species is poisonous in the United States (seen in Arizona).]
S/S of chigger bites	*intensely pruritic red lesions with sharply demarcated borders*
S/S of scabies (human itch mite)	*in adults, they burrow between the webs of the fingers and produce intense pruritus* [It is treated with lindane.]

Table 8–2. CHEMICAL AND DRUG INJURIES *Continued*

Most Common...	Answer and Explanation
clinical findings associated with *Pediculus humanis capitis* (head louse) infestations	*eggs called "nits" on the hair shafts* [Benzene hexachloride is used in treatment, but is very toxic. Current recommendations are to manually remove them with special combs.]
clinical findings associated with *Pediculus humanis corporis* (body louse) infestations	*lice are not attached to the skin surface; eggs are found in crease areas of the body* [Benzene hexachloride is used in treatment.]
infestation in which the louse looks like a crab under magnification	*infestation of Phthirus pubis (pubic louse)* [Benzene hexachloride is used in treatment.]
COD due to a venomous bite	*anaphylaxis secondary to a bee sting*
insect bite causing painful vesicular lesions that necrose	*fire ant bites*
poisonous snake envenomation in the United States	*rattlesnake envenomation* [Hematologic problems and local tissue swelling and necrosis are the primary problems. Rattlesnakes, copperheads, and water moccasins are pit vipers. The coral snake (red and yellow colors abut each other) is a type of cobra whose venom has a potent neurotoxin.]
complication associated with the treatment of rattlesnake envenomations	*serum sickness after using horse serum antivenin*
poisonous lizard in the United States	*Gila monster in the Southwestern United States*

Table continued on following page

Table 8–2. CHEMICAL AND DRUG INJURIES *Continued*

Question: In which of the following tissue sites do both alcohol excess and cigarette smoking directly produce significant disease?
(A) Liver
(B) Lungs
(C) Pancreas
(D) Bladder
(E) Kidneys

Answer: (C): Pancreatic adenocarcinoma is increased in smokers and in alcoholics, in the latter as a result of chronic pancreatitis. The liver is most affected by alcohol, while the bladder (transitional cancer), lungs (cancer), and kidneys (cancer) are more affected by smoking. Other common sites are heart (CAD) with smoking and congestive cardiomyopathy with alcohol), and mouth (cocarcinogens for squamous cancer).

AcAc = acetoacetic acid, ALA = δ-aminolevulinic acid, ALT = alanine aminotransferase, AMI = acute myocardial infarction, AST = aspartate aminotransferase, ATN = acute tubular necrosis, BAL = British anti-Lewisite, β-OHB = β-hydroxybutyric acid, CAD = coronary artery disease, CNS = central nervous system, COD = cause of death, COPD = chronic obstructive pulmonary disease, cyanmetHb = cyanmethemoglobin, DVT = deep vein thrombosis, EDTA = ethylenediaminetetraacetic acid, FCC = fibrocystic change, FEP = free erythrocyte protoporphyrin, FR = free radical, GERD = gastroesophageal reflux disease, GGT = γ-glutamyltransferase, GI = gastrointestinal, GSH = glutathione, Hb = hemoglobin, HBV = hepatitis B virus, HIV = human immunodeficiency virus, IV = intravenous, metHb = methemoglobin, NADH = nicotinamide-adenine dinucleotide (reduced form), PaO$_2$ = partial pressure of arterial oxygen, Pb = lead, PID = pelvic inflammatory disease, P$_{osm}$ = osmolar pressure, RBC = red blood cell, SER = smooth endoplasmic reticulum, S/S = signs and symptoms, THC = Δ9-tetrahydrocannabinol, TIBC = total iron binding capacity, VLDL = very low density lipoprotein.

CHAPTER

NEOPLASIA

CONTENTS

Table 9–1. NOMENCLATURE, TUMOR PROPERTIES, INVASION, METASTASIS, SURGICAL PATHOLOGY

Most Common...	Answer and Explanation
contributory factor responsible for cancer in the United States	*cigarette smoking* [Cancer is the second most common COD in the United States.]
name applied to benign tumors derived from glands	*adenomas* (e.g., a follicular adenoma of the thyroid)
name applied to benign tumors with a cauliflower-like appearance	*polyps* (e.g., adenomatous polyp of the colon)
name applied to malignant tumors derived from epithelium	*carcinomas* [Carcinomas are designated squamous (e.g., squamous cell carcinoma of the skin), adenocarcinoma (e.g., glands; breast adenocarcinoma), or transitional epithelium (e.g., bladder cancer).]
name applied to malignant tumors derived from connective tissue	*sarcomas* (e.g., smooth muscle [leiomyosarcoma], adipose [liposarcoma])
secondary descriptor applied to a hard tumor	*scirrhous* [When a tumor incites a fibroblastic response around areas of invasion, it is called *desmoplasia*.]
secondary descriptor applied to a soft tumor	*medullary* (e.g., medullary carcinoma of the breast and thyroid)

Table continued on following page

Table 9–1. NOMENCLATURE, TUMOR PROPERTIES, INVASION, METASTASIS, SURGICAL PATHOLOGY *Continued*

Most Common...	Answer and Explanation
secondary descriptor applied to a tumor with ducts exuding necrotic material	*comedo* (e.g., comedocarcinoma of the breast)
sarcoma in children and in adults	*embryonal sarcoma* and *malignant fibrous histiocytoma*, respectively
benign soft tissue tumor	*lipoma*
cancer derived from the bone marrow	*leukemia*, which is a malignancy derived from hematopoietic cells [There are no benign hematopoietic tumors.]
cancer derived from the lymph nodes	*malignant lymphoma* [Non-Hodgkin's lymphoma is more common than Hodgkin's lymphoma.]
mixed tumor [tumor with two different cell types derived from the same cell layer]	*mixed tumor of the parotid gland* [The majority are benign.]
site for teratomas [tumor derived from all three germ cell layers]	*ovaries in females* and *testicles in males*
tumor in newborns	*sacrococcygeal teratoma*
germ cell tumor [totipotential tumors]	*teratoma*
benign and malignant tumor derived from trophoblastic tissue	*hydatidiform mole* and *choriocarcinoma*, respectively [Moles consist of a neoplastic chorionic villus lined by syncytiotrophoblast and cytotrophoblast. Choriocarcinoma is composed entirely of malignant syncytiotrophoblast and cytotrophoblast.]
neuroglial tumor	*astrocytoma in the brain* [Other neuroglial tumors are oligodendrogliomas and ependymomas.]

Table 9–1. NOMENCLATURE, TUMOR PROPERTIES, INVASION, METASTASIS, SURGICAL PATHOLOGY *Continued*

Most Common...	Answer and Explanation
tumor of embryonic origin ("blastoma") in children	**neuroblastoma,** a malignant tumor of neuroblasts in the adrenal medulla [Other examples include *Wilms' tumor* (nephroblastoma), *hepatoblastoma, retinoblastoma* of the eye, and *medulloblastoma* in the cerebellum.]
derivation of APUD tumors [**a**mine **p**recursor **u**ptake and **d**ecarboxylation]	*neural crest* and *neuroectoderm* (e.g., small cell carcinoma of the lung, carcinoid tumors, neuroblastoma)
EM finding in APUD tumors	*neurosecretory granules*
tumor-like condition	*hamartoma,* which is an overgrowth of tissue normally present in that tissue [Examples: bronchial hamartomas, hyperplastic polyps, Peutz-Jeghers polyps]
site for choristoma, or heterotopic rest [normal tissue in a foreign location]	*pancreatic tissue in the wall of the stomach*
distinction between a benign and a malignant tumor	*capacity to metastasize to another site*
examples of tumors whose metastatic potential is based on size	*renal adenocarcinoma* (>3 cm malignant, <2 cm benign), *carcinoid tumors* (>2 cm can metastasize, <2 cm usually do not metastasize)
benign tumor without a capsule	*leiomyoma of the uterus* [A *dermatofibroma* on the lower leg is another example.]
malignant tumor with a capsule	*follicular carcinoma of the thyroid* [*Renal adenocarcinomas* have an incomplete capsule.]
type of mitotic spindle associated with malignancy	*atypical mitotic spindle* (e.g., tripolar, tetrapolar)
benign tumor that metastasizes	*invasive mole,* which is a benign trophoblastic tumor

Table continued on following page

Table 9–1. NOMENCLATURE, TUMOR PROPERTIES, INVASION, METASTASIS, SURGICAL PATHOLOGY *Continued*

Most Common...	Answer and Explanation
malignant tumor that does not metastasize	*basal cell carcinoma* [It infiltrates tissue but rarely metastasizes.]
carcinomas that are blood vessel invaders	*renal adenocarcinoma, follicular carcinoma of the thyroid, hepatocellular carcinoma* [Carcinomas usually start as lymphatic invaders and end up in blood vessels.]
sarcomas that are lymphatic invaders	*rhabdomyosarcomas* [Sarcomas are normally blood vessel invaders.]
site of metastasis for carcinomas	*regional lymph nodes*
site of metastasis for sarcomas	*lungs*
cell cycle characteristics of malignant tumors	*longer cell cycle than the parent tissue* [More cells stay in the cell cycle than normal cells, hence they accumulate. This is often due to inactivation of the p53 suppressor gene, which codes for factors that modulate the kinases that control the movement from one phase of the cycle to the next.]
nuclear abnormalities present in malignant cells	**increased nuclear to cytoplasmic ratio,** *hyperchromatic* (increased synthesis of DNA), *irregular nuclear borders, large irregular nucleoli* (increased synthesis of RNA)
Pap stain finding in squamous cancers	*deeply eosinophilic cytoplasm owing to the presence of keratin*
metabolic characteristics of malignant cells	characteristic features include: *anaerobic glycolysis, degradative enzymes, lack of cohesiveness* (reason they exfoliate well in obtaining of Pap smears), *lack of contact inhibition in culture* (pile up on each other), *immortality in culture, loss of their surface ABO antigens, transplantability into susceptible animals*
number of doubling times before tumors are clinically detectable	*30 doubling times*, which is equivalent to 10^9 cells, 1 gram of tissue, volume of 1 mL

Table 9–1. NOMENCLATURE, TUMOR PROPERTIES, INVASION, METASTASIS, SURGICAL PATHOLOGY *Continued*

Most Common...	Answer and Explanation
DNA study abnormalities in highly aggressive malignancies	*aneuploid* (uneven multiple of 23 chromosomes) and *increased S phase* (measure of the number of malignant cells in the proliferating pool)
cause of psammoma bodies in tumors	*apoptosis (individual cell death) of tumor cells with dystrophic calcification* (e.g., meningiomas, papillary carcinomas of the thyroid, serous cystadenocarcinomas of the ovary
growth factors involved in the invasion of tissue by malignant cells	*transforming growth factor-α and -β, and fibroblast growth factors,* which stimulate angiogenesis (new blood vessel formation) and production of collagen
receptors on tumor cells that assist in their movement through tissue	*laminin receptors,* which are important in cell-cell adhesion, cell–basement membrane adhesion, and cell–extracellular matrix adhesion
cancer with perineural invasion	*prostate cancer* [This aids in its spread through the prostate and out into the capsule.]
cause of peau d'orange [surface of the skin is dimpled and looks like an orange]	*inflammatory carcinoma of the breast* [Peau d'orange is due to plugging of the subcutaneous lymphatics by tumor emboli with subsequent lymphedema.]
types of metastasis	**lymphatic,** *hematogenous, seeding* (spreading of tumor within body cavities, e.g., peritoneal cavity)
sites for seeding	**peritoneal cavity** in patients with ovarian, GI, or pancreatic cancers and the *subarachnoid space* in patients with GBM or medulloblastoma
sign indicating seeding in the pelvic cavity of a woman	*induration of the pouch of Douglas,* which is located posterior to the uterus and anterior to the rectum
initial site in a lymph node of carcinomatous spread	*subcapsular sinus*

Table continued on following page

Table 9–1. NOMENCLATURE, TUMOR PROPERTIES, INVASION, METASTASIS, SURGICAL PATHOLOGY *Continued*

Most Common...	Answer and Explanation
location in bone for metastasis	*vertebral column*, owing to the Batson vertebral venous plexus, which connects with the vena cava
organ metastasized to	*lymph nodes* (e.g., breast cancer)
malignancy and primary malignancy of the lymph nodes	*metastasis* (breast primary) and *malignant lymphoma* (nodular poorly differentiated B cell type), respectively
malignancy and primary malignancy of the lungs	*metastasis* (breast primary) and *adenocarcinoma*, respectively
malignancy and primary malignancy of the brain	*metastasis* (lung primary) and *GBM*, respectively
malignancy and primary malignancy of the liver	*metastasis* (lung primary) and *hepatocellular carcinoma*, respectively
malignancy and primary malignancy of the bone	*metastasis* (breast primary) and *multiple myeloma*, respectively
primary site for metastasis to Virchow's node [left supraclavicular node]	*stomach adenocarcinoma*
primary site for osteoblastic metastasis	*prostate cancer* [Radiodense loci are noted on plain films.]
cancer metastatic to the adrenal glands	*primary lung cancer*
enzyme elevated in osteoblastic metastases	*alkaline phosphatase* (sign of osteoblastic activity)
malignancies that produce purely osteolytic metastases	*lung, kidney* [Lytic metastases produce lucencies in bone on plain films.]

Table 9–1. NOMENCLATURE, TUMOR PROPERTIES, INVASION, METASTASIS, SURGICAL PATHOLOGY *Continued*

Most Common...	Answer and Explanation
initial management step in breast and thyroid masses	*fine needle aspiration*
histochemical stain used to identify malignant lymphomas	*leukocyte common antigen* (CD45)
histochemical stains used to identify carcinomas	*epithelial membrane antigen* and *cytokeratin*
histochemical stain used to identify APUD tumors	*S100 antigen*
histochemical stain used to identify tumors of muscle origin	*desmin*
histochemical stain used to identify tumors of vascular origin	*factor VIII–related antigen*
histochemical stain used to identify tumors of histiocytic origin	*CD1 antigen*
EM finding in tumors of vascular origin	*Weibel-Palade bodies*, which contain von Willebrand's factor
EM finding in tumors of melanocytic origin	*melanosomes*
EM finding in tumors of histiocytic origin	*Birbeck's granules* (Langerhans' granules; look like a tennis racket)
EM finding in skeletal muscle	*thick and thin myofilaments*

Table continued on following page

Table 9–1. NOMENCLATURE, TUMOR PROPERTIES, INVASION, METASTASIS, SURGICAL PATHOLOGY *Continued*

Most Common...	Answer and Explanation
EM finding in epithelial tumors	*tonofilaments*

Question: In which of the following sites is the primary malignant tumor most commonly of squamous origin? **SELECT 2**
- (A) Lung
- (B) Esophagus
- (C) Pancreas
- (D) Liver
- (E) Thyroid
- (F) Larynx

Answers: (B), (F): Most esophageal and laryngeal cancers are squamous in origin. All the other sites listed have adenocarcinoma as the most common primary tumor type.

COD = cause of death, EM = electron microscopy, GBM = glioblastoma multiforme, GI = gastrointestinal.

Table 9–2. ONCOGENESIS, GRADE AND STAGE, HOST-TUMOR RELATIONSHIPS, TUMOR-HOST RELATIONSHIPS, TUMOR MARKERS, TUMOR EPIDEMIOLOGY

Most Common...	Answer and Explanation
genes producing cancer	*oncogenes,* which derive from proto-oncogenes [Proto-oncogenes are involved in the growth process.]
function of suppressor genes	control unregulated cell growth
suppressor gene associated with cancer	**p53 suppressor gene on chromosome 17,** which codes for proteins that control kinases involved in the movement of cells through the cell cycle [Other suppressor genes are the *Rb-1 gene* (retinoblastoma; chromosome 13), *APC suppressor gene* (adenomatous polyposis coli; chromosome 5), *NF-1 and NF-2* (neurofibromatosis; chromosome 17 and 22, respectively).]
multistep process involved in oncogenesis	*initiation* (irreversible mutation) → *promotion* (growth enhancement) → *progression* (subdivision of tumor cells into special functions)

Table 9–2. ONCOGENESIS, GRADE AND STAGE, HOST-TUMOR RELATIONSHIPS, TUMOR-HOST RELATIONSHIPS, TUMOR MARKERS, TUMOR EPIDEMIOLOGY *Continued*

Most Common...	Answer and Explanation
general groups of proto-oncogenes involved in the growth process	*growth factor synthesis* (e.g., *sis*), *growth factor receptor* (*erb*-B2/*neu*), *membrane-associated protein kinases* (e.g., *src*), *membrane-related guanine triphosphate (GTP)–binding proteins* (e.g., *ras*), *cytoplasmic protein kinases* (e.g., *raf*), *transcription regulators in the nucleus* (e.g., c-*myc*)
oncogenes involved in cancer	**p53 suppressor gene** (colorectal, breast, lung, and CNS cancers) and *ras oncogene* (lung, colon, pancreas, leukemia, ovarian cancers) [The former is inactivated and the latter activated by point mutations.]
methods of activating proto-oncogenes to oncogenes (initiation)	structural activation: *point mutation* (e.g., *ras* oncogene), *translocation producing an abnormal gene* (e.g., t9;22 of the *abl* oncogene in CML). Increase in function: *gene amplification* (e.g., *erb*-B2/*neu* oncogene), *translocation leading to an abnormal activity* (e.g., t8;14 of the c-*myc* oncogene in Burkitt's lymphoma), *translocation leading to inactivation of the apoptosis gene* (e.g., t14;18 of the *bcl*-2 oncogene in B cell follicular lymphomas), *inactivation of suppressor genes* (e.g., inactivation of p53, inactivation of Rb-1 producing retinoblastoma)
AD syndrome associated with inactivation of the p53 suppressor gene	*Li-Fraumeni multicancer syndrome* with an increased incidence of breast cancer, sarcomas, brain tumors, and leukemia
AD syndrome associated with inactivation of the *APC* suppressor gene	**familial polyposis** and *Gardner's syndrome* (colon polyps + benign soft tissue tumors)
AD syndrome associated with inactivation of the *NF-1* and *NF-2* suppressor genes	*neurofibromatosis, type I and II*, respectively
carcinogenic agents	*chemicals* (80–90%), particularly those in cigarette smoke

Table continued on following page

Table 9–2. ONCOGENESIS, GRADE AND STAGE,
HOST-TUMOR RELATIONSHIPS,
TUMOR-HOST RELATIONSHIPS, TUMOR
MARKERS, TUMOR EPIDEMIOLOGY *Continued*

Most Common...	Answer and Explanation
test utilized to establish the mutagenicity of chemicals	*Ames test* [In this test, *Salmonella* bacteria that are unable to synthesize histidine are placed on a histidine-free culture plate, which also includes the chemical in question and liver microsomes to convert the chemical into a carcinogen. If the *Salmonella* can grow on the media, the chemical must have initiated a mutational event.]
chemical carcinogens that induce transitional carcinoma of the bladder	**polycyclic hydrocarbons in cigarette smoke,** *aniline dyes, cyclophosphamide, benzidine, phenacetin*
chemical carcinogens that induce angiosarcoma of the liver	*vinyl chloride, arsenic, Thorotrast* (mnemonic: VAT)
chemical carcinogens that induce primary lung cancer	**polycyclic hydrocarbons,** *uranium (radon gas), asbestos, chromium, arsenic, nickel, cadmium*
chemical carcinogens that induce hepatocellular carcinoma	**aflatoxins (especially in association with HBV),** *oral contraceptives, Thorotrast, alcohol*
chemical carcinogens that induce leukemia	*benzene, alkylating agents* (also malignant lymphoma)
chemical carcinogens that induce esophageal cancer	*polycyclic hydrocarbons, nitrosamines, alcohol*
chemical carcinogens that induce squamous cancer	**polycyclic hydrocarbons** (cervix, larynx, lung, oral pharynx), *arsenic* (skin), *tar/soot/oils* (skin), *immunosuppressive agents* (skin), *chewing tobacco* (mouth; verrucous type)
chemical carcinogens that induce pancreatic adenocarcinoma	**polycyclic hydrocarbons,** *alcohol* (via production of chronic pancreatitis)

**Table 9-2. ONCOGENESIS, GRADE AND STAGE,
HOST-TUMOR RELATIONSHIPS,
TUMOR-HOST RELATIONSHIPS, TUMOR
MARKERS, TUMOR EPIDEMIOLOGY** *Continued*

Most Common...	Answer and Explanation
chemical carcinogen that induces clear cell adenocarcinoma of the vagina	*diethylstilbestrol* (DES)
oncogenic viruses associated with leukemia/lymphoma	**EBV** (primary CNS lymphoma, polyclonal lymphoma, Burkitt's lymphoma), *HTLV-1* (adult T cell leukemia), *HTLV-2* (? hairy cell leukemia), *HIV* (primary CNS lymphoma)
oncogenic virus associated with nasopharyngeal carcinoma	*EBV*
oncogenic viruses associated with hepatocellular carcinoma	**HBV,** *HCV*
oncogenic virus associated with Kaposi's sarcoma	*herpesvirus 8*
oncogenic virus associated with cervical and anal squamous cell carcinoma	*HPV types* **16,** *18, 31*
radiation-induced cancer	**leukemia** [Other common radiation-induced cancers are *papillary carcinoma of the thyroid,* lung cancer (radon gas from uranium), *breast cancer, angiosarcoma of the liver* (Thorotrast), *UVB-light–induced cancers* (*basal cell carcinoma,* squamous cell carcinoma, malignant melanoma), *osteogenic sarcoma.*]
AR disease associated with skin cancer from UV radiation	*xeroderma pigmentosum* [It is a deficiency of DNA repair enzymes.]

Table continued on following page

Table 9–2. ONCOGENESIS, GRADE AND STAGE, HOST-TUMOR RELATIONSHIPS, TUMOR-HOST RELATIONSHIPS, TUMOR MARKERS, TUMOR EPIDEMIOLOGY *Continued*

Most Common...	Answer and Explanation
bacteria associated with cancer	Helicobacter pylori *is associated with gastric adenocarcinoma and low-grade mucosa-associated primary malignant lymphomas of the stomach*
term applied to squamous cancers originating in burn scars or keloids	*Marjolin's ulcers*
type of cancer associated with scars in the lungs	*adenocarcinoma*
type of cancer developing in chronic sinus tracts draining out to the skin	*squamous cell carcinoma*
cancer associated with immunosuppressive therapy	*squamous cell carcinoma of the skin*
type of PUD associated with cancer	*gastric ulcers* (<3%) [Duodenal ulcers are never associated with cancer.]
terms applied to grading of cancer [grade refers to how closely the tumor resembles its parent tissue]	*low grade* (well differentiated), *intermediate grade* (moderately well differentiated), and *high grade* (poorly differentiated, anaplastic)
elements involved in staging a cancer	*tumor size* (T), *lymph node status* (N), *presence or absence of other metastatic spread* (M) [Stage is more important than grade in prognosis.]
host defenses against cancer	*cellular immunity* (cytotoxic CD_8 T cells), *macrophages, natural killer cells, ADCC*
tumor mechanisms for evading host defenses	*shedding antigens, forming immunocomplexes with cytotoxic antibodies, stimulating CD_8 T suppressor cells to inhibit cellular immunity, coating themselves with platelets*

Table 9–2. ONCOGENESIS, GRADE AND STAGE, HOST-TUMOR RELATIONSHIPS, TUMOR-HOST RELATIONSHIPS, TUMOR MARKERS, TUMOR EPIDEMIOLOGY *Continued*

Most Common...	Answer and Explanation
chemical factor associated with cachexia due to cancer	*tumor necrosis factor-α secreted from host macrophages and cancer cells*
anemia associated with cancer	**anemia of chronic inflammation** [Other anemias include *iron deficiency* (colorectal cancer), *autoimmune hemolytic anemia* (e.g., CLL), *microangiopathic hemolytic anemia* from tumor emboli in vessels, *myelophthisic anemia* (metastasis to the marrow), *marrow suppression* by radiation and chemotherapy.]
cause of a leukoerythroblastic peripheral smear [presence of immature WBCs and RBCs]	*metastasis to the bone marrow,* most commonly due to breast cancer [Metastasis to the marrow pushes hematopoietic elements into the peripheral blood (immature WBCs, nucleated RBCs.]
coagulation abnormality in cancer	*hypercoagulability,* owing to an increase in certain coagulation factors (e.g., fibrinogen and factors V and VIII), release of tissue thromboplastin, thrombocytosis, decreased liver synthesis of antithrombin III and protein C
overall COD in cancer patients	*infections,* often secondary to gram-negative sepsis
malignancies associated with fever not related to infection	**Hodgkin's disease** (Pel-Ebstein fever), *renal adenocarcinoma, osteogenic sarcoma*
paraneoplastic syndrome [syndrome often predating the onset of cancer]	**hypercalcemia secondary to secretion of a PTH-like peptide** [Metastasis to the marrow producing hypercalcemia by stimulating osteoclastic activity is not an example of a paraneoplastic syndrome, since it is a direct effect of the tumor.]
cause of the Eaton-Lambert syndrome [myasthenia gravis–like syndrome]	*small cell carcinoma of the lung* [Unlike true myasthenia, the eyes are not usually involved, muscle strength increases with exercise, and Tensilon does not improve muscle function.]

Table continued on following page

**Table 9–2. ONCOGENESIS, GRADE AND STAGE,
HOST-TUMOR RELATIONSHIPS,
TUMOR-HOST RELATIONSHIPS, TUMOR
MARKERS, TUMOR EPIDEMIOLOGY** *Continued*

Most Common...	Answer and Explanation
cancer associated with Sweet's syndrome [fever, neutrophilic leukocytosis, and a red papular rash]	*acute leukemia*
phenotypic markers for gastric adenocarcinoma	*Leser-Trelat sign* (multiple outcroppings of seborrheic keratosis) and *acanthosis nigricans* (black lesion usually located in the axilla)
cancer associated with pulmonary osteoarthropathy [clubbing and periosteal inflammation]	*primary lung cancer*
cancer associated with superficial migratory thrombophlebitis (Trousseau's sign)	*pancreatic adenocarcinoma*
collagen vascular disease associated with an underlying cancer	*dermatomyositis/polymyositis* (increased incidence of primary lung cancer)
renal disease associated with cancer	*nephrotic syndrome due to diffuse membranous glomerulonephritis*
cancer associated with hyponatremia or ectopic Cushing's syndrome	*small cell carcinoma of the lung with ectopic secretion of ADH and ACTH,* respectively
cancer associated with hypercalcemia or secondary polycythemia	*renal adenocarcinoma with ectopic secretion of PTH and erythropoietin,* respectively
cancer associated with hypoglycemia or secondary polycythemia	*hepatocellular carcinoma with ectopic secretion of an insulin-like factor and erythropoietin,* respectively

Table 9–2. ONCOGENESIS, GRADE AND STAGE, HOST-TUMOR RELATIONSHIPS, TUMOR-HOST RELATIONSHIPS, TUMOR MARKERS, TUMOR EPIDEMIOLOGY *Continued*

Most Common...	Answer and Explanation
cancer associated with secretion of calcitonin or ACTH	*medullary carcinoma of the thyroid* [Calcitonin is an excellent screen for the tumor.]
cancers associated with secretion of β-hCG	*gestationally derived trophoblastic tumors* (e.g., moles and choriocarcinoma), *testicular cancer with trophoblastic tissue* [Syncytiotrophoblast secretes the hormone.]
cancers associated with hypercalcemia due to secretion of a PTH-like peptide	*primary squamous cancer of the lungs, renal adenocarcinoma*, and *breast cancer*
cancers associated with secondary polycythemia	**renal adenocarcinoma** (also in association with von Hippel-Lindau disease and cerebellar hemangioblastomas), *Wilms' tumor, hepatocellular carcinoma*
tumor associated with excessive release of serotonin	*carcinoid tumor arising in the terminal ileum with metastasis to the liver producing the carcinoid syndrome*
cancers associated with secretion of AFP	**hepatocellular carcinoma** and *endodermal (yolk sac) sinus tumors in the ovaries or testicles* [AAT is also increased in hepatocellular carcinomas.]
tumor markers ordered in the evaluation of testicular tumors	*AFP* and β-*hCG*
tumor markers for multiple myeloma	**Bence-Jones protein** (light chains) in the urine and β$_2$-*microglobulin*
tumor marker for surface-derived ovarian cancers	*CA 125*
tumor markers for small cell carcinoma of the lung	**CEA**, *neuron-specific enolase, bombesin*
tumor marker for prostate cancer	*prostate-specific antigen* (PSA)

Table continued on following page

Table 9–2. ONCOGENESIS, GRADE AND STAGE, HOST-TUMOR RELATIONSHIPS, TUMOR-HOST RELATIONSHIPS, TUMOR MARKERS, TUMOR EPIDEMIOLOGY *Continued*

Most Common...	Answer and Explanation
tumor markers for breast cancer	*CEA* and *CA 15-3*
tumor marker for colorectal cancer	*CEA*
tumor markers for pancreatic carcinoma	**CA 19-9** and *CEA*
enzyme that is commonly elevated in malignant lymphomas	*LDH, particularly the LDH₃ isoenzyme fraction*
cancers in decreasing order of incidence in men	**prostate,** *lung, colorectal*
cancers in decreasing order of incidence in women	**breast,** *lung, colorectal*
cancer mortalities in decreasing order in men	**lung,** *prostate, colorectal*
cancer mortalities in decreasing order in women	**lung,** *breast, colorectal* [Colorectal cancer is the second most common cancer killer in men and women.]
cancers that are decreasing in incidence in the United States	*stomach, cervix* (due to Pap screens), *endometrial*
cancers that are increasing in incidence in the United States	*breast* (due to early detection by mammogram), *prostate* (due to detection by PSA), *lung* (particularly in women), *multiple myeloma, malignant lymphoma, pancreatic carcinoma* [In general, cancer is more common in blacks than whites.]
cancer that is increasing at the fastest rate around the world	*malignant melanoma* [Australia is the #1 country for malignant melanomas.]

Table 9–2. ONCOGENESIS, GRADE AND STAGE, HOST-TUMOR RELATIONSHIPS, TUMOR-HOST RELATIONSHIPS, TUMOR MARKERS, TUMOR EPIDEMIOLOGY *Continued*

Most Common...	Answer and Explanation
cancer in Southeast China	*nasopharyngeal carcinoma secondary to EBV* [In Northern China, esophageal cancer is more common.]
cancer in Japan	**stomach adenocarcinoma** (due to food preserved by smoking) [*HTLV-1* adult T cell leukemia/lymphoma are also common.]
cancer in the Far East	*hepatocellular carcinoma secondary to HBV and enhanced by aflatoxins*
malignant lymphoma in Africa	*Burkitt's lymphoma due to EBV*
cancer prevented by immunization	*hepatocellular carcinoma due to HBV* [Vaccination not only reduces liver cancer risk but risk for contracting HDV as well.]
cancer in the Far East that is related to α-thalassemia	*choriocarcinoma* [Hb Bart's disease (deletion of all 4α-globin chains) is associated with spontaneous abortions, which in turn predispose to choriocarcinoma.]
cancers associated with parasitic diseases	*cholangiocarcinoma* due to Clonorchis sinensis and *squamous cancer of the bladder* due to Schistosoma hematobium
chromosome instability syndromes that predispose to cancer	*ataxia-telangiectasia* (AR; malignant lymphoma), *Bloom's syndrome* (AR; acute leukemia), *Fanconi's syndrome* (AR; acute leukemia)
SXRs associated with cancer	*Wiskott-Aldrich syndrome* (B and T cell immunodeficiency, eczema, thrombocytopenia, malignant lymphoma), *sex-linked lymphoproliferative syndrome due to EBV* (malignant lymphoma)
trisomy associated with acute leukemia	*Down syndrome* (trisomy 21)
chromosome disorder associated with ovarian cancer	*Turner's syndrome* (45 XO) has an increased risk of dysgerminoma, especially if a Y chromosome is present (e.g., mosaic with XO/XY genotype)

Table continued on following page

Table 9–2. ONCOGENESIS, GRADE AND STAGE, HOST-TUMOR RELATIONSHIPS, TUMOR-HOST RELATIONSHIPS, TUMOR MARKERS, TUMOR EPIDEMIOLOGY *Continued*

Most Common...	Answer and Explanation
components of the MEN-I syndrome (AD)	*pituitary tumors, parathyroid adenomas, and pancreatic tumors* (usually Zollinger-Ellison syndrome)
components of the MEN-IIa and IIb syndromes (AD)	MEN-IIa: *medullary carcinoma of the thyroid, parathyroid adenoma, and pheochromocytoma* MEN-IIb: same as IIa except there is no parathyroid adenoma and there are *mucosal neuromas in the lips*
AD polyp syndrome associated with ovarian tumors	*Peutz-Jeghers syndrome* is associated with sex cord tumors with annular tubules
AD syndrome associated with tumors and/or hamartomas in the CNS, heart, and kidneys	*tuberous sclerosis* has hamartomatous lesions in the brain (hamartomas of glial elements), heart (rhabdomyoma), and kidneys (angiomyolipoma, a hamartoma)
AD syndrome associated with acoustic neuromas and meningiomas	*neurofibromatosis*
precursor lesion for squamous cancer of the skin	*actinic keratosis*
precursor lesions for squamous cancer in the oral cavity	**erythroplakia** (e.g., erythematous lesions) and *leukoplakia* (white lesions)
precursor lesion for distal adenocarcinoma of the esophagus	*Barrett's esophagus* (glandular metaplasia)
precursor lesion for gastric adenocarcinoma	*intestinal metaplasia* (goblet cells and Paneth cells in the stomach mucosa as a reaction to *H. pylori*–induced chronic atrophic gastritis)
precursor lesion for colorectal cancer	*adenomatous polyps*

Table 9–2. ONCOGENESIS, GRADE AND STAGE, HOST-TUMOR RELATIONSHIPS, TUMOR-HOST RELATIONSHIPS, TUMOR MARKERS, TUMOR EPIDEMIOLOGY *Continued*

Most Common...	Answer and Explanation
precursor lesion for gallbladder cancer	*gallstones*
precursor lesion for clear cell adenocarcinoma of the vagina	*vaginal adenosis secondary to DES*
precursor lesion for cervical cancer	*cervical dysplasia*
precursor lesion for endometrial cancer	*endometrial hyperplasia*
precursor lesion for breast cancer	*atypical ductal hyperplasia*
precursor lesion for vulvar cancer	*hypertrophic vulvar dystrophy* (HPV relationship)
inflammatory bowel disease associated with cancer	*ulcerative colitis*, particularly if over 10 years' duration
genetic precursor lesion for colorectal cancer	*familial polyposis*
precursor lesion for medullary carcinoma of the thyroid	*C cell hyperplasia*, particularly in MEN IIa and IIb

Question: Which of the following carcinogens is associated with primary cancer of the skin, liver, and lungs?
(A) Asbestos
(B) Estrogen
(C) Arsenic
(D) Polycyclic hydrocarbons
(E) EBV

Answer: (C): Arsenic is associated with squamous cancer of the skin, angiosarcoma of the liver, and primary cancer of the lungs. None of the other carcinogens listed have this spectrum of cancer.

AAT = α₁-antitrypsin, ACTH = adrenocorticotropic hormone, AD = autosomal dominant, ADCC = antibody-dependent cellular cytotoxicity, ADH = antidiuretic hormone, AFP = alpha-fetoprotein, AR = autosomal recessive, CEA = carcinoembryonic antigen, CLL = chronic lymphocytic leukemia, CML = chronic myelogenous leukemia, CNS = central nervous system, COD = cause of death, DES = diethylstilbestrol, EBV = Epstein-Barr virus, Hb = hemoglobin, HBV = hepatitis B virus, hCG = human chorionic gonadotropin, HCV = hepatitis C virus, HDV = hepatitis D virus, HIV = human immunodeficiency virus, HPV = human papilloma virus, HTLV = human T cell lymphotropic virus, LDH = lactate dehydrogenase, MEN = multiple endocrine neoplasia, PTH = parathormone, PUD = peptic ulcer disease, RBC = red blood cell, SXR = sex-linked recessive, UV = ultraviolet, WBC = white blood cell.

CHAPTER

10

CARDIOVASCULAR PATHOLOGY

CONTENTS

Table 10–1. HISTORY AND PHYSICAL EXAM

Most Common...	Answer and Explanation
symptom of heart failure	*dyspnea* (the sensation of difficulty with breathing)
symptom of ischemic heart disease (IHD)	*chest pain*
cause of wheezing in left heart failure (LHF)	*peribronchiolar edema producing small airway constriction* (cardiac asthma)
cause of calf claudication [pain at rest or with exercise]	*atherosclerotic peripheral vascular disease* (PVD)
type of heart failure associated with dependent pitting edema	*right heart failure* (RHF) [Blood builds up behind the failed heart, in this case the venous system, with subsequent increase in hydrostatic pressure and pitting edema.]
valvular lesion associated with syncope with exercise and angina with exercise	*aortic stenosis* [Owing to stenosis of the valve, the stroke volume is decreased, hence not enough blood enters the cerebral vessels. LVH also imposes a need for oxygen, hence predisposing to exertional angina.]
factor responsible for the systolic blood pressure	*stroke volume* (SV), which is the amount of blood ejected from the heart during systole

Table continued on following page

175

Table 10–1. HISTORY AND PHYSICAL EXAM *Continued*

Most Common...	Answer and Explanation
factor responsible for the diastolic blood pressure	*total peripheral resistance* (TPR) [It is expressed in Poiseuille's equation as follows: 8 n $l/\pi r^4$, where n = viscosity of blood, l = length of the vessel, and r = radius of the arteriole. The peripheral arterioles are the resistance vessels. The amount of blood remaining in the arterial tree during diastole represents the diastolic blood pressure.]
sites for auscultation of the MV, AV, TV, and PV	*apex of the heart for the MV, second right ICS for the AV, left parasternal border for the TV,* and the *second left ICS for the PV*
heart sound corresponding with the carotid pulse	*S1 heart sound*
cause of S1	*closure of the MV and TV in systole* (valves make noise when they close) [It is accentuated with a short PR interval or early mitral stenosis.]
cause of S2	*closure of the AV and PV during diastole* [Normally, there is a split during inspiration and a single sound during expiration as blood is drawn into the right heart, with inspiration causing the PV to close later than the AV.]
cause of a paradoxical S2 [where P2 comes before A2 and the split occurs during expiration rather than inspiration]	*LBBB* [This causes delayed activation of the left side of the heart, so the AV closes later than the PV. Early closure of P2 can also produce the same finding.]
cause of fixed splitting of S2 [A2 and P2 remain split on expiration and inspiration.]	*left to right shunting of blood* (e.g., ASD) [A constant increase in volume of blood moving into the right heart causes the PV to remain open for much longer periods of time.]
cause of an accentuated A2	*essential hypertension*
cause of an accentuated P2	*pulmonary hypertension*

Table 10–1. HISTORY AND PHYSICAL EXAM *Continued*

Most Common...	Answer and Explanation
cause of an S3	*it corresponds with blood rushing into a volume-overloaded ventricle, causing vibration of the valves and ventricular wall* (e.g., early LHF) [It is normal in patients <40 years old and abnormal in those >40 years old.]
cause of an S4	*increased resistance to blood flow into the ventricle in late diastole* (e.g., LVH)
cause of a systolic ejection click	*MVP as the MV balloons into the left atrium* [The click is closer to S1 with anxiety or standing up, owing to decreased venous return to heart. It is closer to S2 with lying down or clenching the fists, owing to increased return of blood to the heart.]
cause of an OS	*mitral stenosis*, as the nonpliable valve finally opens in diastole with increased left atrial pressure [The closer the OS is to S2, the worse the stenosis.]
cause of a pathologic murmur	*structural disease* (e.g., aortic stenosis)
cause of a physiologic murmur	*anemia*, due to decreased viscosity of blood and increased rapidity of blood flow through the PV
cause of an innocent murmur	*turbulent pulmonary artery blood flow during systole, heard most often in children* [It is a low-grade (1–2) murmur, which is best heard with the patient supine and disappears with sitting or standing up.]
grade of murmur heard without a stethoscope	*grade 6 on a scale of 1–6*
heart sound that is absent with atrial fibrillation	*S4*, since it is due to atrial contraction

Table continued on following page

Table 10–1. HISTORY AND PHYSICAL EXAM *Continued*

Most Common...	Answer and Explanation
murmurs heard during systole	*aortic/pulmonic stenosis and mitral/tricuspid regurgitation* [Stenosis murmurs are due to problems with opening the valve, hence aortic and pulmonic valve stenoses are best heard in systole and have an ejection type of pattern (crescendo/decrescendo). Regurgitation murmurs are due to problems with closing the valves, hence mitral and tricuspid regurgitation murmurs occur during systole when they close. They are characteristically pansystolic.]
murmurs heard in diastole	*aortic/pulmonic regurgitation and mitral/tricuspid stenosis* [The AV and PV close in diastole, hence they are high-pitched blowing murmurs heard right after S2. MV and TV open in diastole, hence they have an OS followed by a mid-diastolic rumble of blood as it rushes into the ventricles.]
effects of a Valsalva maneuver	*jugular neck vein distention and decrease in cardiac output,* since less blood enters the right side of the heart.
cause of a parasternal heave	*RVH* [The right ventricle is behind the sternum, so enlargement produces a left parasternal heave. This commonly occurs with pulmonary hypertension.]
cause of a laterally displaced PMI	*LVH* [In addition, there is a sustained PMI during systole.]
cause of LVH	*essential hypertension,* owing to the ventricle contracting against an increased afterload (increased TPR)
cause of a pericardial knock	*constrictive pericarditis* [Owing to the small amount of room for expansion of the heart chamber. When the chambers fill with blood they bump into the thickened parietal pericardium, producing a knock. This is not heard with a pericardial effusion, since the chambers are unable to fill properly.]
cause of a pericardial friction rub	*fibrinous pericarditis* secondary to an AMI, uremia, rheumatic fever [It is a scratchy sound with three components.]

Table 10–1. HISTORY AND PHYSICAL EXAM *Continued*

Most Common...	Answer and Explanation
valvular cause of a narrow pulse pressure	*aortic stenosis* [The pulse pressure is the difference between the systolic and the diastolic pressure. Owing to a decreased SV in aortic stenosis, the systolic pressure is decreased, therefore decreasing the pulse pressure.]
valvular cause of an increased pulse pressure	*aortic regurgitation* [As blood leaks back into the LV through the incompetent valve during diastole, there is volume overload of the LV with a subsequent increase in the SV (Frank-Starling forces). Loss of blood in the arterial tree during diastole lowers the TPR, hence the diastolic pressure is also lowered. An increase in SV and decrease in TPR increases the pulse pressure.]
cause of an increase in systolic blood pressure in the elderly	*loss of elasticity of the aorta*
cause of a bounding ("water hammer") pulse	*increase in pulse pressure* (e.g., aortic regurgitation, severe anemia, hyperthyroidism)
valvular cause of a weak pulse	*aortic stenosis*
cause of a bisferiens pulse [pulse with a double systolic peak]	*idiopathic hypertrophic subaortic stenosis*
cause of pulsus paradoxus [drop in blood pressure >10 mm Hg during inspiration]	*restricted filling of the right heart* (e.g., pericardial effusion, decreased lung compliance in severe bronchial asthma), *with concomitant reduction in the stroke volume from the LV*
cause of Kussmaul's sign	*restricted filling of the right heart* (e.g., pericardial effusion, decreased lung compliance in severe bronchial asthma, tricuspid stenosis) [Normally, the jugular veins collapse on inspiration as the negative intrathoracic pressure draws blood into the right heart. With restricted right heart filling, the blood regurgitates back into the neck veins on inspiration.]

Table continued on following page

Table 10–1. HISTORY AND PHYSICAL EXAM *Continued*

Most Common...	Answer and Explanation
JVP corresponding with S1	*c wave*, which corresponds with RV contraction and bulging of the closed TV into the RA
JVP corresponding to RA contraction	*a wave*, which is the late diastolic contraction of the RA [It is a positive wave that precedes the c wave.]
JVP that disappears with atrial fibrillation	*a wave*, since it corresponds with RA contraction
cause of the x wave	*negative wave corresponding to the downward drag on the closed TV as blood is emptied into the PA*
cause of the v wave	*positive wave due to filling of the RA during systole while the TV is closed*
cause of the y wave	*negative wave corresponding with diastole and the opening of the TV with blood emptying into the RV*
cause of a cannon a wave	**TV stenosis,** *RVH, PS* as the RA contracts against increased resistance
cause of a giant c-v wave	*TV regurgitation with regurgitation of the blood up into the RA during systole*

Question: A 54-year-old man has a prominent A2, an S4 heart sound, no murmurs, and lateral displacement of the PMI with increased amplitude during systole. You expect the patient has which of the following?
(A) Mitral stenosis
(B) Essential hypertension
(C) Aortic stenosis
(D) Mitral valve prolapse
(E) Coarctation of the aorta

Answer: (B): In essential hypertension, LVH results in an S4 heart sound, lateral displacement of the PMI, and increased amplitude. A2 is accentuated owing to increased tension on the valve during diastole with accentuation of A2. All of the other choices is associated with accentuation of A2. All of the other choices have characteristic heart murmurs as well.

A2 = second aortic sound, AMI = acute myocardial infarction, ASD = atrial septal defect, AV = aortic valve, ICS = intercostal space, JVP = jugular venous pulse, LBBB = left bundle branch block, LV = left ventricle, LVH = left ventricular hypertrophy, MV = mitral valve, MVP = mitral valve prolapse, OS = opening snap, P2 = second pulmonic sound, PA = pulmonary artery, PMI = point of maximal impulse,

PS = pulmonary stenosis, PV = pulmonic valve, RA = right atrium, RV = right ventricle, RVH = right ventricular hypertrophy, S1 = first heart sound, S2 = second heart sound, S3 = third heart sound, S4 = fourth heart sound, TV = tricuspid valve.

Table 10–2. LIPID DISORDERS

Most Common...	Answer and Explanation
lipid fraction increased after eating a fatty meal	*chylomicrons,* which contain ~85% TG from the saturated fat in the diet [This is the reason why patients must fast for an accurate lipid profile. CH and HDL are not affected, since chylomicrons have a low percentage of these fractions.]
lipid fraction containing endogenously synthesized TG	*VLDL,* which contains 55% TG and ~18% CH
lipid fraction from which LDL is derived in the peripheral blood	*VLDL* [Capillary lipoprotein lipase, enhanced by insulin, removes TG from the VLDL to form IDL and eventually LDL.]
lipoprotein fraction that serves as a reservoir of apolipoproteins	*HDL* (it is the circulating reservoir for apolipoproteins CII and E) [Other functions: it removes CH from foam cells and delivers it to the liver for its disposal.]
enzyme that converts chylomicrons and VLDL into remnants	*capillary lipoprotein lipase,* which is activated by apo CII and insulin. [It removes FAs and glycerol from these fractions (decreases TG content) and changes chylomicrons into chylomicron remnants and VLDL into IDL and then LDL.]
apoproteins that differentiate chylomicrons from VLDL	*apo B48 is attached to chylomicrons in the intestinal cell and apo B100 to VLDL in the hepatocyte* [Both fractions also have apo CII and apo E.]

Table continued on following page

Table 10–2. LIPID DISORDERS *Continued*

Most Common...	Answer and Explanation
fate of FAs removed from chylomicrons and VLDL	*FAs enter adipose cells, where they combine with glycerol 3-PO₄ (glycerol kinase) to form TG for storage* [Insulin enhances the uptake of glucose in adipose cells, so that glycerol 3-PO₄, the carbohydrate backbone of TG, is available for TG synthesis. Insulin inhibits hormone-sensitive lipase in the adipose cell to prevent lipolysis, while glucagon and its counter-regulatory hormones activate it to use fatty acids for fuel.]
fate of glycerol removed from chylomicrons and VLDL	*glycerol is only metabolized in the liver and is converted into glycerol 3-PO₄, which can then be used to synthesize VLDL in the fed state or converted into DHAP and used as an intermediate for gluconeogenesis in the fasting state*
functions of CH	*cell membrane lipid, steroid synthesis in the adrenal, sex-hormone synthesis in the ovaries and testes, bile salt/acid synthesis, vitamin D synthesis*
effects of CH when it is internalized by a cell	*prevents further LDL receptor synthesis, inhibits 3-hydroxy-3-methylglutaryl (HMG)-Co reductase to prevent further synthesis of CH, and activates acyl-CoA acyltransferase, which esterifies the CH*
test used to screen for primary prevention of CAD	*CH and HDL* [Primary prevention is for someone who does not have a history of CAD.]
test used to screen for secondary prevention of CAD	*LDL* [Secondary prevention is for someone who has already had CAD or a stroke.]
formula used to calculate LDL	*LDL = CH − HDL − TG/5* [TG/5 equals the VLDL fraction.]
diuretics that adversely alter lipids	*thiazide diuretics and β-blockers, both of which increase TG and decrease HDL*
effect of primary hypothyroidism and the nephrotic syndrome on lipids	*hypercholesterolemia*, the former by decreasing LDL receptor synthesis and the latter by increasing CH synthesis in the liver
effect of DM on lipids	*increase in CH, TG, VLDL, and LDL, and a decrease in HDL*

$LDL = CH - HDL - TG/5$

Table 10–2. LIPID DISORDERS *Continued*

Most Common...	Answer and Explanation
CH value selected as medically significant for CAD	*CH ≥240 mg/dL* [A value <200 mg/dL is considered acceptable.]
LDL value selected as medically significant for CAD	*LDL ≥160 mg/dL* [A value <130 mg/dL is considered acceptable for primary prevention and <100 mg/dL for secondary prevention.]
HDL value selected as medically significant for CAD	*<35 mg/dL* [A value >60 mg/dL is a negative risk factor for CAD, indicating that it has a beneficial effect in preventing CAD.]
factors that increase the HDL concentration	**female sex** (estrogen effect), *exercise, weight loss, mild alcohol intake*
TG value selected as medically significant for CAD	*TG >1000 mg/dL* [A value <200 mg/dL is acceptable. An increase in TG is an independent risk factor for CAD.]
function of lipoprotein (a)	*it enhances atherosclerosis* by combining LDL with an inhibitor of plasminogen, decreasing the production of plasmin, which normally lyses fibrin clots, contributing to plaque formation
"good" and "bad" apolipoproteins	*apo A is good*, since it accompanies HDL, and *apo B is bad*, since apo B100 accompanies LDL
cause of a supranate [floats on the surface] in plasma left in a refrigerator overnight at 4°C	*chylomicrons*, the fraction with the lowest density (amount of protein)
cause of an infranate [settles beneath the surface] in plasma left in a refrigerator overnight at 4°C	*VLDL*, owing to its slightly higher density (more protein) than chylomicrons [CH does not increase plasma turbidity.]
major risk factors for CAD	**age >45 in a man and >55 in a woman** (age is the most important factor), *family history of premature CAD or stroke, hypertension, smoking, DM, HDL <35 mg/dL*, and *LDL ≥160 mg/dL*
hyperlipoprotein-emia	*type IV hyperlipoproteinemia*, due to decreased catabolism of VLDL

Table continued on following page

Table 10–2. LIPID DISORDERS *Continued*

Most Common...	Answer and Explanation
hyperlipoprotein-emia associated with tendon xanthomas (e.g., Achilles' tendon)	*familial hypercholesterolemia*, an AD disease with absent LDL receptors
genetic type of type II hyperlipoproteinemia	*polygenic hypercholesterolemia* (probable multifactorial inheritance)
clinical findings in abetalipoprotein-emia (AD)	*it is associated with absence of apo B lipoproteins, resulting in very low CH levels; clinical findings include hemolytic anemia, malabsorption, and retinitis pigmentosum*

Question: In an adult, the most common cause of turbidity of plasma submitted for a lipid profile and formation of a supranate in the tube after refrigeration at 4°C is which of the following?
(A) A defect in capillary lipoprotein lipase
(B) An LDL receptor defect
(C) A defect in clearing VLDL
(D) Absence of apo B lipoprotein
(E) A non-fasting patient

Answer: (E): Chylomicrons represent diet-derived TG. Type I hyperlipoproteinemia (choice A) is the only choice listed that has a primary increase in chylomicrons (supranate); however, it is rare and seen in children. Hence, not fasting before collection of the sample is the most likely explanation.

AD = autosomal dominant, apo = apolipoprotein, CAD = coronary artery disease, CH = cholesterol, DM = diabetes mellitus, DHAP = dihydroxyacetone phosphate, FA = fatty acid, HDL = high-density lipoprotein, IDL = intermediate-density lipoprotein, LDL = low-density lipoprotein, TG = triglyceride, VLDL = very low density lipoprotein.

Table 10–3. VESSEL DISORDERS

Most Common...	Answer and Explanation
cause of arteriosclerosis [hardening of the arteries]	*atherosclerosis*, which primarily affects elastic and muscular arteries
primary lesions in atherosclerosis	*fatty streak* initially (reversible) and the *fibrous plaque*, representing the advanced lesion that commonly undergoes dystrophic calcification and ulceration, and serves as a

Table 10–3. VESSEL DISORDERS *Continued*

Most Common...	Answer and Explanation
Continued	site for hemorrhage and thrombosis [An Ornish diet (pure vegan, high fiber, low saturated fat diet) can reverse complicated plaques.]
location of fatty streaks and fibrous plaques	*intima*
initiating event in atherosclerosis	*endothelial cell damage* from products in **cigarette smoke** (e.g., carbon monoxide), *increased LDL, turbulence, immunologic injury, increased plasma homocysteine levels*
cause of an increase in plasma homocysteine levels	*folate deficiency* (see Chapter 11 Hematology tables)
cells that become foam cells in a fatty streak	*smooth muscle cells* (SMCs) that have migrated to the intima and endocytosed CH with their LDL receptors and *scavenger macrophages* that have engulfed CH without using receptors
cells involved in forming a fibrous plaque	*endothelial cells* (produce oxidized LDL), *SMCs* (foam cells, produce collagen), *macrophages* (foam cells, release chemotactic factors for SMCs, release growth factors for SMC hyperplasia), *platelets* (release growth factors for SMC hyperplasia), *CD$_8$ T lymphocytes* (release cytokines)
functions of oxidized LDL [LDL free radical]	*more atherogenic than native LDL* [It is chemotactic to monocytes, cytotoxic, a stimulant for growth factor release, and immunogenic.]
antioxidants that neutralize oxidized LDL	*vitamin E, vitamin C, beta-carotenes*
sites for atherosclerosis in descending order	**abdominal aorta,** *coronary artery, popliteal artery, descending thoracic aorta, internal carotid*
complications of atherosclerosis in the abdominal aorta	**aneurysm formation,** *embolization, bowel infarction, renovascular hypertension*

Table continued on following page

Table 10–3. VESSEL DISORDERS *Continued*

Most Common...	Answer and Explanation
complications of atherosclerosis in the peripheral vascular system	*gangrene, claudication*
complications of atherosclerosis in the coronary artery	**angina,** *AMI, sudden cardiac death, chronic ischemic heart disease*
complications of atherosclerosis in the circle of Willis	**cerebral infarction,** *laminar necrosis of neurons leading to cerebral atrophy, aneurysms*
complications of atherosclerosis in the internal carotid artery	**TIA,** *atherosclerotic stroke, embolic stroke*
complication of atherosclerosis in the renal artery	*renovascular hypertension,* the most common cause of secondary hypertension
complications of atherosclerosis in the superior mesenteric artery	**thrombosis,** *embolization* leading to small bowel infarction and ischemic colitis
types of arteriolosclerosis	**hyaline** and *hyperplastic arteriolosclerosis* [Hyaline arteriolosclerosis is the small vessel disease of DM and hypertension. Hyperplastic arteriolosclerosis is noted in malignant hypertension.]
complication associated with Mönckeberg's medial calcification of muscular arteries	*none,* since it is a benign, degenerative disease of old age that does not produce occlusive disease
aneurysm [weakening with outpouching of the vessel]	*abdominal aortic aneurysm* [It is most common in men >55 years of age. Popliteal artery aneurysms are also present in ~50% of cases.]
complication of an abdominal aortic aneurysm	*rupture,* which is most dependent on the size of the aneurysm

Table 10–3. VESSEL DISORDERS *Continued*

Most Common...	Answer and Explanation
test used to identify an abdominal aortic aneurysm	*ultrasonography,* which is the gold standard test
clinical triad associated with rupture of an abdominal aortic aneurysm	*sudden onset of left flank pain, hypotension, pulsatile mass in the abdomen*
cause and complication of a popliteal artery aneurysm	*atherosclerosis* and *embolization,* respectively [They also commonly thrombose, leading to gangrene and the need for amputation. Angiography is the diagnostic test of choice.]
cause, site, and complication of a berry aneurysm	*congenital absence of the internal elastic membrane and muscle wall at the bifurcation of the anterior communicating artery with the anterior cerebral artery* [They have the potential for rupture, leading to a subarachnoid hemorrhage.]
cause, site, and complication of a mycotic aneurysm	*septic embolization* (fungal or bacterial) *to the aorta* with the potential for *thrombosis* and *rupture*
fungi associated with invasive vasculitis	*Mucor, Aspergillus, Candida* (mnemonic: MAC)
bacteria associated with invasive vasculitis	*Pseudomonas aeruginosa* and *Bacteroides fragilis*
cause of an aneurysm of the arch of the aorta	*dissecting aortic aneurysm* [In the past, tertiary syphilis was the most common cause.]
manifestation of tertiary syphilis	*aortic arch aneurysm* owing to vasculitis of the vasa vasorum (endarteritis obliterans with a very characteristic plasma cell infiltrate) and weakening of the vessel wall.
cause of a dissecting aortic aneurysm	**elastic tissue fragmentation** and *cystic medial necrosis* in the middle and outer layer of the aorta

Table continued on following page

Table 10–3. VESSEL DISORDERS *Continued*

Most Common...	Answer and Explanation
predisposing event leading to a dissection of the aorta	*hypertension,* which supplies a shearing force on the structurally weak aorta, leading to an intimal tear [Other associations include Marfan's syndrome (most common COD), Ehlers-Danlos syndrome (most common COD), copper deficiency, pregnancy.]
type of dissecting aortic aneurysm	**type A, which involves the ascending aorta** [*Type B aneurysms* begin below the ligamentum arteriosum.]
COD in a dissecting aortic aneurysm	*rupture into the pericardial sac* [Other rupture sites are the mediastinum, peritoneum, or re-entry into the aorta, creating a double-barreled aorta.]
presentation and initial step in diagnosis of a dissecting aortic aneurysm	*acute onset of severe chest pain in association with hypertension* (hypertension is uncommon in an AMI). A *chest radiograph will show widening of the aortic knob.* [Arteriography is the gold standard confirmatory test, although transesophageal ultrasonography is replacing it in some institutions. Aortic regurgitation and heart failure may also occur.]
initial management step in treating a dissecting aortic aneurysm	*lower the blood pressure with nitroprusside to prevent further dissection*
cause and site for transection of the aorta	*car accident with transection of the aorta distal to the ligamentum arteriosum* [It may also be the site of a false aneurysm, owing to blood clot collecting around the transected vessel.]
cause of an AV fistula [abnormal communication between an artery and vein]	**surgical creation of an AV fistula for renal dialysis** [*Trauma secondary to a knife wound* is the most common pathologic cause. Another cause is Paget's disease of bone.]
cardiovascular complication of an AV fistula	*high output cardiac failure,* owing to bypassing of the microcirculation with increased venous return to the heart

Table 10–3. VESSEL DISORDERS *Continued*

Most Common...	Answer and Explanation
cardiovascular effect of compressing the proximal artery leading into an AV fistula	*sinus bradycardia* [This is called Branham's sign.]
causes of the thoracic outlet syndrome [abnormal compression of the arteries, veins, or nerves in the neck]	*cervical rib, spastic scalenus anticus muscle, positional changes in the neck and arms*
S/S of the thoracic outlet syndrome	*pain, paresthesias, or numbness in the distribution of the ulnar nerve*
screening test to document thoracic outlet syndrome	*demonstrating weakening of the radial pulse with abduction of the arm and the head turned to the side of the lesion (Adson's test)* [A bruit is frequently heard over the subclavian artery. Percussion over the brachial plexus may reproduce the symptoms (Tinel's test). Arteriography confirms the lesion.]
cause of the subclavian steal syndrome	*proximal obstruction of the first portion of the subclavian artery leading to reversal of blood flow in the vertebral artery and cerebral ischemia to supply blood in the arm*
sign of small vessel vasculitis [sometimes designated leukocytoclastic vasculitis]	*palpable purpura* owing to immunocomplex deposition (type III hypersensitivity) in the wall of post-capillary venules with activation of complement (C5a in particular) leading to chemotaxis of neutrophils to the area with destruction of the vessel
clinical presentation for vasculitis involving muscular arteries	*vessel thrombosis with infarction*
clinical presentation for vasculitis involving the elastic arteries	*lack of a pulse* (Takayasu's giant cell arteritis involving the subclavian artery), *stroke, blindness*
vasculitis in adults	*temporal arteritis,* which is a granulomatous vasculitis involving the temporal artery and extracranial vessels

Table continued on following page

Table 10–3. VESSEL DISORDERS *Continued*

Most Common...	Answer and Explanation
presentation of temporal arteritis	**headache along the course of the temporal artery,** *jaw claudication, polymyalgia rheumatica* (pain and morning stiffness), *blindness*
lab test used to screen for temporal arteritis	*ESR,* since inflammation should increase the ESR [A positive clinical history and increased ESR is sufficient to start the patient on corticosteroids (prevent permanent blindness). A temporal artery biopsy is performed to confirm the diagnosis.]
vasculitis in children	*Henoch-Schönlein purpura (HSP),* which is a small vessel vasculitis involving post-capillary venules
S/S for HSP	**palpable purpura limited to the buttocks and lower extremity,** *abdominal pain* (sometimes with GI bleed), *hematuria with RBC casts* (glomerulonephritis), *polyarthritis*
vasculitis associated with HBV	*polyarteritis nodosa* (PAN) [It is a male dominant IC vasculitis involving muscular arteries (lesions are in different stages of development, acute or chronic). ~30–40% of patients have HBV surface antigenemia. "Nodosa" refers to the focal aneurysm formation (may be palpable) of the vessel owing to destruction and weakening of the vessel wall.]
S/S of PAN	**fever with multisystem disease involving the kidneys** (most common site; vasculitis and GN; hematuria, RBC casts), *coronary vessels* (thrombosis, aneurysm formation), *liver, GI tract* (bowel infarction), *skin* (painful nodules with ulceration) [The lungs are not usually involved.]
lab findings in PAN	**p-ANCA** (p refers to perinuclear staining), *neutrophilic leukocytosis, eosinophilia, HBV surface antigenemia*
vasculitis associated with HCV	*cryoglobulinemic vasculitis,* which is a necrotizing vasculitis involving IC deposition of cryoglobulins (cold-precipitating IgM antibodies) and complement in vessels within the skin (Raynaud's phenomenon) and glomeruli (GN, vasculitis)

Table 10–3. VESSEL DISORDERS *Continued*

Most Common...	Answer and Explanation
S/S of Churg-Strauss vasculitis	*associated with granulomatous vasculitis in the respiratory tract vessels, allergic rhinitis, bronchial asthma, and peripheral eosinophilia*
vasculitis associated with male smokers	*thromboangiitis obliterans* (Buerger's disease) [It involves the arteries, veins, and nerves of the digital vessels in the upper and lower extremities. Vessels thrombose, leading to gangrene that often requires amputation. Unlike Raynaud's phenomenon, the pulse is absent owing to vessel thrombosis, not vasospasm. Early cessation of smoking prevents the disease.]
cause of an AMI in children	*Kawasaki's disease* [It produces a coronary artery vasculitis with thrombosis. Mucosal inflammation, a desquamating rash, lymphadenopathy, and swelling of the hands and feet are also observed. The cause is unknown.]
vasculitis producing an absent pulse	*Takayasu's arteritis* [It involves the aortic arch vessels and is most commonly seen in Asian women <50 years old. Upper extremity claudication, unequal blood pressures between the upper and lower extremity (opposite of a coarctation), blindness, and strokes may also occur.]
vasculitis producing a saddle nose deformity	*Wegener's granulomatosis* (WG) [It is a necrotizing granulomatous vasculitis involving upper and lower respiratory tract (sinuses, nose, nasopharynx, lungs [nodular densities]), and kidneys (GN). Inflammation in the nose destroys the cartilage, resulting in a saddle nose deformity.]
lab findings in WG	**c-ANCA,** *neutrophilic leukocytosis, eosinophilia*
treatment for WG	*cyclophosphamide,* [It produces dramatic results. Complications include hemorrhagic cystitis and transitional cell carcinoma of the bladder.]

Table continued on following page

Table 10–3. VESSEL DISORDERS *Continued*

Most Common...	Answer and Explanation
vasculitis progressing to a malignant lymphoma	*lymphomatoid granulomatosis* [It is similar to WG except for the absence of upper respiratory disease and its predilection for progressing to a malignant lymphoma.]
initial manifestation of PSS and CREST syndrome	*Raynaud's phenomenon* [It is a vasospastic disease involving the digital vessels that produces color changes (white to blue to red). In PSS and CREST syndrome (calcinosis, Raynaud's, esophageal motility dysfunction, sclerodactyly, telangiectasia), the digital vessels eventually become fibrosed. Other causes of Raynaud's include Takayasu's arteritis, cold agglutinin disease, cryoglobulinemia, ergot poisoning, and Buerger's disease.]
IC vasculitis findings in infective endocarditis	bacterial antigens combine with antibodies and activate the complement system to produce a small vessel vasculitis, which includes *Roth's spot* (retinal vasculitis with a red lesion and a white center), *Janeway's lesions* (painless hemorrhages on the hands), and *Osler's nodes* (painful areas of hemorrhage on the hands or feet); *glomerulonephritis* may also occur
organism producing a small vessel vasculitis and meningitis	*Neisseria meningitidis*
organism producing a small vessel vasculitis and septic arthritis	*Neisseria gonorrhoeae* when it disseminates via the blood stream [The vasculitis localizes to the hands, wrists, and feet. The septic arthritis is usually in the knee.]
organism transmitted by a tick that produces a vasculitis	*Rickettsia rickettsiae*, which produces Rocky Mountain spotted fever [The "spots" are where small vessels have ruptured in the skin owing to invasion of endothelial cells by the organism. The spots progress from the hands to the trunk.]
organism that produces a vasculitis leading to a painless ulcer	*Treponema pallidum*, the cause of syphilis [The pathogenesis of all the lesions in primary (painless ulcer), secondary (skin lesions), and tertiary syphilis (tabes dorsalis leading to a neuropathic joint) is a vasculitis caused by invasion of the vessels by the organism (endarteritis obliterans).]

Table 10–3. VESSEL DISORDERS *Continued*

Most Common...	Answer and Explanation
organism producing a vasculitis leading to a serum sickness–like disease and hepatitis	**HBV** and *HCV*
location for a port wine stain (PWS; nevus flammeus) at birth	*face* [A PWS is a vascular malformation that is flat and grows proportionately with the patient without regressing, unlike a capillary hemangioma, which is raised and does undergo regression with time.]
PWS distributed in the ophthalmic division of the trigeminal nerve	*Sturge-Weber syndrome* (SWS) [It is also associated with mental retardation and a vascular defect in the leptomeninges on the ipsilateral side that can bleed or be the focus for epileptic seizures.]
AD hereditary vascular disease	*hereditary hemorrhagic telangiectasia, or Osler-Weber-Rendu disease* [It is associated with small aneurysmal telangiectasias on the skin and mucous membranes (which produce nosebleeds and GI bleeds).]
location for a pyogenic granuloma in pregnancy	*gingiva* [These are pedunculated benign masses that grow rapidly, ulcerate, and bleed owing to the presence of inflammatory granulation tissue.]
cause of spider angiomas on the skin	*hyperestrinism secondary to* **pregnancy** *or cirrhosis of the liver* (liver cannot metabolize estrogen) [They are AV fistulas.]
treatment of capillary hemangiomas on the face in newborns	*no treatment,* since they regress with time
S/S of von Hippel-Lindau disease (AD disease)	*associated with cavernous hemangiomas in the cerebellum, skin, and eyes and an increased risk for renal adenocarcinoma*
cause of Kaposi's sarcoma (KS) in AIDS	*herpesvirus 8* [KS is the most common cancer in AIDS and is a malignancy of endothelial cells.]
genetic disease associated with lymphangiomas (cystic hygromas)	*Turner's syndrome* (45 XO) [Lymphangiomas are most commonly located in the neck and produce the classic webbed neck noted in these patients.]

Table continued on following page

Table 10–3. VESSEL DISORDERS *Continued*

Most Common...	Answer and Explanation
location for angiosarcomas	*liver in association with exposure to vinyl chloride, arsenic, or Thorotrast* (mnemonic: VAT)
cause of lymphangiosarcoma in the United States	*chronic lymphedema secondary to radiation after modified radical mastectomy* [The arm is edematous (nonpitting edema).]
cause of phlebothrombosis [thrombosis of a vein without inflammation]	*stasis of blood flow*, most commonly in the patients who are post partum or post operative (particularly hip and pelvic surgery)
initial site for development of a venous thrombus	*valve cusps* [Initially, it is a platelet thrombus, but as it propagates, it is made up of a mixture of RBCs and fibrin from activation of the coagulation system (red clot).]
location for phlebothrombosis	**deep saphenous veins of the calf** followed by the *femoral, popliteal,* and *iliac veins*
serious complication of a DVT in the lower extremity	*pulmonary embolism with the potential for infarction* [Most emboli arise from thrombi that have propagated up into the popliteal, **femoral,** and iliac veins from thrombosis that began in the deep saphenous vein of the calf.]
test used to document a DVT	*duplex ultrasonography* (a modification of Doppler ultrasonography) [Invasive venography is the gold standard test.]
initial anticoagulant used in treating a DVT	*low-dose heparin,* which immediately anticoagulates the patient along with warfarin, which requires 3–5 days before the patient is fully anticoagulated.
cause of thrombophlebitis [inflammation of the superficial veins of the legs]	*varicose veins* [It is identified by the presence of pain, heat, and tenderness along the course of a superficial vein. Other causes include inflammation due to IV catheters, IV drug abuse, or trauma.]
cancer associated with migratory superficial thrombophlebitis	*pancreatic carcinoma* [It is called Trousseau's sign and is a paraneoplastic syndrome that underscores the thrombogenic state associated with cancer.]
cause of primary varicose veins in the legs	*congenital absence of venous valves* (particularly the sentinel valve in the common femoral vein) [Pregnancy is a common precipitating event.]

Table 10–3. VESSEL DISORDERS *Continued*

Most Common...	Answer and Explanation
causes of secondary varicose veins	*vessel damage* (e.g., thrombophlebitis), *vessel obstruction* (e.g., DVT)
cause of stasis dermatitis [post-phlebitic syndrome] around the ankles	*DVT* [Venous blood in the legs flows from the superficial system through penetrating branches to the deep venous system and back to the heart. Around the ankles, blood flows back into the superficial system, hence a proximal DVT leads to increased pressures around the vessels in the ankles, resulting in edema (first sign), hemorrhage (hemosiderin deposition), and ulceration.]
cause of the superior vena caval syndrome	*obstruction of the superior vena cava from invasion by a primary small cell carcinoma of the lung* [The patient's face, neck, and shoulders are congested and jugular veins distended.]
organism producing acute lymphangitis	***group A Streptococcus*** and *Staphylococcus aureus* to a lesser extent
parasitic disease associated with lymphedema	filariasis due to *Wuchereria bancrofti*
pathologic cause of a chylous effusion in the pleural cavity	*malignant lymphoma* [True chylous effusions have mature lymphocytes and chylomicrons containing TG. A surgical mishap is also a common cause.]
cause of a pseudochylous effusion in the pleural cavity	*rheumatoid arthritis involving the lungs* [A pseudochylous effusion is milky, but, unlike a true chylous effusion, it is not lymphatic fluid but an inflammatory exudate containing neutrophils and CH.]

Question: Which of the following vascular diseases is most likely secondary to IC deposition in the vessel wall?
(A) Abdominal aortic aneurysm
(B) Berry aneurysm
(C) Buerger's disease
(D) Polyarteritis nodosa
(E) Hyaline arteriolosclerosis

Answer: (D): PAN is an IC disease involving muscular arteries. Choice (A) is most commonly due to atherosclerosis, (B) a congenital defect, (C) a cell-mediated immune reaction, and (E) nonenzymatic glycosylation in DM or insudation of proteins into the vessel wall in essential hypertension.

AD = autosomal dominant, AIDS = acquired immunodeficiency syndrome, AMI = acute myocardial infarction, ANCA = antineutrophil cytoplasmic antibody, AV = arteriovenous, CH = cholesterol, DM = diabetes mellitus, DVT = deep venous thrombosis, ESR = erythrocyte sedimentation rate, GI = gastrointestinal, GN = glomerulonephritis, HBV = hepatitis B virus, HCV = hepatitis C virus, IC = immunocomplex, IV = intravenous, LDL = low-density lipoprotein, PSS = progressive systemic sclerosis, RBC = red blood cell, S/S = signs and symptoms, TG = triglyceride, TIA = transient ischemic attack.

Table 10–4. HYPERTENSION, HYPERTROPHY, HEART FAILURE

Most Common...	Answer and Explanation
condition for which patients receive a prescription in the United States	*essential hypertension*
cause of hypertension	*essential hypertension* (~95%) [The blood pressure must be ≥140/90 mm Hg on at least three separate readings on three separate occasions.]
condition for which a reduction in mortality will be seen due to control of hypertension	**stroke** followed by *CAD*
factors predisposing to hypertension	**sodium intake, genetic predisposition,** *obesity* (increased intravascular volume), *sedentary life-style, race* (black > white) [An increase in intracellular Na^+ concentration in the SMCs of the peripheral resistance vessels with opening up of calcium channels with a subsequent increase in vessel tone and resistance is one of the most popular theories.]
alteration in plasma renin activity (PRA) in elderly hypertensives and blacks with hypertension	*decreased PRA,* indicating an excess in intravascular volume with suppression of renin release
alteration in PRA in young hypertensives	*increased PRA,* indicating sympathetic over-activity

Table 10–4. HYPERTENSION, HYPERTROPHY, HEART FAILURE *Continued*

Most Common...	Answer and Explanation
alteration in PRA in most hypertensives	*normal PRA*
target organ adversely affected by hypertension	**heart** (LVH, ischemic heart disease) [Other target organs include the *kidneys* (nephrosclerosis) and the *CNS* (hypertensive intracerebral bleeds, infarctions).]
small vessel disease associated with hypertension	*hyaline arteriolosclerosis* due to insudation of plasma proteins into the vessel wall from increased intravascular pressure
drug of abuse producing hypertension	*cocaine,* which stimulates the sympathetic nervous system
effect of alcohol and cigarette smoking on BP	*hypertension* due to stimulation of catecholamine release
S/S of hypertension	**pulsating suboccipital headache occurring early in the morning and subsiding before noon,** *dizziness, blurry vision, sweating, chest pain, dyspnea* [Most patients are asymptomatic.]
cardiovascular findings in hypertension	*accentuated S4, LVH* (concentric hypertrophy; increased amplitude of the PMI, laterally displaced PMI), *early systolic ejection click*
cause of a falsely elevated BP in elderly patients	*atherosclerotic involvement of the brachial artery leading to noncompressibility by the sphygmomanometer cuff*
COD in hypertension	**AMI** followed by *stroke* and *renal failure*
cause of systolic hypertension [systolic pressure >160 mm Hg and a normal diastolic pressure]	*decreased compliance of the aorta secondary to atherosclerosis*
effect on BP if the cuff is too short or too narrow	*false elevation of the BP*

Table continued on following page

Table 10–4. HYPERTENSION, HYPERTROPHY, HEART FAILURE *Continued*

Most Common...	Answer and Explanation
initial tests in the work-up of hypertension	*CBC* (R/O polycythemia or anemia), *serum electrolytes* (R/O primary aldosteronism), *fasting blood glucose* (R/O DM and pheochromocytoma), *urinalysis* (R/O primary renal disease; e.g., proteinuria), *serum BUN and creatinine* (R/O renal disease), *serum uric acid* (R/O urate nephropathy), *serum CH and HDL* (primary prevention screen for CAD), *ECG* (R/O LVH, ischemia), *chest radiograph* (evaluate the heart and lungs)
life-style modification that has the greatest effect on lowering BP	**weight reduction** (diet high in fiber and low in saturated fats, plus exercise) [Other life-style modifications include *reducing alcohol intake, cessation of smoking, reducing salt intake*, and *increasing the intake of potassium, calcium*, and *magnesium*.]
antihypertensive agents used in treating blacks	**diuretics** and *calcium channel blockers*
antihypertensive agents used in treating elderly patients	*diuretics*
antihypertensive agents that may precipitate bronchial asthma	β-*blockers*
antihypertensive agents associated with cough and angioedema	*ACE inhibitors*
cause of secondary hypertension	*renovascular hypertension due to atherosclerotic occlusion of the proximal renal artery in elderly men* (increased renin hypertension) [Fibromuscular hyperplasia is the most common cause in women.]
S/S of renovascular hypertension	**abrupt onset of severe, uncontrolled hypertension that is resistant to standard medical therapy,** *presence of an abdominal bruit, renal failure associated with use of an ACE inhibitor*

Table 10–4. HYPERTENSION, HYPERTROPHY, HEART FAILURE *Continued*

Most Common...	Answer and Explanation
screening test for renovascular hypertension	**captopril (ACE inhibitor) plus a radionuclide scan of the kidneys, which reveals a small kidney with delayed emptying** [A *captopril stimulation test* shows a marked increase in PRA activity over baseline owing to block of the inhibitory effect of AT II on renin release.]
confirmatory test for renovascular hypertension	*renal arteriography and evaluation of PRA from the affected and unaffected renal vein* [The latter should show an increase in PRA activity on the affected side and suppression of PRA on the unaffected side due to suppression of renin release by AT II.]
lab findings and S/S suggesting primary aldosteronism	*severe muscle weakness* (hypokalemia) associated with *diastolic hypertension, normal to high serum Na⁺, hypokalemia,* and *metabolic alkalosis*
S/S of a pheochromocytoma	*sustained hypertension in a patient with excessive sweating, anxiety,* and *headaches*
screening tests for a pheochromocytoma	**24-hour urine for metanephrine** (most sensitive test) and *vanillylmandelic acid* (VMA)
retinal changes in hypertension	*narrowing of arterioles, AV nicking* (thickened arteriole compresses the underlying vein), *thickening of the arterioles* (copper [early] and silver [later] wiring), *hemorrhage, aneurysms, soft exudates* (infarction), *hard exudates* (increased vessel permeability), *papilledema* (increased intracranial pressure)
cause of LVH	*essential hypertension*
types of LVH	**concentric** (secondary to an increase in afterload; e.g., aortic stenosis, increased peripheral resistance) and *dilatation with hypertrophy* (hypertrophy secondary to volume overload [increase in preload], e.g., aortic and mitral regurgitation, left-to-right shunts with increased return of blood to the left heart)
cause of physiologic hypertrophy of the heart	*athletic conditioning* [Hypertrophy increases the force of contraction, thereby increasing the SV and the ejection fraction (SV/ LVEDV).]

Table continued on following page

Table 10–4. HYPERTENSION, HYPERTROPHY, HEART FAILURE *Continued*

Most Common...	Answer and Explanation
cause of RVH	**pulmonary hypertension** (concentric) [Other causes include *left-to-right shunt with volume overloading* (dilated; e.g., VSD), pulmonic stenosis (concentric).]
cause of cor pulmonale [PH + RVH from primary lung disease or primary pulmonary vascular disease]	**COPD from smoking** [Other causes include *cystic fibrosis, restrictive lung diseases* (e.g., sarcoidosis), *primary PH, chronic hypoxemia of noncardiac origin* (e.g., high-altitude resident).]
cause of LHF	**AMI** [Other causes include *ischemic heart disease, cardiomyopathies, myocarditis, valvular disease, essential hypertension.*]
cause of RHF	**LHF** [Blood builds up behind the failed left heart causing an increase in afterload that the right heart must contract against. Other causes include *right-sided valvular disease, cor pulmonale, cardiomyopathies, myocarditis, pulmonary embolus.*]
cause of acute RHF	*large pulmonary embolus* producing right heart strain and failure
heart sound associated with left and right heart failure	*S3* [This is due to volume overload in the failed ventricle and blood rushing into the overfilled chamber.]
murmur associated with left and right heart failure	*mitral and tricuspid regurgitation,* respectively [Volume overload of the failed ventricle dilates the valve ring, producing regurgitation murmurs.]
symptom of LHF	*dyspnea* [It is secondary to stimulation of the juxtacapillary J receptors in the interstitium, which are innervated by the vagus nerve. Stimulation of the nerve fibers by fluid in the interstitium results in termination of the inspiratory effort before inspiration is fully completed.]
cause of pillow orthopnea and PND	*LHF* [These symptoms occur at night and are due to increased venous return to the heart while the patient is supine. The left heart is unable to handle the extra load and blood refluxes back into the lungs, producing dysp-

Table 10–4. HYPERTENSION, HYPERTROPHY,
HEART FAILURE *Continued*

Most Common...	Answer and Explanation
Continued	nea that may cause the patient to wake up gasping for breath (PND). Placing pillows under the head improves ventilation by reducing venous return to the right heart (pillow orthopnea).]
lab finding in LHF	*prerenal azotemia* [Owing to a decrease in cardiac output and GFR, there is a disproportionate increase in the proximal tubule reabsorption of urea. Since creatinine is not reabsorbed in the kidneys, it is only slightly increased from the reduction in GFR. The BUN to creatinine ratio (normally 10:1) is 15:1 or higher (e.g., 60 mg/dL BUN to 2 mg/dL creatinine). The most common cause of prerenal azotemia is LHF.]
chest radiograph finding in LHF	**prominent congestion of blood in the upper lobes** (first sign) [Other changes include *perihilar congestion* ("bat-wing" configuration), *Kerley B lines* (septal edema at the costophrenic angle), and *patchy interstitial and alveolar infiltrates representing pulmonary edema.*]
sign in RHF	**jugular neck vein distention** [Other signs include *S3 heart sound, TV regurgitation from dilatation of the TV ring* (this produces a giant c-v wave and pulsation of the liver during systole), *hepatojugular reflux* due to *hepatic congestion* (hepatomegaly; nutmeg liver), *dependent pitting edema, ascites, cyanosis* (increased amount of time for tissue to extract oxygen).]
lab findings in RHF	*hyponatremia* due to a hypotonic gain of fluid from the kidneys (see Chapter 5) and *prerenal azotemia* from a decrease in cardiac output.
nonpharmacologic treatment for LHF and RHF	**restrict salt and water intake,** *rotating tourniquets to reduce preload*
pharmacologic treatment of heart failure	*diuretics* (reduce preload), *ACE inhibitors* (reduce afterload by blocking synthesis of AT II and reduce preload by blocking release of aldosterone), *digitalis glycosides* (if diuretics

Table continued on following page

**Table 10–4. HYPERTENSION, HYPERTROPHY,
HEART FAILURE** *Continued*

Most Common...	Answer and Explanation
Continued	and ACE inhibitors do not work; positive inotropic agent), *oxygen,* β-*blockers* (chronic CHF)
cause of systolic dysfunction [problem in LV contractility]	**AMI** [Others include *congestive cardiomyopathy* and *chronic ischemic heart disease.*]
cause of diastolic dysfunction [decreased LV compliance; it does not fill properly]	**severe LVH** [Others include *hypertrophic cardiomyopathy* and *restrictive cardiomyopathy* (e.g., amyloid heart).]
cause of high output failure [normal to increased cardiac output] secondary to increased contractility	*hyperthyroidism* [An increase in contractility increases the SV, which increases the systolic BP.]
cause of high output failure due to decreased blood viscosity	*severe anemia* [An increase in viscosity decreases the TPR and increases venous return to the heart, thereby increasing cardiac output.]
causes of high output failure due to vasodilatation of peripheral resistance vessels	**endotoxic shock** (release of anaphylatoxins C3a and C5a, release of nitric oxide from damaged endothelial cells) [Others include *thiamine deficiency, AV fistula,* and *Paget's disease of bone* (increased vascularity in the soft bone matrix).]

Question: Which of the following differentiates LHF from RHF?
(A) Orthopnea
(B) Neck vein distention
(C) Congestive hepatomegaly
(D) Dependent pitting edema
(E) Decreased cardiac output

Answer: (A): Orthopnea is a sign of LHF and occurs at night when the patient sleeps and venous return to the heart increases. The failed left heart is unable to handle the increased load and blood backs up into the lungs, producing dyspnea that is relieved by putting pillows under the head, sitting, or standing up. Choices (B), (C), and (D) are signs of RHF. Decreased cardiac output is present in both conditions.

ACE = angiotensin converting enzyme, AMI = acute myocardial infarction, AT II = angiotensin II, AV = arteriovenous, BP = blood pressure, BUN = blood urea nitrogen, CAD = coronary artery disease, CBC = complete blood cell count, CH = cholesterol, CHF = congestive heart failure, CNS = central nervous system, COD = cause of death, COPD = chronic obstructive pulmonary disease, DM = diabetes mellitus, ECG = electrocardiogram, GFR = glomerular filtration rate, HDL = high-density lipoprotein, LHF = left heart failure, LV = left ventricle, LVEDV = left ventricular end-diastolic volume, LVH = left ventricular hypertrophy, PH = pulmonary hypertension, PMI = point of maximal impulse, PND = paroxysmal nocturnal dyspnea, RHF = right heart failure, R/O = rule out, RVH = right ventricular hypertrophy, S3 = third heart sound, S4 = fourth heart sound, SMC = smooth muscle cell, SV = stroke volume, S/S = signs and symptoms, TPR = total peripheral resistance, TV = tricuspid valve, VSD = ventricular septal defect.

Table 10–5. CONGENITAL HEART DISEASE

Most Common...	Answer and Explanation
source of fetal oxygen	*placenta* [Unoxygenated fetal blood travels by two umbilical arteries to the placenta, where it is oxygenated. One umbilical vein returns the oxygenated blood to the fetal heart, which pumps it into the systemic circulation.]
shunt directing blood from the fetal PA into the Ao	*ductus arteriosus* (DA) [It redirects the oxygenated fetal blood from the PA into the Ao. PA vessels are thickened by smooth muscle cell (SMC) proliferation, which obstructs blood flow through the nonaerated lungs. The DA redirects the blood back into the Ao.]
cause of functional closure of the DA	*loss of the vasodilating effect of prostaglandin produced by the placenta after delivery*
cause of reduction in fetal PA resistance to blood flow after birth	*increase in PaO_2* [This causes a rapid loss of the SMCs in the pulmonary vessels, hence facilitating blood flow through the lungs for oxygenation.]
heart disease in children	*CHD* [The incidence is higher in premature newborns.]
cause of CHD	*unknown* (~90%) [A minority are due to multifactorial inheritance, chromosomal disorders, and maternal factors. The majority are shunts.]
type of acyanotic left-to-right shunt	**ventricular septal defect (VSD)** [Others include *atrial septal defect (ASD)* and *patent ductus arteriosus (PDA).*]

Table continued on following page

Table 10–5. CONGENITAL HEART DISEASE *Continued*

Most Common...	Answer and Explanation
site for a VSD	*membranous portion of the septum* (75–80%; endocardial cushion defect) [The majority close spontaneously.]
VSD associations	*trisomy 18, trisomy 13, cri-du-chat* (partial deletion of chromosome 5)
late complication of left-to-right shunts	*Eisenmenger's syndrome* [It refers to reversal of a left-to-right shunt to a right-to-left shunt owing to development of PH from volume overload of the right heart. It is also called *cyanosis tardive* (late-onset cyanosis).]
type of ASD	*ostium secundum type* (patent foramen ovale; endocardial cushion defect)
CHD discovered in adults	*ASD* [It is more frequent in females and may present with atrial arrhythmias, PH, or right-to-left shunts.]
S2 finding in an ASD	*fixed splitting of S2,* owing to delayed closure of the PV from increased left-to-right shunting
CHD in Down syndrome	*atrioventricular septal defect* (endocardial cushion defect) [It is an ASD + VSD with a common valve. Heart disease is most responsible for increased early mortality in Down syndrome.]
CHD in the fetal alcohol syndrome	**ASD,** VSD [Heart disease is the least common malformation in the syndrome.]
cause of a PDA	**persistent hypoxemia** [Others: *acidosis* or *prematurity.* It is an isolated defect in 75% of affected newborns and represents a defect in the sixth aortic arch. It is increased in congenital rubella.]
late complication of a PDA	*Eisenmenger's syndrome with differential cyanosis* [This occurs because unoxygenated blood enters the Ao below the subclavian artery (the lower extremity is cyanotic and the upper extremity is pink).]
murmur associated with PDA	*machinery murmur* (to and fro murmur)
method of nonsurgically closing a patent DA	*indomethacin* (inhibits prostaglandin synthesis)

Table 10–5. CONGENITAL HEART DISEASE *Continued*

Most Common...	Answer and Explanation
genetic disease associated with a preductal coarctation	*Turner's syndrome* [A preductal coarctation is immediately symptomatic at birth. It is less common than an adult coarctation.]
congenital valvular disease associated with a postductal coarctation	*bicuspid aortic valve* (25%) [A coarctation is due to a defect in the media of the Ao. It is more common in men than women and develops later in life.]
S/S in a postductal coarctation	*hypertension in the upper extremities and diminished blood pressure in the lower extremities* [Other findings include greater muscular development in the upper than the lower extremities, systolic murmur heard between the scapulas, leg claudication with exercise (ischemia), and diastolic hypertension (reduced renal blood flow).]
chest radiograph findings in a postductal coarctation	*rib notching* due to erosion of bone by dilated collateral intercostal arteries and a *"figure of 3" sign* (pre- and poststenotic dilatation of the Ao)
complication in cyanotic CHD	**secondary polycythemia** (hypoxemia is a stimulus for erythropoietin release) [Others include *infective endocarditis, metastatic abscesses* (particularly cerebral abscesses).]
cyanotic CHD	**tetralogy of Fallot** [The components of a tetralogy are subpulmonic valve stenosis, RVH, VSD, and an overriding Ao. Other cyanotic CHDs include *transposition of the great vessels, truncus arteriosus* (common trunk for the Ao and PA), *tricuspid atresia* (accompanied by an ASD), *total anomalous pulmonary venous return* (oxygenated blood empties into the right heart).]
defect in tetralogy of Fallot that determines the presence or absence of cyanosis	*subpulmonic valve stenosis* [If the stenosis is not great, some blood is directed to the lungs for oxygenation and less through the VSD. A high degree of stenosis directs most of the unoxygenated blood through the VSD (cyanosis).]
disease associated with transposition of the great vessels	*maternal diabetes mellitus* [In a transposition, the Ao empties the RV (unoxygenated blood) and the PA empties the LV (oxygen-

Table continued on following page

Table 10–5. CONGENITAL HEART DISEASE *Continued*

Most Common...	Answer and Explanation
Continued	ated blood). Three shunts are usually present: PDA, ASD, VSD. Oxygenated blood passes from the LA to the RA through the ASD where it mixes with the unoxygenated blood returning to the right heart. It is pumped into the systemic circulation by the Ao. Some of the blood passes through the VSD and is pumped by the PA into the lungs for oxygenation. The PDA redirects blood from the Ao to the PA for oxygenation in the lungs.]
CHD associated with a step-up of oxygen in the RA, RV, and PA	*ASD*
CHD associated with a step-up of oxygen in the PA	*PDA*
CHD associated with a step-up of oxygen in the RV and PA	*VSD*
CHD associated with a step-down of oxygen in the LV and Ao	*tetralogy of Fallot*
complication secondary to a postductal coarctation	**AV regurgitation** (dilatation of the valve ring) [Others include *congenital berry aneurysm* (increased pressure in the cerebral vessels), *dissecting aortic aneurysm, infective endocarditis.*]

Question: Which of the following CHDs are most often associated with secondary polycythemia? **SELECT 3**
  (A) VSD
  (B) ASD
  (C) PDA
  (D) Transposition of the great vessels
  (E) Coarctation of the aorta
  (F) Tetralogy of Fallot
  (G) Anomalous pulmonary venous return

Answers: (D), (F), (G): Secondary polycythemia is a feature of cyanotic CHD, so a transposition of the great vessels, tetralogy, and anomalous pulmonary venous return are correct choices. All the other CHDs listed are acyanotic.

Ao = aorta, AV = aortic valve, CHD = congenital heart disease, LA = left atrium, LV = left ventricle, PA = pulmonary artery, PaO$_2$ = partial pressure of arterial oxygen, PH = pulmonary hypertension, PV = pulmonic valve, RA = right atrium, RV = right ventricle, RVH = right ventricular hypertrophy, S2 = second heart sound, S/S = signs and symptoms.

Table 10–6. ISCHEMIC HEART DISEASE

Most Common...	Answer and Explanation
COD in the United States	*AMI*
symptom of IHD	**angina pectoris** [Other signs of IHD include *AMI, sudden cardiac death* (SCD; death within 1 hour of chest pain), *chronic IHD,* and *cardiac arrhythmias.*]
cause of CAD	**atherosclerosis** [Less common causes include vasculitis, embolization, vasospasm.]
distribution of the LAD coronary artery	*supplies the anterior wall of the LV and anterior two thirds of the IVS* [It is the most common vessel thrombosed in an AMI complicated by complete heart block, owing to the location of the bundles in the anterior one third of the IVS.]
distribution of the RCA	*supplies the posterior-inferior wall of the LV, right ventricle (RV), and posterior one third of the IVS*
coronary artery supplying the atrioventricular node and posteromedial papillary muscle in the LV	*RCA* [It is the most common vessel thrombosed in an AMI associated with sinus bradycardia, papillary muscle dysfunction/rupture, and right ventricular infarction.]
distribution of the LCA coronary artery	*supplies the lateral wall of the LV*
autopsy finding in SCD	**severe coronary artery atherosclerosis** [Occlusive thrombi are not usually present. Other causes of SCD include *mitral valve prolapse* (MVP), *Marfan's syndrome, hypertrophic cardiomyopathy, aortic stenosis,* short QT interval, *conduction system defects, cocaine abuse.*]

Table continued on following page

Table 10–6. ISCHEMIC HEART DISEASE *Continued*

Most Common...	Answer and Explanation
site in the myocardium susceptible to ischemia	*subendocardium,* which is furthest away from the epicardial surface
ECG manifestation of subendocardial ischemia	*ST depression*
ECG manifestation of transmural ischemia	*ST elevation*
screening test to determine the source of chest pain	*stress ECG* [Positive tests are often followed by a coronary angiogram.]
type of angina pectoris and the stress ECG finding	**exertional angina** (ST depression) [Other types: *Prinzmetal's* (ST elevation), *unstable angina* (usually ST depression; a stress ECG is not usually performed). Exertional angina is chest pain with exercise that is relieved by rest, while unstable angina normally occurs at rest. Both types have occlusive atherosclerotic disease. Prinzmetal's angina is due to vasospasm secondary to the release of thromboxane A_2 from platelet thrombi.]
procedure performed in the United States for the treatment of occlusive CAD	*angioplasty* [It has a higher rate of recurrence than coronary artery bypass grafting (CABG).]
vessels used in the CABG procedure	*internal mammary artery* and *saphenous veins* [The former have a 90% patency rate after 10 years, while the latter only have a 70–80% patency rate after 10 years, owing to "arterialization" of the vessels, fibrosis, and occlusion.]
vessel thrombosed in an AMI	**LAD** followed by the *RCA* and *LCA*
time of day for an AMI to occur	*early morning*
clinical findings in a Q wave infarction	*usually transmural, associated with a coronary thrombosis, large size, and increased early mortality*

Table 10–6. ISCHEMIC HEART DISEASE *Continued*

Most Common...	Answer and Explanation
clinical findings of a non–Q wave infarction	usually subendocardial, with coronary thrombosis (30% of cases), small size, and increased risk of SCD within several months
effects of an AMI on compliance and contractility	*infarcted muscle is less compliant than normal muscle and has less contractility*
cause of reperfusion injury of cardiac muscle in an AMI	*FR injury to injured cells by oxygen FRs and calcium secondary to thrombolytic therapy*
G/M findings in the heart 24 hours post-AMI	*pallor (pale infarct) after 12 hours; coagulation necrosis begins after 6 hours*
time after an AMI that the muscle is most subject to rupture	*between 3 and 7 days when the muscle is softest* [The infarcted muscle has a well-demarcated yellow discoloration; myocardial fibers are disappearing; and macrophages are migrating into the necrotic tissue.]
S/S distinguishing an AMI from angina	*crushing pain lasting >30–45 minutes and not relieved by nitroglycerin; radiation of pain down the ulnar aspect of the left arm, into the left shoulder or jaw; pain associated with sweating* (diaphoresis) *and nausea and vomiting*
complication in an AMI	**arrhythmias** (ventricular extrasystoles) [Other complications in descending order are *LHF, cardiogenic shock, cardiac rupture.*]
AMI associated with mural thrombosis	*anterior AMI* (LAD thrombosis) [Mural thrombi are mixed "venous" and arterial clots. There is a danger of embolization, hence the need for anticoagulation with heparin, warfarin, and aspirin.]
cerebral artery embolized to in an AMI	*middle cerebral artery* leading to an embolic stroke (hemorrhagic infarction)
cause of cardiac tamponade in an AMI	*rupture of the anterior free wall of the LV during the 3rd to 10th day*
cause of a mitral regurgitation murmur in an AMI	**LHF** (dilatation of the MV ring) followed by *posteromedial papillary muscle dysfunction* (RCA thrombosis)

Table continued on following page

Table 10–6. ISCHEMIC HEART DISEASE *Continued*

Most Common...	Answer and Explanation
cause of reappearance of CK-MB after 3 days	*reinfarction* [This occurs in ~10% of patients.]
cause of a friction rub during the first week of an AMI	*transmural infarction* with increased vessel permeability leading to fibrinous pericarditis
late complication of an AMI	*ventricular aneurysm* [They begin developing after 2 weeks.]
cause of a precordial bulge during systole in a patient with a past history of an AMI	*ventricular aneurysm on the free wall of the LV*
complication associated with a ventricular aneurysm	**LHF** [This complication correlates with how much of the LV is involved by the aneurysm. *Thromboembolization* also occurs. Rupture rarely occurs, since the aneurysm is composed of scar tissue.]
S/S of Dressler's syndrome	*it is an autoimmune pericarditis* (fibrinous type) *that produces fever, pericarditis, and arthralgias a few weeks post-AMI*
COD in an AMI	*ventricular tachycardia leading to ventricular fibrillation and death*
S/S of a RV infarction	*hypotension, jugular venous distention, and preserved LV function* [They are due to thrombosis of the RCA.]
sequential ECG findings in a transmural AMI	*peaked T waves* (area of ischemia), *ST segment elevation* (area of injury), *symmetric T wave inversion* (area of ischemia), *Q wave* (area of infarction)
ECG findings in an anterior AMI (LAD thrombosis)	*Q waves in leads V1 through V4*
ECG findings in an inferior AMI (RCA thrombosis)	*Q waves in leads II, III, and aVF*
CK isoenzyme in cardiac tissue	**CK-MM** (~85%) followed by *CK-MB* (10–15%) [CK-MB increases in 4–6 hours, peaks in 24 hours, and disappears by 1.5–3 days.]

Table 10–6. ISCHEMIC HEART DISEASE *Continued*

Most Common...	Answer and Explanation
LDH isoenzymes in cardiac tissue	$LDH_1 > LDH_2$ [Normally, LDH_2 is $>$ than LDH_1; however, in an AMI, LDH_1 is $> LDH_2$ (LDH flip). The LDH_1/LDH_2 flip peaks in 48–72 hours and disappears in 7–10 days. It is most useful for AMIs >24 hours old.]
cause of an LDH_1/LDH_2 flip and an increase in LDH_5	*an AMI with an LDH_1/LDH_2 flip and RHF secondary to LHF with congestive hepatomegaly, which is responsible for the increase in LDH_5*
time sequence of elevation of troponin-I in an AMI	*initially increases in 2–6 hours, peaks in 15–24 hours, and returns to normal in 7 days* [Since it appears earlier and lasts longer than CK-MB, it is replacing LDH isoenzymes for AMIs >3 days old.]
time frame for beginning fibrinolytic therapy in an AMI	*within 4–6 hours of an AMI*
factor determining the prognosis in an AMI	*the degree of LV dysfunction* [This is evaluated with measurement of the ejection fraction by echocardiography.]
microscopic findings in CIHD	*patchy fibrosis of the cardiac muscle owing to long-term ischemia* [This results in diastolic dysfunction, heart failure, and death.]

Question: Absence of an auscultatory abnormality would **MOST LIKELY** be associated with which of the following?
(A) A ventricular aneurysm
(B) Dressler's syndrome
(C) Posteromedial papillary muscle dysfunction
(D) Congestive heart failure
(E) Ventricular premature beats

Answer: (A): Ventricular aneurysms produce a precordial bulge during systole, but no abnormal heart sounds or murmurs are usually noted. Choice (B) is associated with a pericardial friction rub; choice (C), a murmur of mitral regurgitation; choice (D), an S3 and bibasilar rales in the lungs; and choice (E), a skipped beat.

AMI = acute myocardial infarction, CAD = coronary artery disease, CIHD = chronic ischemic heart disease, CK = creatine kinase, COD = cause of death, ECG = electrocardiogram, FR = free radical, G/M = gross and microscopic, IHD = ischemic heart disease, IVS = interventricular septum, LAD = left anterior descending, LCA = left circumflex artery,

LDH = lactate dehydrogenase, LHF = left heart failure, LV = left ventricle, MV = mitral valve, RCA = right coronary artery, RHF = right heart failure, S3 = third heart sound, S/S = signs and symptoms.

Table 10–7. VALVULAR HEART DISEASE

Most Common...	Answer and Explanation
valvular heart disease	*mitral valve prolapse* (MVP)
valvular heart disease due to immunologic damage of the valve	*rheumatic heart disease* (RHD) [Immunologic damage is due to cross-reactivity of antibodies directed against group A streptococci M protein with antigens also present in host tissue (e.g., heart, synovial tissue). The initiating infection is usually a pharyngitis.]
valve involved and initial valvular abnormality in RHD	*mitral valve (MV) leading to mitral regurgitation* [Warty, nonembolic vegetations develop along the line of closure of the valve. The aortic valve (AV) is the second most common valve involved and the pulmonic valve (PV) the least common valve involved.]
myocardial lesion noted at autopsy	*Aschoff body* [It consists of a collection of Anitschkow histiocytes and multinucleated giant cells surrounded by fibrinoid necrosis.]
initial manifestation of RHD	**migratory asymmetric polyarthritis** (75% of cases) [Other findings include *carditis* (35% of cases), *chorea* (10% of cases), *subcutaneous nodules* (10% of cases), and *erythema marginatum* (10% of cases). These are called the Jones criteria for the diagnosis of acute rheumatic fever.]
COD in acute rheumatic fever	*myocarditis leading to heart failure*
chronic valvular disease in RHD	*mitral stenosis* [Recurrent attacks of rheumatic fever lead to thickening of the valve, interadherence of valve leaflets (narrows the orifice), and shortening of the chordae tendineae. Dystrophic calcification is common. The valve orifice has a fish-mouth appearance when viewed from the left atrium (LA).]
COD in chronic RHD	*heart failure secondary to mitral stenosis*

Table 10–7. VALVULAR HEART DISEASE *Continued*

Most Common...	Answer and Explanation
cardiac signs in mitral stenosis	*accentuation of S1, OS* as the valve gives way to atrial pressure, *mid-diastolic rumble* best heard at the apex [Over time, mitral stenosis leads to heart failure, pulmonary hypertension (PH; increased P2), and RVH (parasternal heave).]
cause of dysphagia for solids in mitral stenosis	*LA enlargement* [This chamber is the most posteriorly located chamber and can push on the esophagus.]
cause of hemoptysis in mitral stenosis	*pulmonary congestion* [Rust-colored sputum (alveolar macrophages with hemosiderin) is common.]
arrhythmia in mitral stenosis	*atrial fibrillation secondary to dilatation of the LA* [There is a danger of clot formation and embolization, hence the reason for anticoagulating the patient.]
immune diseases associated with sterile valvular vegetations	**RHD** and *SLE* (Libman-Sacks endocarditis [10–20%]) [The latter disease has warty vegetations scattered over the valves and valve structures.]
valvular disease associated with malignancy	*nonbacterial (sterile) thrombotic endocarditis* (marantic vegetations) [This complication most commonly occurs on the MV in patients with mucinous carcinomas of the colon, pancreas, or lungs. It is a paraneoplastic syndrome (see Chapter 9).
organism producing infective endocarditis (IE)	*Streptococcus viridans*
valve involved in IE	*MV* [The vegetations are bulky and friable, hence the common occurrence of embolization.]
organism producing IE in an IV drug abuser	*Staphylococcus aureus* [The TV, MV, and AV are commonly involved. *S. aureus* colonizes normal as well as abnormal valves.]
immunocomplex findings in IE	*Roth's spot* in the retina, *splinter hemorrhages* of the nails, *Osler's nodes* (painful nodules on the hands and feet), *Janeway's lesions* (painless lesions on the hands and feet), and glomerulonephritis [The majority of these lesions represent immunocomplex-mediated small vessel vasculitis.]

Table continued on following page

Table 10–7. VALVULAR HEART DISEASE *Continued*

Most Common...	Answer and Explanation
cause of hematuria in IE	*immunocomplex-mediated glomerulonephritis*
sign of IE	*fever from bacteremia* (cultures positive in ~95% of cases) [Changing murmurs are uncommon.]
organism producing IE in a patient with colon cancer	*Streptococcus bovis*
organism associated with IE in valve prostheses	*Staphylococcus epidermidis*, a coagulase-negative organism
organism producing IE after dental or upper respiratory procedures	*Streptococcus viridans* [Amoxicillin is usually prescribed 1 hour before the procedure.]
organism producing IE after a GI or GU procedure	*Enterococcus*
cause of MVP	*myxomatous degeneration* leading to redundant valve leaflets
cause of sudden death in Marfan's syndrome	*MVP* [Both Marfan's syndrome and Ehlers-Danlos syndrome have an increased incidence of MVP.]
clinical presentation of MVP	*most cases are asymptomatic* and are discovered incidentally on physical exam [Most MVPs are present in tall, thin women. An AD inheritance pattern is noted in some cases.]
cardiac signs in MVP	*midsystolic ejection click followed by a mid-to late systolic murmur of mitral regurgitation* [The MV leaflets prolapse into the LA like a parachute during systole.]
effect of standing or anxiety on the click and murmur of MVP in relation to S1	*the click and murmur occur closer to S1* owing to decreased venous return associated with standing and reduced diastolic filling in patients who are anxious [Lying down or sustained hand grip exercises move the click and murmur closer to S2.]
complications associated with MVP	*palpitations, chest pain, fatigue, rupture of the chordae* (acute mitral regurgitation), *sudden cardiac death, IE*

Table 10–7. VALVULAR HEART DISEASE *Continued*

Most Common...	Answer and Explanation
treatment used for symptomatic MVP	β-*blockers* or *calcium channel blockers*
cause of mitral valve regurgitation	*MVP* [Other causes are RHD, IE, and CHF.]
cause of aortic stenosis	*congenital bicuspid aortic valve* (>50% of cases) [The murmur is a systolic ejection type murmur that radiates into the carotid arteries.]
valvular lesion associated with syncope and angina with exercise	*aortic stenosis* [The former problem secondary to reduced cardiac output and the latter from concentric hypertrophy of the LV and the need for oxygen with exercise.]
valvular lesion associated with microangiopathic hemolytic anemia	*aortic stenosis* [RBCs hitting the dystrophically calcified valve are damaged (produces schistocytes [fragmented RBCs]), leading to an intravascular hemolysis. Serum haptoglobin is decreased (complexes with free Hb and is removed by macrophages) and hemosiderin is present in the urine.]
cause of aortic regurgitation	**chronic RHD** [Other causes include *IE* (especially in IV drug abusers), *dissecting aortic aneurysm, coarctation of the aorta, ankylosing spondylitis.*]
cause of an Austin Flint murmur	*aortic regurgitation* [It is secondary to blood dripping onto the anterior MV leaflet during diastole. It indicates severe regurgitant disease.]
cardiac findings in aortic regurgitation	*high-pitched blowing murmur after S2 leading to LV dilatation and hypertrophy* [Other findings include a wide pulse pressure (increased SV) and signs of a hyperdynamic circulation (e.g., water hammer pulse).]
cause of tricuspid stenosis	*chronic RHD*, usually in association with mitral stenosis
S/S in tricuspid stenosis	*heart murmur similar to mitral stenosis except that it increases in inspiration, giant a wave in the JVP*
cause of tricuspid regurgitation	*RHF owing to stretching of the ring from RV dilatation* [Less common causes include carcinoid syndrome and IE.]

Table continued on following page

Table 10–7. VALVULAR HEART DISEASE *Continued*

Most Common...	Answer and Explanation
S/S in tricuspid regurgitation	*pansystolic murmur that increases with inspiration, giant c-v wave in the JVP, hepatic pulsation during systole*
cause of pulmonic stenosis	**congenital** (e.g., subvalvular stenosis in tetralogy of Fallot) or *acquired* (e.g., carcinoid heart disease)
cause of pulmonic regurgitation	*RHF with dilatation of the ring* [It may also occur with PH. It is sometimes called the Graham-Steell murmur.]
valve abnormalities in carcinoid heart disease	*tricuspid regurgitation* and *pulmonic stenosis* secondary to the fibrogenic effect of serotonin
valve involved in RHD, IE, prolapse, and nonbacterial thrombotic endocarditis	*MV*

Question: Atrial dilatation without ventricular hypertrophy or dilatation would most likely be associated with which of the following?
   (A) Aortic stenosis
   (B) Mitral regurgitation
   (C) Pulmonic stenosis
   (D) Mitral stenosis
   (E) MVP

Answer: (D): Mitral and tricuspid stenoses are associated with atrial dilatation without ventricular hypertrophy or dilatation. Choices (A) and (C) are associated with ventricular hypertrophy alone, choice (B) with hypertrophy and dilatation, and choice (E) is usually not associated with either hypertrophy or dilatation.

AD = autosomal dominant, CHF = congestive heart failure, COD = cause of death, GI = gastrointestinal, GU = genitourinary, Hb = hemoglobin, IV = intravenous, JVP = jugular venous pulse, LV = left ventricle, OS = opening snap, RBC = red blood cell, RHF = right heart failure, RV = right ventricle, RVH = right ventricular hypertrophy, S1 = first heart sound, S2 = second heart sound, SLE = systemic lupus erythematosus, S/S = signs and symptoms, SV = stroke volume, TV = tricuspid valve.

Table 10–8. MYOCARDIAL AND
PERICARDIAL DISORDERS

Most Common...	Answer and Explanation
cause of myocarditis	*viral infection, usually Coxsackie B*
parasitic disease causing myocarditis	*Chagas' disease due to Trypanosoma cruzi [Trichinella spiralis* (trichinosis) may also invade cardiac tissue.]
toxin associated with myocarditis	*diphtheria exotoxin* produced by *Corynebacterium diphtheriae*
collagen vascular diseases associated with myocarditis	*progressive systemic sclerosis, rheumatoid arthritis*
cause of drug-induced myocarditis	*doxorubicin* [Others include *tricyclic antidepressants,* α*-interferon, cyclophosphamide.*]
type of cardiomyopathy	*congestive cardiomyopathy* [It presents with both left and right heart failure with dilation of all chambers.]
cause of congestive cardiomyopathy	*previous viral myocarditis* [Other causes include *post partum, alcohol* (direct toxic effect or thiamine deficiency), *drugs* (see above), *cocaine, hypothyroidism.*]
cardiomyopathy associated with sudden cardiac death	*hypertrophic cardiomyopathy* [This is secondary to abnormalities in the conduction system in the asymmetrically hypertrophied IVS. It is also associated with syncope with exercise and angina-like aortic stenosis.]
cause of the obstruction in hypertrophic cardiomyopathy	*the anterior leaflet of the MV is drawn against the asymmetrically hypertrophied IVS in systole*
drugs used in treating hypertrophic cardiomyopathy	**β-blockers** *and calcium channel blockers* [These drugs decrease myocardial contractility, which increases LVEDV and cardiac output. Maneuvers that increase venous return to the heart improve the cardiac output (e.g., squatting, lying down). Positive inotropic agents like digitalis reduce the cardiac output by increasing the degree of obstruction. Factors that reduce venous return to the heart (e.g., venodilators, Valsalva maneuver) also reduce cardiac output.]

Table continued on following page

Table 10–8. MYOCARDIAL AND
PERICARDIAL DISORDERS *Continued*

Most Common...	Answer and Explanation
method for diagnosing hypertrophic cardiomyopathy	*echocardiography* [This study demonstrates the asymmetric IVS and abnormal MV motility. There is a sharp upstroke of the carotid pulse.]
cause of restrictive cardiomyopathy in children	*endocardial fibroelastosis* (thick endocardial tissue) with an associated hypoplastic left heart [Endomyocardial biopsies are necessary to confirm the diagnosis. Heart transplantation is required. Other causes include Pompe's glycogenosis and mucopolysaccharidoses.]
causes of restrictive cardiomyopathy in adults	*amyloidosis* (low voltage ECG, conduction disturbances), *iron overload* (e.g., hemochromatosis)
cardiac tumor in adults	*cardiac myxoma* [Most arise in the LA where they may embolize or produce syncope.]
cardiac tumor in children	*rhabdomyoma* [These occur in tuberous sclerosis (AD disease with mental retardation) in 30–50% of cases.]
cancer of the heart	*metastatic disease from a primary in the lung*
cause of pericarditis	*a viral infection, most commonly secondary to Coxsackie B*
causes of fibrinous pericarditis	*uremia, transmural AMI, SLE, RHD, Dressler's syndrome* (autoimmune pericarditis following an AMI), *rheumatoid arthritis*
collagen vascular disease associated with pericarditis	*SLE* [Pericarditis is the most common cardiac manifestation of SLE.]
S/S of pericarditis	*precordial chest pain, friction rub*, and *effusion*
cause of constrictive pericarditis worldwide	*tuberculosis* [In the United States, prior open heart surgery is the most common cause. The mean pressures in all cardiac chambers are equally elevated.]
cause of a pericardial knock	*constrictive pericarditis* [As the chambers fill up with blood, they come in contact with the wall of the thickened pericardium.]
S/S of a pericardial effusion	*hypotension, elevated JVP*, and *muffled heart sounds* [This is called Beck's triad. Kussmaul's sign (distended JVPs with inspiration)

Table 10–8. MYOCARDIAL AND
PERICARDIAL DISORDERS *Continued*

Most Common...	Answer and Explanation
Continued	and pulsus paradoxus (decrease in blood pressure during inspiration) are also noted. Unlike constrictive pericarditis, all the chambers have restricted filling throughout diastole.]
test used to document a pericardial effusion	*echocardiogram* [A chest radiograph reveals a "water bottle" configuration.]
treatment of cardiac tamponade [effusion that compromises normal filling]	*pericardiocentesis*

Question: Which of the following has the greatest effect on increasing cardiac output in hypertrophic cardiomyopathy?
- (A) Digitalis
- (B) Venodilators
- (C) β-Blockers
- (D) Valsalva maneuver
- (E) Standing up

Answer: (C): β-Blockers decrease contractility of the heart, thereby increasing preload in the LV, which separates the anterior leaflet of the MV from the asymmetric IVS. All the other choices either enhance obstruction by increasing myocardial contraction (choice A) or reducing venous return to the heart (choices B, D, and E).

AD = autosomal dominant, AMI = acute myocardial infarction, ECG = electrocardiogram, IVS = interventricular septum, JVP = jugular venous pulse, LA = left atrium, LV = left ventricle, LVEDV = left ventricular end-diastolic volume, MV = mitral valve, RHD = rheumatic heart disease, SLE = systemic lupus erythematosus, S/S = signs and symptoms.

CHAPTER

11

RESPIRATORY PATHOLOGY

CONTENTS

Table 11–1. HISTORY, PHYSICAL EXAM, AND LAB EVALUATION OF THE RESPIRATORY SYSTEM USING PULMONARY FUNCTION TESTS

Most Common...	Answer and Explanation
symptom of respiratory disease	*dyspnea* (difficulty with breathing) [It may be secondary to problems with the work of breathing (e.g., reduced lung compliance) or the stimulation for breathing (e.g., stimulation of the J receptors).]
cause of cough	*postnasal discharge*
cause of hemoptysis [coughing up blood]	*chronic bronchitis* [Next most common causes are *pneumonia* and *cancer.*]
causes of massive hemoptysis [>1000 mL/d]	*TB, bronchiectasis, cancer, aspergilloma* (fungus ball)
cause of chest pain of respiratory origin	*pleuritis* secondary to pneumonia or pulmonary infarction [It refers to a sharp inspiratory pain.]
types of breathing alterations	*tachypnea* (rapid, shallow breathing; 16–25/minute) and *hyperpnea* (rapid, deep breathing; Kussmaul's breathing in DKA)

Table continued on following page

Table 11–1. HISTORY, PHYSICAL EXAM, AND LAB EVALUATION OF THE RESPIRATORY SYSTEM USING PULMONARY FUNCTION TESTS *Continued*

Most Common...	Answer and Explanation
types of cyanosis [dusky blue appearance]	*peripheral and central cyanosis* [The former is due to redistribution of oxygenated blood (e.g., cold, hypovolemic shock; skin is cyanotic but mucous membranes are normal). The latter refers to dusky skin and mucous membranes and indicates either intrapulmonary or cardiac shunting.]
ABG abnormality associated with cyanosis	*decreased SaO_2* (<80%; percentage of heme groups occupied by O_2) [The amount of deoxygenated Hb is the primary determinant of cyanosis.]
cause of stridor [high-pitched inspiratory/ expiratory sound]	*upper airway obstruction* [It may be due to food (cafe coronary), epiglottitis (*Haemophilus influenzae*), laryngotracheobronchitis (parainfluenza virus).]
cause of wheezing [musical sounds on inspiration/ expiration]	*small airway obstruction* (nonrespiratory [terminal] bronchioles) [It may be due to asthma, pulmonary edema, bronchiolitis.]
site for normal airway resistance	*segmental bronchi* [The airflow is turbulent.]
site for laminar air flow	*terminal bronchioles*
cause of crackles (rales)	*reduced compliance in the small airways or alveoli* due to fluid or fibrosis
cause of gurgles (rhonchi)	*airflow through liquids of different viscosities,* as in pulmonary edema, bronchitis, bacterial pneumonia
signs of lung consolidation	*decreased percussion, increased tactile fremitus* (vibration on the chest wall), *egophony* (e sounds like a)
cause of hyperresonance of the lungs	**increased AP diameter** (e.g., emphysema) and *pneumothorax* (e.g., collapse of the lungs)
cause of clubbing [bulbous enlargement of the end of the fingers or toes]	**pulmonary disease** (e.g., bronchiectasis, cystic fibrosis), *cyanotic CHD, GI disease*

Table 11–1. HISTORY, PHYSICAL EXAM, AND LAB EVALUATION OF THE RESPIRATORY SYSTEM USING PULMONARY FUNCTION TESTS *Continued*

Most Common...	Answer and Explanation
method of measuring volumes and capacities (more than one volume) in the lungs	*spirometry* [Spirometry cannot directly measure the RV (volume left over after maximal expiration) or TLC (amount of air in a fully expanded lung), which is measured with a nitrogen or helium washout method.]
outpatient method of evaluating the FVC [total amount of air expelled after a maximal inspiration]	*peak expiratory flow meter*
method of measuring the diffusing capacity [DL; evaluates gas exchange]	*diffusion capacity using carbon monoxide (DL_{CO}).* [It is dependent on CO reaching the alveoli (decreased with $\dot{V}/\dot{Q}$ mismatches), CO crossing the alveolar–capillary interface (decreased with fibrosis and fluids), and CO binding to Hb in RBCs (decreased with PE owing to less perfusion of the capillaries.]
effect of restrictive lung disease [fibrosis at the alveolar–capillary interface] on compliance and elasticity	*compliance is decreased* (cannot fill the lungs with air) and *elasticity is increased* (increased expulsion of air from the lungs due to increased recoil) [All lung volumes and capacities are reduced. The FEV_{1sec} (amount of air expelled in 1 second after maximal inspiration) and FVC are decreased, but the FEV_{1sec} to FVC ratio is increased, since both parameters are often the same, owing to increased elasticity.]
effect of obstructive lung disease [air trapping on expiration] on compliance and elasticity	*compliance is increased* (elastic support is damaged) and *elasticity is decreased* (elastic support is damaged) [Hence, the RV and TLC are increased, while the other volumes and capacities are decreased (compressed by the increase in RV). The FEV_{1sec}, FVC, and FEV_{1sec} to FVC ratio are all decreased.]
cause of an alveolar-arterial gradient [A-a gradient; difference between the PaO_2 and PaO_2] in the lungs	*ventilation without perfusion* (e.g., atelectasis; this produces intrapulmonary shunting) [Other causes: *perfusion without ventilation* (e.g., pulmonary embolus; increases dead space), *diffusion abnormalities* (e.g., interstitial fibrosis). Right-to-left shunts in the heart also increase the A-a gradient.]

Table continued on following page

Table 11-1. HISTORY, PHYSICAL EXAM, AND LAB EVALUATION OF THE RESPIRATORY SYSTEM USING PULMONARY FUNCTION TESTS Continued

Most Common...	Answer and Explanation
formula used to calculate the A-a gradient	PaO_2 = % oxygen (713) − $PaCO_2/0.8$ [Using normal values: PaO_2 = 0.21 (713) − 40/0.8 = 100 mm Hg]
causes of hypoxemia [low PaO_2] and a normal A-a gradient	depression of the respiratory center in the medulla (e.g., barbiturates, CNS injury) and chest bellows dysfunction (e.g., paralyzed diaphragm)

Question: Which of the following differentiates restrictive from obstructive lung disease?
(A) Tidal volume
(B) Vital capacity
(C) FEV_{1sec}
(D) FVC
(E) FEV_{1sec} to FVC ratio

Answer: (E): The FEV_{1sec} to FVC ratio is increased in restrictive disease, since elasticity is increased, and decreased in obstructive disease, since elasticity is decreased. All the other parameters are decreased in both disorders. Tidal volume is the volume of air entering and leaving the lungs with quiet respiration.

ABG = arterial blood gas, AP = anteroposterior, CHD = congenital heart disease, CNS = central nervous system, DKA = diabetic ketoacidosis, DL = diffusion capacity, DL_{CO} = diffusion capacity using carbon monoxide, FEV_{1sec} = forced expiratory volume in 1 second, FVC = forced vital capacity, GI = gastrointestinal, Hb = hemoglobin, $PaCO_2$ = partial pressure of carbon dioxide, PaO_2 = partial pressure of arterial oxygen, PAO_2 = partial pressure of alveolar oxygen, PE = pulmonary embolism, SaO_2 = oxygen saturation, RBC = red blood cell, RV = residual volume, TB = tuberculosis, TLC = total lung capacity, $\dot{V}/\dot{Q}$ = ventilation/perfusion.

Table 11-2. UPPER RESPIRATORY DISORDERS

Most Common...	Answer and Explanation
cause of nasal polyps	**allergic disease** (adults) [Other causes: triad asthma (aspirin sensitivity leading to asthma), and cystic fibrosis (children)]
site and organism involved in acute sinusitis	maxillary sinus and Streptococcus pneumoniae [Amoxicillin is the most commonly used drug.]

Table 11–2. UPPER RESPIRATORY DISORDERS *Continued*

Most Common...	Answer and Explanation
sinus infection responsible for orbital cellulitis in children	*ethmoid sinusitis* [The infection extends into the orbit (proptosis of the eye, weak eye movements) and may involve the cavernous sinus (danger of thrombosis).]
cause of saddle nose deformity	*Wegener's granulomatosis* [It is a necrotizing granulomatous vasculitis involving the nasal cavity, sinuses, upper airway, lungs, and kidneys.]
malignancy of the nasal cavity and paranasal sinuses	*squamous cell carcinoma*
malignancy associated with woodworking	*adenocarcinoma of the nasal cavity*
neuroendocrine tumor of the nasal cavity	*olfactory neuroblastoma*
malignant tumor of the nasopharynx	*nasopharyngeal carcinoma* [It has a causal relationship with EBV and commonly metastasizes to the cervical lymph nodes.]
cause of laryngeal cancer	*squamous cell carcinoma,* most commonly secondary to **smoking** and *alcohol* (both have an additive effect) [The *supraglottic area* (above the false vocal cords) is the most common site. *Hoarseness* is the most common symptom.]
cause of acute epiglottitis in children	*Haemophilus influenzae* [Epiglottitis is declining owing to *H. influenzae* immunization.]
radiographic finding in acute epiglottitis	*lateral radiograph of the neck reveals swelling of the epiglottis resembling a thumbprint* ("thumbprint sign")
radiographic finding in croup (laryngotracheobronchitis) in children	*lateral radiograph of the neck reveals narrowing of the airway below the true vocal cords, which appear like a church steeple* ("steeple sign")
type of inflammation in diphtheria	*pseudomembranous inflammation* [It produces a toxin-induced damage of the mucosa. *Corynebacterium diphtheriae* is a gram-positive bacillus. Vaccination is the most important means of prevention.]

Table continued on following page

Table 11–2. UPPER RESPIRATORY DISORDERS *Continued*

Most Common...	Answer and Explanation
COD in diphtheria	*cardiac dysfunction* [It is secondary to toxin inhibition of protein synthesis and impaired fatty acid synthesis.]
cause of vocal cord polyps	*voice abuse,* hence the name "singer's nodules"
cause of squamous papillomas of the vocal cord in adults and children	*HPV types 6 and 11* [It is contracted while passing through an infected birth canal. There is a risk for squamous carcinoma of the larynx.]

Question: The most common cancer in the upper respiratory tract has its origin from which of the following?
(A) Glandular cells
(B) Neuroendocrine cells
(C) Neural crest tissue
(D) Squamous epithelium
(E) Transitional epithelium

Answer: (D): Squamous cancers (not adenocarcinomas) are the over-all most common cancers of the upper respiratory tract. Olfactory neuroblastomas are of neural crest origin and are considered neuroendocrine tumors. Transitional tumors are most commonly located in the bladder.

COD = cause of death, EBV = Epstein-Barr virus, HPV = human papilloma virus.

Table 11–3. ATELECTASIS, ASPIRATION, PNEUMOTHORAX, VASCULAR DISORDERS

Most Common...	Answer and Explanation
cause of atelectasis [collapse of alveoli]	*obstruction of small airways by mucus plugs with resorption of air from the alveoli* [Other causes include *compression of lung* by an intrapulmonary mass or pleural effusion, *lack of surfactant* (RDS, ARDS).]
gross appearance of atelectasis	*bluish-gray depression of the lung* [This causes elevation of the ipsilateral diaphragm due to loss of lung mass.]
S/S in atelectasis	*fever* (not related to infection), *cyanosis* (if widespread), *dyspnea, elevation of the diaphragm,* and *inspiratory lag on the affected side*

Table 11–3. ATELECTASIS, ASPIRATION, PNEUMOTHORAX, VASCULAR DISORDERS *Continued*

Most Common...	Answer and Explanation
cause of fever in the first 24–48 hours after surgery	*atelectasis*
cause of RDS	*decrease in pulmonary surfactant* (lecithin, or phosphatidyl choline) [Surfactant decreases alveolar surface tension, which keeps alveoli from collapsing on expiration.]
cell producing surfactant	*type II pneumocytes* [Maximal amounts of surfactant are present after 35 weeks of gestation.]
method (gold standard) used to measure surfactant	*measurement of the lecithin to sphingomyelin (L/S) ratio by TLC* [An L/S ratio >2 indicates pulmonary maturity.]
method of increasing surfactant production in the newborn prior to birth	*treating the mother with glucocorticoids,* which enhances surfactant synthesis by the fetus [Thyroxine also increases surfactant synthesis but is not used for this purpose.]
cause of RDS	*prematurity* [Other causes include *maternal diabetes mellitus* (fetal insulin in response to maternal hyperglycemia inhibits surfactant synthesis), *Cesarean section* (less stress-induced release of cortisol by the fetus).]
pathophysiologic effect of RDS	*massive intrapulmonary shunting* from atelectasis [Positive end-expiratory pressure (PEEP) therapy keeps the alveoli open after expiration. Intrapulmonary shunts show very little PaO_2 response after the administration of 100% oxygen. Hyaline membranes from increased vessel permeability to protein contribute to a diffusion defect.]
clinical and lab findings in RDS	*dyspnea soon after birth* and *central cyanosis;* a chest radiograph reveals a "ground glass" appearance; *respiratory acidosis, severe hypoxemia*, and an *increased A-a gradient* are present
oxygen FR injuries in RDS	*retinopathy of prematurity* (blindness) and *bronchopulmonary dysplasia* (repair of injured lung by fibrosis)

Table continued on following page

Table 11–3. ATELECTASIS, ASPIRATION, PNEUMOTHORAX, VASCULAR DISORDERS *Continued*

Most Common...	Answer and Explanation
non-oxygen FR–related complications of RDS	*intraventricular hemorrhage, PDA* (persistent hypoxemia), *necrotizing enterocolitis* (ischemic necrosis with bowel invasion by bacteria)
cause of ARDS	*gram-negative sepsis* [Other causes: *aspiration of gastric contents, pneumonia, severe trauma, acute pancreatitis*]
pathophysiologic abnormality in ARDS	*massive intrapulmonary shunting* from atelectasis [Atelectasis is due to neutrophil-related injury of type II pneumocytes. Immigration of neutrophils into the alveoli through the pulmonary capillaries produces leaky capillaries and exit of a protein-rich edema fluid forming hyaline membranes.]
cause of spontaneous pneumothorax	*rupture of a subpleural bulla at the apex of the lung* [Most patients are tall, slender individuals who have recurrent disease. In most cases, the cause of the subpleural bullae are unknown. Other causes include Marfan's syndrome, paraseptal emphysema, iatrogenic (insertion of a subclavian catheter), ruptured esophagus.]
S/S in a spontaneous pneumothorax	*sudden onset of severe pleuritic chest pain with dyspnea;* there is *hyperresonance to percussion, absent tactile fremitus, ipsilateral tracheal deviation,* and *elevation of the hemidiaphragm*
signs of a tension pneumothorax	*similar to spontaneous pneumothorax except there is bulging of intercostal muscles, depression of the diaphragm, and tracheal deviation to the contralateral side* [Air enters the pleural cavity on inspiration but cannot exit. Insertion of a needle into the pleural space is life-saving.]
body position for aspiration into the posterobasal segment of the RLL	*sitting or standing*
body position for aspiration into the superior segment of the RLL	*lying down on the back*

Table 11–3. ATELECTASIS, ASPIRATION, PNEUMOTHORAX, VASCULAR DISORDERS *Continued*

Most Common...	Answer and Explanation
body position for aspiration into the right middle lobe and/or posterior segment of the RUL	*lying down on the right side*
body position for aspiration into the lingula of the left lung	*lying down on the left side*
cause of meconium aspiration	*post-term infant (>42 weeks) with fetal asphyxia*
causes of aspiration of gastric contents	*trauma patients who are unconscious* [Other causes: *postanesthesia, stroke patients*]
cause of endogenous lipoid pneumonia	*obstruction of an airway by tumor* [Cholesterol-laden alveolar macrophages behind the obstruction provide a golden color to the lung tissue.]
site of origin of pulmonary emboli (PE)	*proximal deep veins of the thigh* (**femoral,** iliac, popliteal) [Most of these are the result of propagation of a venous clot from the deep saphenous veins of the calf.]
cause of a PE	*postoperative state* (particularly hip surgery) [Other causes: *post partum, CHF, malignancy, oral contraceptives*]
cause of acute cor pulmonale [right ventricular strain]	*large pulmonary embolus blocking the majority of PA orifices* (saddle embolus)
initial pathophysiologic effect of a PE	*perfusion defect leading to increased dead space* [After 48 hours, atelectasis occurs, leading to an intrapulmonary shunt.]
initial S/S of a PE	*tachypnea* and *dyspnea* [Pleuritic chest pain, cough, leg pain (DVT), hemoptysis, fever, and wheezing also occur.]
complications of a PE	**hemorrhagic infarction** (10–15% of cases; more likely with pre-existing lung disease), *secondary PH* (loss of the capillary bed over time)

Table continued on following page

Table 11–3. ATELECTASIS, ASPIRATION, PNEUMOTHORAX, VASCULAR DISORDERS *Continued*

Most Common...	Answer and Explanation
radiographic findings in a PE	*pleural effusion* [Other findings: *area of hypovascularity* (Westermark's sign), *wedge-shaped density* (Hampton's sign). A *perfusion scan* is the first step in the work-up. A *pulmonary angiogram* is the gold standard study (performed in equivocal cases).]
lab and ECG abnormalities in a PE	*respiratory alkalosis, PaO$_2$ <80 mm Hg* (90%), *increased A-a gradient, ECG with RV strain pattern (S$_1$Q$_3$T$_3$).*
cardiac causes of PH [PA pressure >25 mm Hg]	*mitral stenosis, left-to-right shunts* (e.g., VSD)
pulmonary cause of PH	*COPD* [Other causes: *ILD, recurrent small pulmonary emboli, chronic hypoxemia* (e.g., high altitude), *idiopathic, hyperviscosity* (e.g., polycythemia vera)]
G/M features of PE	*atherosclerosis of the PA, intimal fibrosis and medial smooth muscle hypertrophy, angiomatoid lesions* (interlacing small blood channels)
S/S of PH	*accentuation of P2, left parasternal heave* (RVH), *paradoxical split of S2* (PV closes early)
cause of cor pulmonale [PH + RVH resulting from primary PH or primary lung disease]	*COPD* [Other causes: *CF, ILD*]
radiographic findings in Wegener's granulomatosis	*nodular densities in the lungs secondary to granulomatous vasculitis* (angiocentric masses)

Table 11–3. ATELECTASIS, ASPIRATION, PNEUMOTHORAX, VASCULAR DISORDERS *Continued*

Question: Which of the following would most likely be a cause of secondary PH?
  (A) PE
  (B) ARDS
  (C) Wegener's granulomatosis
  (D) Pneumothorax
  (E) RDS

Answer: (A): Recurrent pulmonary emboli with destruction of the vascular bed are associated with secondary PH. None of the other choices would be expected to result in PH.

A-a = alveolar-arterial, ARDS = adult respiratory distress syndrome, CF = cystic fibrosis, CHF = congestive heart failure, COPD = chronic obstructive pulmonary disease, DVT = deep venous thrombosis, ECG = electrocardiogram, FR = free radical, G/M = gross and microscopic, ILD = interstitial lung disease, P2 = pulmonic component of the second heart sound, PA = pulmonary artery, PDA = patent ductus arteriosus, PH = pulmonary hypertension, PV = pulmonary valve, RDS = respiratory distress syndrome, RLL = right lower lobe, RUL = right upper lobe, RV = right ventricle, RVH = right ventricular hypertrophy, S/S = signs and symptoms, S2 = second heart sound, TLC = thin layer chromatography, VSD = ventricular septal defect.

Table 11–4. RESPIRATORY TRACT INFECTIONS

Most Common...	Answer and Explanation
cause of a typical community-acquired pneumonia	*Streptococcus pneumoniae (Pneumococcus), a gram-positive lancet-shaped diplococcus* [Typical pneumonias have a sudden onset, high fever, productive cough, and signs of consolidation in the lungs.]
cause of an atypical community-acquired pneumonia	*Mycoplasma pneumoniae* [Atypical pneumonias have an insidious onset, low-grade fever, nonproductive cough, and an interstitial pattern in the lungs.]
types of typical pneumonia	**bronchopneumonia** (bronchitis leading to patchy areas of pneumonia) and *lobar pneumonia*
test ordered in the initial evaluation of pneumonia	*Gram stain of sputum* [It is usually accompanied by a *chest radiograph* and *CBC*. A CBC in typical pneumonia reveals absolute neutrophilic leukocytosis and left shift.]

Table continued on following page

Table 11–4. RESPIRATORY TRACT INFECTIONS *Continued*

Most Common...	Answer and Explanation
complications associated with a typical pneumonia	*septicemia* [Others: *lung abscesses, empyema* (pus in the pleural cavity)]
cause of nosocomial [hospital-derived] typical pneumonias	*Escherichia coli* [Others: *Pseudomonas aeruginosa, Staphylococcus aureus.* These organisms initially colonize the airways and then spread into the lungs.]
cause of the common cold	*rhinovirus* [School children are the primary reservoir.]
cause of bronchiolitis and pneumonia in children	*respiratory syncytial virus* (RSV)
viral cause of increased morbidity/ mortality in people >55 years of age	*influenzavirus* [The egg-based vaccine is recommended for patients >65 years of age, immunocompromised patients, and those with underlying cardiac, lung, or hepatic disease.]
serious early complication of rubeola	*pneumonia* [Warthin-Finkeldey multinucleated giant cells are noted in the lungs at autopsy.]
cause of pneumonia in handlers of psittacine birds (parakeets, parrots)	*Chlamydia psittaci,* which produces psittacosis
Chlamydia species associated with atypical pneumonia in adults	*Chlamydia pneumoniae*
cause of bilateral conjunctivitis and pneumonia in a newborn infant	*Chlamydia trachomatis* [These complications usually occur after 1 week. The pneumonia is not associated with fever and produces a bronchiolitis picture with wheezing and a staccato cough.]
cause of pneumonia in a person with exposure to sheep manure	*Coxiella burnetii* [It is the cause of Q fever. This disease may occur in dairy farmers, veterinarians, and those who clean up sheep, goat, or cattle manure.]
cause of tension pneumothorax in a patient with CF	*Staphylococcus aureus* [It is often associated with pneumonias that develop tension pneumatocysts in the pleura, which may rupture and produce a tension pneumothorax.]

Table 11–4. RESPIRATORY TRACT INFECTIONS *Continued*

Most Common...	Answer and Explanation
nosocomial pneumonia associated with transmission by respiratory therapy	*Pseudomonas aeruginosa* [It is a water-loving, gram-negative bacterium.]
cause of pneumonia in nursing homes	*Klebsiella pneumoniae,* a fat, gram-negative rod
cause of pneumonia and abscess formation in an alcoholic	*Klebsiella pneumoniae*
cause of pneumonia where water coolers are present	*Legionella pneumophila* [It is a gram-negative rod. It is a water-loving bacterium that frequently contaminates water coolers. A Dieterle silver stain is the best way to directly visualize the bacteria.]
organism producing pneumonia that is partially acid fast and a gram-positive filamentous bacterium	*Nocardia asteroides*
cause of pneumonia anticipated in earthquakes in Southern California	*Coccidioides immitis* [Earthquakes shake up dust, which contains the arthrospores of the fungus. The Southwest is the most common location for this fungus.]
cause of pneumonia associated with exposure to pigeons	*Cryptococcus neoformans* [Pigeons commonly congregate under bridges, in warehouses, and on top of air conditioners outside windows.]
cause of pneumonia associated with cave explorers	*Histoplasma capsulatum* [Birds, other than pigeons, and bats are potential agents for transmission of the fungus. The Midwest is the most common location for this fungus].
systemic fungal infection	*histoplasmosis*
fungus associated with hemoptysis, asthma, and pneumonia	*Aspergillus fumigatus* [It often colonizes abandoned TB cavities (fungus ball; hemoptysis); is a mold associated with asthma; and produces a hemorrhagic pneumonia with infarctions (vessel invader).]

Table continued on following page

Table 11–4. RESPIRATORY TRACT INFECTIONS *Continued*

Most Common...	Answer and Explanation
AIDS-defining pneumonia	*Pneumocystis carinii* [It is best treated with trimethoprim/sulfamethoxazole. Prophylaxis begins when the CD_4 T helper count is ≤200 cells/μL.]
fungal pneumonia associated with broad-based budding yeasts	*Blastomyces dermatitidis*
location for primary TB	*subpleural location in the upper part of the lower lobes or lower part of the upper lobes of lung*
worldwide COD due to an infectious disease	*TB*
cause of secondary of TB	*reactivation of a previous primary TB site*
site of reactivation of TB	*apex of the lungs where the oxygen concentration is highest*
extrapulmonary site for TB	*kidneys*
complications of TB in the lungs	*miliary spread in the lungs* (invasion into the bronchus or PA), *systemic miliary spread* (invasion of the pulmonary vein), *scar carcinoma* (usually an adenocarcinoma), *massive hemoptysis, bronchiectasis* (most common cause worldwide), *secondary amyloidosis*
type of TB in AIDS	*Mycobacterium avium-intracellulare*
atypical mycobacteria that produce lung disease	***Mycobacterium avium-intracellulare*** and *Mycobacterium kansasii*
parasitic diseases involving the lungs	*larval phases of ascaris, hookworms, and strongyloides when they migrate through the lungs; lung tapeworm (Paragonimus westermani); pulmonary infarctions due to Dirofilaria immitis; pleurocavitary disease in Entamoeba histolytica*

Table 11–4. RESPIRATORY TRACT INFECTIONS *Continued*

Most Common...	Answer and Explanation
cause of pulmonary abscesses	*aspiration of infected oropharyngeal material or infected teeth* [Other causes include pneumonias associated with *Staphylococcus aureus* and *Klebsiella pneumoniae*.]

Question: Pneumonia in a military recruit who has low-grade fever, flu-like symptoms, and bullous myringitis is most likely due to which of the following:
(A) Influenzavirus
(B) *Mycoplasma pneumoniae*
(C) *Chlamydia pneumoniae*
(D) *Streptococcus pneumoniae*
(E) Respiratory syncytial virus

Answer: (B): The history suggests an atypical pneumonia and the presence of crowded conditions, and bullous myringitis specifically points to *M. pneumoniae* over the other choices listed.

AIDS = acquired immunodeficiency syndrome, CBC = complete blood cell count, CF = cardiac failure, COD = cause of death, PA = pulmonary artery, TB = tuberculosis.

Table 11–5. OBSTRUCTIVE AND RESTRICTIVE LUNG DISEASES, LUNG CANCER, MEDIASTINAL DISORDERS, DISEASES OF THE PLEURA

Most Common...	Answer and Explanation
cause of ILD	*pneumoconioses* (dust diseases) [Other causes include *sarcoidosis, hypersensitivity pneumonitides, drugs, noninfectious interstitial pneumonias, collagen-vascular diseases, alveolar filling disorders*.]
cause of "black lung" disease	*inhalation of anthracotic pigment* [Alveolar macrophages containing the pigment are coughed up in sputum (called "dust cells").]
complication of CWP	*simple CWP* (nodular fibrotic opacities <1 cm) [Other complications: *progressive massive fibrosis* (PMF; opacities >1 cm; incapacitating disease), *centrilobular emphysema in the upper lobes, predisposition for TB but not lung cancer, cor pulmonale, Caplan syndrome* (rheumatoid lung disease + CWP)]

Table continued on following page

Table 11–5. OBSTRUCTIVE AND RESTRICTIVE LUNG DISEASES, LUNG CANCER, MEDIASTINAL DISORDERS, DISEASES OF THE PLEURA *Continued*

Most Common...	Answer and Explanation
complication of silicosis [inhalation of silicon dioxide; foundry workers; sandblasters]	*nodulation in the lung* (fibrotic nodules with quartz crystals) [Other complications: *"egg shell" calcification of hilar lymph nodes, Caplan syndrome, PMF, increased incidence of TB, not cancer.*]
cause of ferruginous bodies in sputum	*inhalation of asbestos minerals (chrysotile and crocidolite), which become coated by iron*
complication of asbestosis [roofers, pipefitters, old insulation]	*primary lung cancer* (smoking enhances this complication) [Other complications: *pleural plaques* (most common pleural lesion), *mesothelioma* (no smoking relationship).]
cause of farmer's lung [hypersensitivity pneumonitis]	*inhalation of thermophilic actinomycetes* [It begins as a localized Arthus reaction (type III IC disease) and progresses to granuloma formation (type IV]).]
cause of silo filler's disease [hypersensitivity pneumonitis]	*inhalation of nitrous oxide fumes*
cause of bagassosis [hypersensitivity pneumonitis]	*exposure to moldy sugar cane*
cause of "Monday morning blues"	*byssinosis, referring to exposure to cotton, hemp, or linen in the textile industry* [Reactions occur when patients return to work on Monday.]
long-term effect of noninfectious interstitial pneumonias [fibrosing alveolitis; DIP, UIP, LIP]	*Hamman-Rich lung* [Diffuse interstitial fibrosis leaves the alveoli fibrosed and the proximal terminal bronchioles dilated (honeycomb effect). A chest radiograph reveals "ground glass" opacification.]
noninfectious granulomatous lung disease	*sarcoidosis* [It is more common in blacks than whites and primarily targets the lungs. It is a noncaseating granulomatous disease.]

**Table 11–5. OBSTRUCTIVE AND RESTRICTIVE LUNG
DISEASES, LUNG CANCER, MEDIASTINAL DISORDERS,
DISEASES OF THE PLEURA** Continued

Most Common...	Answer and Explanation
S/S in sarcoidosis	*tachypnea/dyspnea* [Other S/S include *fever, uveitis, cranial nerve palsies, lacrimal and salivary gland enlargement, granulomatous hepatitis, myocarditis, diabetes insipidus.*]
radiographic findings in sarcoidosis	*bilateral hilar node lymphadenopathy* ("potato nodes"), *reticulonodular densities*
lab findings in sarcoidosis	*increased ACE* [Other findings include *hypercalcemia* (lymphocytes in granulomas synthesize 1-α-hydroxylase → hypervitaminosis D), *hypercalciuria* (renal stones), *polyclonal gammopathy, cutaneous anergy* (decreased CD_4 helper cells), *positive Kveim test* (intradermal injection of sarcoid antigens).]
drugs causing ILD	*amiodarone, bleomycin, busulfan, cyclophosphamide, methotrexate, methysergide, nitrofurantoin*
collagen vascular diseases producing ILD	*PSS* [Others: *RA* (nodules, effusions, Caplan's syndrome), *SLE*]
ILD associated with hemoptysis and renal failure	*Goodpasture's syndrome* [It begins in the lungs and usually progresses into the kidneys, leading to renal failure. Anti-basement membrane antibodies are produced against the pulmonary and glomerular capillaries.]
cause of COPD	*cigarette smoking* [10–15% of smokers develop COPD.]
types of COPD	*CB/emphysema* [Other types: *bronchial asthma, bronchiectasis, CF*]
type of COPD that is a clinical diagnosis	*CB* [It is defined as productive cough for at least 3 months for 2 consecutive years.]
sites and microscopic findings in CB	*segmental bronchi* (increased mucus production, gland hyperplasia, goblet cell hyperplasia, squamous metaplasia), *terminal bronchioles* (primary site of obstruction; goblet cell metaplasia, mucus plugs, smooth muscle hypertrophy, fibrosis)

Table continued on following page

Table 11–5. OBSTRUCTIVE AND RESTRICTIVE LUNG DISEASES, LUNG CANCER, MEDIASTINAL DISORDERS, DISEASES OF THE PLEURA *Continued*

Most Common...	Answer and Explanation
pathophysiologic abnormality in CB	*V̇/Q̇ mismatch* [Since it is more centrally located than emphysema, a much larger area of gas exchange is involved, which leads to respiratory acidosis and hypoxemia.]
site of damage in emphysema	*respiratory unit consisting of the respiratory bronchioles, alveolar ducts, and alveoli*
site of damage of centrilobular emphysema	*elastic tissue destruction of the respiratory bronchioles in the upper lobe* (most common type of emphysema) [Smoking and CWP are the most common causes.]
site of damage of panacinar emphysema	*elastic tissue destruction of the entire respiratory unit in the lower lobes* [AAT deficiency due to smoking (chemicals denature AAT) and an AR disease are the most common causes.]
site of damage of paraseptal emphysema	*elastic tissue damage of the alveolar duct and alveoli* [Subpleural blebs commonly occur, which can be the cause of a spontaneous pneumothorax.]
cause of irregular emphysema	*scar tissue causing localized cystic spaces*
changes in the lungs in old age	*overinflation of the lung with mild obstructive-type PFTs* [It is called senile emphysema but is a normal age-dependent change in the lungs.]
chronic respiratory disease in children	*bronchial asthma* [Bronchial asthma is an episodic, hyper-reactive, reversible, small airway disease (terminal bronchioles). Histologic changes are similar to CB except for an increase in eosinophils in type I hypersensitivity-related asthma.]
cause of bronchial asthma	*exposure to allergens* (type I hypersensitivity) [Other causes: *aspirin* (triad asthma; nonimmunogenic), *cold temperature, exercise, environmental pollutants*]
cause of Curschmann's spirals and Charcot-Leyden crystals in sputum	*bronchial asthma* [The former are due to mucus plugs intermixed with epithelial cells, while the latter are composed of the crystalline material within eosinophils.]

Table 11–5. OBSTRUCTIVE AND RESTRICTIVE LUNG DISEASES, LUNG CANCER, MEDIASTINAL DISORDERS, DISEASES OF THE PLEURA *Continued*

Most Common...	Answer and Explanation
S/S in asthma	*wheezing* [Other S/S: *cough* (common at night), *increased AP diameter.* Respiratory alkalosis occurs first but may progress to respiratory acidosis if bronchospasm is not relieved.]
cause of bronchiectasis	*CF* (in the United States). [Other causes: **TB** (worldwide), *B cell immunodeficiencies, immotile cilia syndrome* (absent dynein arm, situs inversus; Kartagener's syndrome)]
pathophysiologic abnormalities causing bronchiectasis	*obstruction and infection* [Obstruction and infection lead to weakening of the wall and dilatation. Bronchi and bronchioles are filled with pus and extend to the periphery of the lungs.]
S/S in bronchiectasis	*cough productive of copious sputum* [Other S/S: *hemoptysis, fever, cerebral abscess*]
COD in CF	*respiratory failure secondary to pulmonary infections*
respiratory manifestations of CF	*bronchiolitis* (initial infection), *pneumonia* (*Staphylococcus aureus, Haemophilus influenzae, Pseudomonas aeruginosa, Burkholderia cepacia*), *cor pulmonale, bronchiectasis*
COD due to cancer in men and women	*primary lung cancer*
lung cancer	*metastasis from breast cancer*
primary lung cancer	*adenocarcinoma* [Other cancers: *squamous cell carcinoma, small cell carcinoma*]
cause of primary lung cancer	*cigarette smoking* [Other causes include *arsenic, exposure to uranium* (radon gas), *chromates, asbestos, beryllium, vitamin A deficiency.*]
oncogenes involved in small cell cancer	*point mutations leading to inactivation of the p53 suppressor gene and the* ras *oncogene*

Table continued on following page

Table 11–5. OBSTRUCTIVE AND RESTRICTIVE LUNG DISEASES, LUNG CANCER, MEDIASTINAL DISORDERS, DISEASES OF THE PLEURA *Continued*

Most Common...	Answer and Explanation
centrally located primary lung cancers	*squamous and small cell cancer* [These cancers have the greatest relationship with cigarette smoking.]
peripherally located primary lung cancer	*adenocarcinoma* [Bronchioloalveolar cancers have no relationship to smoking, while other types have a slightly greater risk.]
primary lung cancer in non-smokers	*adenocarcinoma*
ectopic hormone–secreting primary lung cancers	**small cell carcinoma** (ACTH [ectopic Cushing's syndrome], ADH [inappropriate ADH syndrome]) and *squamous carcinoma* (PTH-like peptide [hypercalcemia])
primary lung cancer confused with a lobar pneumonia	*bronchioloalveolar carcinoma* [It is derived from nonciliated epithelium (Clara cells).]
cytologic findings in squamous and small cell cancers	*Pap stains reveal deeply eosinophilic staining squamous cells in squamous cell cancers and small, basophilic staining cells in small cell carcinoma*
S/S of primary lung cancer	*cough* [Other S/S: *weight loss, chest pain, hemoptysis*]
site of metastasis of primary lung cancer outside the lungs	*adrenal glands* [Other sites: *liver, brain, bone*]
cause of the superior vena caval syndrome	*primary small cell carcinoma with invasion and compression of the superior vena cava*
cause of the Pancoast syndrome	*primary squamous cell carcinoma* [The syndrome is due to invasion of the brachial plexus (T1 and T2) and cervical sympathetic ganglion, the latter associated with Horner's syndrome (ipsilateral lid lag, miosis, absence of sweating).]
primary lung cancer that is not usually treated by surgery	*small cell carcinoma* [Most of these cancers are already disseminated when initially discovered.]
symptom of lung metastasis	*dyspnea* [Hemoptysis is uncommon.]

Table 11–5. OBSTRUCTIVE AND RESTRICTIVE LUNG DISEASES, LUNG CANCER, MEDIASTINAL DISORDERS, DISEASES OF THE PLEURA *Continued*

Most Common...	Answer and Explanation
primary neuro-endocrine tumor of lung with a low-grade malignant potential	*bronchial carcinoid* [They have no relation-ship to smoking. ~40% metastasize locally. They rarely produce the carcinoid syn-drome.]
overall cause of a solitary coin lesion in the lungs	*granulomatous disease* (e.g., TB, histoplas-mosis) [Most are benign if the patient is <35 years old, whereas most are malignant if the patient is >50 years old. Calcifications and lack of growth are benign features.]
hamartoma in the lungs	*bronchial hamartoma* [They are a localized overgrowth of cartilage and have a "popcorn" type of configuration on a chest radiograph.]
mediastinal compartment involved with disease	*anterior mediastinum* (**thymoma,** *malignant lymphoma*)
tumors in the mediastinum	*neurogenic tumors* (e.g., neuroblastoma in chil-dren, ganglioneuroma in adults), *which are most commonly in the posterior mediastinum*
mediastinal tumor associated with myasthenia gravis and pure RBC aplasia	*thymomas* [They are most commonly located in the anterior mediastinum. Thymic hyper-plasia (germinal follicles composed of B cells that synthesize antibodies against acetylcho-line receptors) is more common than thymo-mas in myasthenia gravis.]
anterior mediastinal tumor in a woman with axillary lymph node enlargement	*nodular sclerosing Hodgkin's disease* [It usu-ally involves a single lymph node group in the axilla, neck, or supraclavicular region + the anterior mediastinum.]
disorder in the middle mediastinum	*pericardial cyst*
lab findings that distinguish a transudate from an exudate in pleural fluid	*it is an exudate if any one of the following are present: PF protein to serum protein ratio >0.5; PF LDH to serum LDH >0.6; PF LDH two thirds the upper limit of normal of the serum LDH* [Values less than the above indi-cate a transudate.]

Table continued on following page

**Table 11–5. OBSTRUCTIVE AND RESTRICTIVE LUNG
DISEASES, LUNG CANCER, MEDIASTINAL DISORDERS,
DISEASES OF THE PLEURA** *Continued*

Most Common...	Answer and Explanation
cause of a pleural effusion	*CHF* (transudate)
cause of PF exudates	*pneumonia* [Other causes: *pulmonary infarction* (hemorrhagic exudate), *cancer* (hemorrhagic exudate)]
PF findings in TB	*exudate with a lymphocyte-dominant cell count*
cause of increased amylase in the PF	**acute pancreatitis** (left-sided PF), *Boerhaave's syndrome*
primary malignancy of pleura	*mesothelioma secondary to asbestos exposure* [They have an extremely poor prognosis and no relation to smoking.]

Question: Which of the following is primarily an obstructive type of lung disease?
  (A) Silicosis
  (B) Sarcoidosis
  (C) CF
  (D) Farmer's lung
  (E) Asbestosis

Answer: (C): CF is primarily an obstructive lung disease, while all the other choices are examples of ILD.

AAT = α-1 antitrypsin, ACE = angiotensin converting enzyme, ACTH = adrenocorticotropic hormone, ADH = antidiuretic hormone, AP = anteroposterior, AR = autosomal recessive, CB = chronic bronchitis, CF = cystic fibrosis, CHF = congestive heart failure, COD = cause of death, COPD = chronic obstructive pulmonary disease, CWP = coal worker's pneumoconiosis, DIP = desquamative interstitial pneumonitis, IC = immunocomplex, ILD = interstitial lung disease, LDH = lactate dehydrogenase, LIP = lymphoid interstitial pneumonitis (common in children with AIDS; ? EBV/HIV-related), PF = pleural fluid, PFT = pulmonary function tests, PSS = progressive systemic sclerosis, PTH = parathyroid hormone, RA = rheumatoid arthritis, RBC = red blood cell, SLE = systemic lupus erythematosus, S/S = signs and symptoms, TB = tuberculosis, UIP = usual interstitial pneumonitis, V/Q̇ = ventilation-perfusion.

CHAPTER

12

HEMATOPATHOLOGY

CONTENTS

Table 12–1. HEMATOPOIESIS

Most Common...	Answer and Explanation
site of hematopoiesis at birth	*bone marrow* [In the fetus, the sequence for hematopoiesis is yolk sac, liver, spleen, and bone marrow by the 5th month.]
stem cell involved in the pathogenesis of aplastic anemia and PRV	*trilineage myeloid stem cell* [Derived from the pluripotential stem cell, this stem cell divides into stem cells producing RBCs, WBCs, and platelets. Suppression of this stem cell leads to aplastic anemia and over-activity to PRV.]
interleukin stimulating hematopoiesis	*IL-3* [It acts directly on the pluripotential stem cell, which divides into a lymphoid stem cell and trilineage myeloid stem cell.]
skull abnormalities noted in severe hemolytic anemias	*owing to expansion of the marrow cavity from enhanced RBC hyperplasia* (e.g., sickle cell anemia), *skull abnormalities include a "chipmunk face" (zygomatic arch), frontal bossing, and a skull radiograph with a "hair on end" appearance*
sites for extramedullary [outside the marrow] hematopoiesis	**spleen** *and liver* [Marrow replacement by fibrosis (myelofibrosis) or hematopoiesis beyond the capacity of the marrow are the most common causes of this alteration.]

Table continued on following page

243

Table 12–1. HEMATOPOIESIS *Continued*

Most Common...	Answer and Explanation
site for erythropoietin synthesis	*kidneys* [There is a minor contribution from the liver. Erythropoietin stimulates marrow erythropoiesis.]
stimuli for accelerated erythropoiesis	*tissue hypoxia secondary to hypoxemia* (low PaO_2) [Other causes: *severe anemia, left-shifted ODC*]
PB finding of accelerated erythropoiesis	*marrow reticulocytes (shift cells; blue discoloration called polychromasia)* [These RBCs contain RNA filaments that are visible with supravital stains. They require 2–3 days to become mature RBCs in the PB.]
cause of ineffective erythropoiesis [destruction of RBCs within the marrow by macrophages]	B_{12} *and folate deficiency* [Other causes include severe thalassemia and myelodysplastic syndrome.]
shape of a mature RBC	*biconcave disk*
biochemical functions in a mature RBC	*anaerobic glycolysis* (lactate is the end-product), *pentose phosphate shunt* (synthesis of glutathione and NADPH), *methemoglobin reductase system* (reduces heme iron from $+3$ to $+2$), *synthesis of 2,3-BPG* (right-shifts the ODC) [They lack mitochondria, nuclei, and class I and II antigens.]
mechanism for removal of senescent, abnormally shaped, or IgG/C3-coated RBCs	*extravascular hemolysis by macrophages in the* **spleen,** *liver* (C3 coated), and *bone marrow* [The end-product of macrophage destruction is unconjugated bilirubin (UCB), which binds to albumin in the PB and is conjugated in the liver.]
end-products of accelerated intravascular hemolysis	*Hb in the plasma and urine, hemosiderin in the urine* from breakdown of Hb in renal tubular cells, *methemalbumin* (methemoglobin bound to albumin)
liver-derived protein that is consumed by intravascular hemolysis	*haptoglobin* [It complexes with free Hb and is removed by macrophages. Low haptoglobin indicates intravascular hemolysis.]
enzyme marker of intravascular hemolysis	*lactate dehydrogenase*

Table 12–1. HEMATOPOIESIS *Continued*

Most Common...	Answer and Explanation
bone marrow calculation representing total erythropoiesis	*myeloid to erythroid ratio* (M/E ratio), which is normally 3:1
PB finding indicating effective erythropoiesis [good marrow response to anemia]	*presence of PB reticulocytes* [Similar to marrow reticulocytes, these reticulocytes also contain RNA filaments. Unlike marrow reticulocytes, they only require 24 hours to become mature RBCs and they are normally colored with the standard Wright-Giemsa stain.]
formula used to correct the reticulocyte count for the degree of anemia	*patient Hct/45 × %reticulocyte count* [For example: Hct 30%, reticulocyte count 15%: 30/45 × 15 = 10%. A good marrow response to anemia is >3%, while a poor response is <2%.]
formula used to calculate the reticulocyte index when marrow reticulocytes are present in the PB	*same formula as above, except the final answer is divided by 2* [Since it is important to determine the 24-hour-old PB reticulocyte count and marrow reticulocytes require 2–3 days to become mature RBCs, their presence falsely increases the overall reticulocyte count (both PB and marrow reticulocytes have RNA filaments), hence the need to further divide the initial count by 2.]
cells in the mitotic, postmitotic, and PB granulocyte pools	*mitotic pool*: myeloblasts, progranulocytes, myelocytes; *postmitotic pool*: metamyelocytes, band and segmented neutrophils; *PB pool*: segmented and band neutrophils (50% circulating and 50% adhering to the endothelium [marginating pool])
enzyme marker of a mature neutrophil	*leukocyte alkaline phosphatase* (LAP)
cause of a left-shifted neutrophil count	*release of the postmitotic pool into the PB by interleukin-1* [Left shift implies a shift to immature neutrophils (>10% bands or younger cells).]
nonpathologic cause of an increased PB marginating pool of granulocytes	*black race* (normal finding) [It produces neutropenia.]

Table continued on following page

Table 12–1. HEMATOPOIESIS *Continued*

Most Common...	Answer and Explanation
cause of a decreased PB marginating pool of granulocytes	*corticosteroids* [Other causes: *catecholamines, lithium, alcohol.* Neutrophilic leukocytosis occurs.]
circulating lymphocytes	*T cells (60–80%), with twice as many CD_4 cells as CD_8 cells.* 10–20% are B cells and 5–10% natural killer cells
platelet markers	*ABO blood groups, PL_{A1} antigens, class I antigens* [They lack Rh antigens.]
Hb at birth	*Hb F* (fetal Hb; 2α 2γ globin chains; 70–90%)
adult Hbs	in decreasing concentration: **Hb A** (2α 2β), *Hb A_2 (2α 2δ), Hb F (2α 2γ)*
Hb disorder resulting in cyanosis	*(deoxyhemoglobin >5 g/dL* [Other causes: *metHb >1.5 g/dL, sulfhemoglobin >0.5 g/dL.*]
rule relating the Hb and Hct	*rule of 3, which states that the Hb $\times$ 3 = Hct*
microcytic anemia with an increased RBC count	α *and* β *thalassemias* [It may be secondary to a left shift in the ODC and erythropoietin stimulation of RBC production.]
RBC index used to classify anemia	*mean corpuscular volume* (MCV) [It is an average size of an RBC passing through an aperture. Anemias are microcytic, normocytic, or macrocytic.]
RBC index paralleling the degree of pallor of an RBC in the PB	*mean corpuscular Hb concentration (MCHC)* [A low MCHC indicates decreased Hb concentration (microcytic anemias) and increased MCHC, an increase in Hb concentration in the RBC (e.g., spherocytes).]
MCV finding in the presence of microcytic and macrocytic RBCs	*normal MCV* [Since the instrument takes an average of the RBCs, the MCV is normal. The RDW is increased (see below).]
use of the RBC distribution width (RDW)	*estimating the degree of variation in RBC sizes* [An increase in the RDW represents significant RBC size variation (anisocytosis); therefore, in the presence of microcytic and macrocytic RBCs, it is increased.]

Table 12–1. HEMATOPOIESIS *Continued*

Most Common...	Answer and Explanation
microcytic anemia with an increase in the RDW	*iron deficiency anemia* [It progresses from a normocytic to microcytic anemia, hence the variation in RBC size.]
effect of phenytoin on WBCs	*produces an atypical (antigenically stimulated) lymphocytosis*
effect of corticosteroids on WBCs	*absolute neutrophilic leukocytosis, lymphopenia,* and *eosinopenia*
stain used for iron	*Prussian blue*
cause of a dry (no cells) bone marrow aspirate	*inadequate placement of the needle* [Pathologic causes include myelofibrosis, leukemia.]

Question: Which of the following would most likely result in an increase in PB reticulocytes? **SELECT 3**
  (A) Aplastic anemia
  (B) Iron deficiency
  (C) B_{12} deficiency
  (D) Blood loss >1 week
  (E) Folate deficiency
  (F) Hemolytic anemia
  (G) Marrow invasion by tumor

Answers: (D), (F), (G): The marrow must be free of disease (stem cells) must be present; no tumor cells pushing cells out) and have adequate raw materials for erythropoiesis (iron, B_{12}, folate). Hence, choices (D), (F), and (G) would increase the PB reticulocyte response while all the other choices would not.

BPG = bisphosphoglycerate, Hb = hemoglobin, Hct = hematocrit, Ig = immunoglobulin, IL-3 = interleukin-3, metHb = methemoglobin, NADPH = nicotinamide-adenine dinucleotide phosphate (reduced form), ODC = oxygen dissociation curve, PaO_2 = partial pressure of oxygen, PB = peripheral blood, PRV = polycythemia rubra vera, RBC = red blood cell, WBC = white blood cell.

Table 12–2. GENERAL ASPECTS OF ANEMIA AND MICROCYTIC ANEMIAS

Most Common...	Answer and Explanation
overall cause of anemia	*iron deficiency anemia due to GI blood loss*
symptom of anemia	*dyspnea with exertion* [Other findings include dizziness, palpitations, insomnia.]
effect of anemia on the O_2 content of blood	*decreased* [The O_2 content is decreased because the Hb concentration is decreased (O_2 content = [1.34 × **Hb**] × SaO_2 + PaO_2). The SaO_2 and PaO_2 are normal (see Chapter 2).]
cause of physiologic anemia in infants	*replacement of RBCs with HbF by RBCs with adult HbA* [The drop occurs primarily between the 2nd and 3rd month in full-term infants.]
mechanism for producing a microcytic anemia	*reduced Hb synthesis* [It causes the developing RBCs in the marrow to undergo extra divisions.]
microcytic anemia	*iron deficiency* [Other causes include *anemia of chronic disease* (ACD), *thalassemia*, and *sideroblastic anemias.*]
effect of iron stores on transferrin synthesis in the liver	*low iron stores increase transferrin synthesis* (binding protein for iron), *whereas high iron stores decrease transferrin synthesis* [Transferrin is measured as the total iron binding capacity (TIBC). It is high in iron deficiency and low in ACD and iron overload diseases.]
effect of intracellular heme [iron + protoporphyrin] on uptake of iron by the developing RBC	*decreased heme increases the uptake of iron, whereas increased heme decreases the uptake of iron*
storage form of iron in macrophages	*ferritin* [A small circulating fraction can be measured, indicating iron stores. Ferritin is also stored in hepatocytes, which require iron for heme in the cytochrome system.]
valence of iron in meat versus vegetables	*in meat, heme iron is* + *2* (ferrous), which is directly reabsorbed in the duodenum; *plant iron is non-heme with a valence of* + *3* (ferric) and must be reduced by ascorbic acid to + 2 for reabsorption in the duodenum.

Table 12–2. GENERAL ASPECTS OF ANEMIA AND MICROCYTIC ANEMIAS *Continued*

Most Common...	Answer and Explanation
effect of pregnancy on iron stores	*without supplements, a woman loses ~500 mg per pregnancy* [Normal iron stores in a woman only amount to ~400 mg.]
microcytic anemias due to a decreased amount of circulating iron	**iron deficiency** (absent iron stores), *ACD* (increased iron stores; iron is blocked in macrophages)
lab findings in iron deficiency	*low serum iron, high TIBC, low % saturation* (iron/TIBC × 100), *low serum ferritin* (single best test), *high RDW* [The laboratory abnormalities occur first (ferritin is the first of these abnormalities), then there is a normocytic, and, finally, a microcytic anemia.]
lab findings in ACD	*low serum iron, decreased TIBC, decreased % saturation, increased ferritin, normal RDW* [The TIBC and ferritin distinguish ACD from iron deficiency.]
causes of iron deficiency in premature infants	*premature delivery* (deprives the fetus of daily iron)
cause of iron deficiency in term newborns	*bleeding Meckel's diverticulum*
cause of iron deficiency in children ~1 year old	*nutritional from drinking too much milk*
cause of iron deficiency in children	*bleeding Meckel's diverticulum*
cause of iron deficiency in women <50 yrs old	*menorrhagia*
cause of iron deficiency in men <50 years old	*peptic ulcer disease*
cause of iron deficiency in men/women >50 years old	*GI cancer*

Table continued on following page

Table 12–2. GENERAL ASPECTS OF ANEMIA AND MICROCYTIC ANEMIAS *Continued*

Most Common...	Answer and Explanation
causes of ACD	**chronic inflammation** (e.g., rheumatoid arthritis), *malignancy* (most common anemia)
cause of koilonychia (spoon nails) and Plummer-Vinson syndrome	*iron deficiency* [Plummer-Vinson syndrome is associated with esophageal webs (dysphagia for solids), and achlorhydria.]
treatment of iron deficiency and ACD	*ferrous sulfate in the former and treating the underlying disease in the latter* (iron is not useful)
microcytic anemia due to a defect in globin chain synthesis	*thalassemia (thal), which most commonly involves either α (α-thal) or β (β-thal) globin chains* [α-Thal occurs in Asians and blacks, while β-thal occurs in blacks, Italians, and Greeks.]
cause of α-thal	*AR disease with gene deletions on chromosome 16* [Four genes control α-globin chain synthesis. *One gene deletion*: normal MCV; *two gene deletions*: mild microcytic anemia; *three gene deletions*: HbH disease (HbH = 4 β chains); *four gene deletions*: Hb Bart's disease (incompatible with life; Hb Bart = 4 γ chains).]
cause of β-thal	*AR disease most commonly due to a splicing defect of β-globin chains on chromosome 11* (splicing defects are most common) [Clinical severity ranges from minor, to intermediate, to major.]
Hb electrophoresis findings in α-thal	*no abnormalities are noted in 1–2 gene deletion types of α-thal* [HbA, A_2, and F all need α chains, hence all are equally decreased. HbH and Hb Bart's can be identified. In mild disease, the iron studies are normal, RDW normal, and RBC counts increased.]
Hb electrophoresis findings in β-thal	*a decrease in HbA and an increase in Hbs A_2 and F* [Since only β chains are decreased, δ and γ chains are normally produced and combine with α chains to form HbA_2 and F, respectively. In mild disease, the iron studies are normal, RDW normal, and RBC counts increased.]

Table 12–2. GENERAL ASPECTS OF ANEMIA AND MICROCYTIC ANEMIAS *Continued*

Most Common...	Answer and Explanation
cause of sideroblastic anemia	*alcohol abuse* [Other causes include pyridoxine (B_6) deficiency (most often due to isoniazid therapy) and Pb poisoning. Sideroblasts refer to excess iron in the mitochondria in developing normoblasts.]
mechanisms producing sideroblastic anemias	*defect in synthesizing heme; iron enters the mitochondria but cannot get out, hence forming ringed sideroblasts* [Alcohol is a mitochondrial poison, therefore disrupting heme synthesis. B_6 is required to synthesize Δ-ALA from glycine and succinyl CoA. Pb denatures chelatase, which combines iron with protoporphyrin. Since heme is decreased, iron readily enters the mitochondria where it is trapped, producing *ringed sideroblasts* (mitochondria encircle the nucleus) and iron overload in the marrow.]
cause of Pb poisoning in children and adults	*children*: eating Pb-based paint or plaster *adults*: incineration of car batteries, working with pottery
S/S of Pb poisoning in children and adults	*children*: Pb poisoning targets the brain (edema, learning defects), bone (densities in the epiphyses), and GI tract (colic; radiographs identify Pb) *adults*: Pb targets peripheral nerves, the gums (Pb line), and the kidneys (proximal renal tubular acidosis, urate nephropathy)
lab findings in Pb poisoning	*high blood Pb level* (best screening and confirmatory test combined); *iron overload*: high serum iron, low TIBC (increased iron stores decrease transferrin synthesis), high % saturation, high serum ferritin; *normal RDW*; *coarse basophilic stippling of RBCs* (Pb denatures ribonuclease, so ribosomes remain in the RBCs); *high FEP* (protoporphyrin increases behind the blocked chelatase)
treatment of Pb poisoning	*EDTA, BAL* [Some clinicians recommend *penicillamine* as well.]
lab findings in sideroblastic anemias other than Pb poisoning	*bone marrow exam demonstrates ringed sideroblasts* (necessary for the diagnosis) and *iron studies are similar to those of Pb poisoning*

Table continued on following page

Table 12–2. GENERAL ASPECTS OF ANEMIA AND MICROCYTIC ANEMIAS *Continued*

Question: Which of the following are **LEAST** useful in differentiating iron deficiency, ACD, α- and β-thal, and Pb poisoning from each other? **SELECT 4**

(A) MCV
(B) Serum ferritin
(C) Hb electrophoresis
(D) RBC count
(E) Bone marrow aspirate
(F) RDW
(G) Peripheral smear exam
(H) FEP
(I) Hb concentration

Answers: (B), (E), (H), (I): The serum ferritin (choice B) is low only in iron deficiency, high in ACD and Pb poisoning, and normal in the mild thalassemias. The MCV (choice A) and Hb concentration (choice I) are low in all microcytic anemias. Hb electrophoresis (choice C) and a high RBC count (choice D) are useful in separating the thalassemias. A bone marrow aspirate (choice E) is not cost effective for any of the microcytic anemias. FEP (choice H) no longer has any use in Pb poisoning and is not useful in any of the other types either. The RDW (choice F) is increased only in iron deficiency.

ALA = aminolevulinic acid, AR = autosomal recessive, BAL = British anti-Lewisite, EDTA = ethylenediaminetetraacetic acid, FEP = free erythrocyte protoporphyrin, GI = gastrointestinal, Hb = hemoglobin, MCV = mean corpuscular volume, PaO$_2$ = partial pressure of arterial oxygen, Pb = lead, RBC = red blood cell, RDW = RBC distribution width, SaO$_2$ = arterial oxygen saturation, S/S = signs and symptoms.

Table 12–3. MACROCYTIC ANEMIAS

Most Common...	Answer and Explanation
cause of macrocytic anemia	*folate deficiency in an alcoholic* [Other causes include B_{12} deficiency, hypothyroidism, toxic effect of alcohol.]
sources of folate and B_{12}	*folate is present in plant and animal products, while B_{12} is only present in animal products* [Both are required for DNA synthesis, so deficiency leads to a large, immature nucleus and a *megaloblastic anemia*.]
drugs interfering with absorption of folate in the jejunum	*phenytoin and birth control pills* [Phenytoin inhibits intestinal conjugase, which must convert folate from its polyglutamate form into a monoglutamate form for absorption in the jejunum. BCPs interfere with the uptake of monoglutamates in the jejunum.]

Table 12–3. MACROCYTIC ANEMIAS *Continued*

Most Common...	Answer and Explanation
factor required for the absorption of B_{12}	*intrinsic factor (IF)* [It is synthesized in the parietal cells of the body and fundus of the stomach. R factor combines with B_{12} to prevent acid destruction. R factor is cleaved off from B_{12} in the duodenum by pancreatic enzymes. IF then binds with B_{12} to form a complex that is reabsorbed in the terminal ileum.]
functions of B_{12} related to folate metabolism	*it cleaves off the methyl group of N^5-methyl FH_4 (circulating form of folate) to form FH_4,* which is used in synthesizing deoxythymidine monophosphate in DNA synthesis [Methyl-B_{12} (cobalamin) transfers the methyl group to homocysteine, which is converted into methionine. A decrease in B_{12} or *folate* increases plasma homocysteine (damages endothelial cells, leading to thrombosis).]
drugs that block dihydrofolate reductase	*methotrexate and trimethoprim* [FH_4 is converted to $N^{5,10}$ methylene FH_4 (substrate specifically required for DNA synthesis; citrovorum factor replaces this substrate), which, in turn, becomes dihydrofolate. Dihydrofolate is reduced by a reductase to FH_4, which is reutilized for DNA synthesis.]
function of B_{12} in propionate metabolism	*propionate (odd chain fatty acid) is converted to propionyl CoA → methylmalonyl CoA → succinyl CoA, the latter reaction requiring B_{12}* [B_{12} deficiency causes a buildup of methylmalonic acid (excellent screening test for B_{12} deficiency only) and propionates, which cause demyelination of the dorsal columns and lateral corticospinal tracts and dementia.]
cause of folate deficiency	*nutritional deficiency* (e.g., *alcohol abuse* [excluding beer, which is rich in folates]) [Other causes: *goat's milk, small bowel disease* (e.g., celiac disease), *drugs* (see above), *overutilization* (e.g., pregnancy, cancer)]
cause of B_{12} deficiency	*pernicious anemia* (PA) [Other causes include *pure vegan diet, fish tapeworm, bacterial overgrowth, chronic pancreatitis, terminal ileal disease* (e.g., Crohn's disease).]
S/S in folate and B_{12} deficiency	*glossitis* (smooth, sore tongue), *signs associated with anemia*

Table continued on following page

Table 12–3. MACROCYTIC ANEMIAS *Continued*

Most Common...	Answer and Explanation
S/S of B_{12} deficiency alone	*sallow complexion, posterior column disease* (decreased vibratory sensation, loss of proprioception), lateral corticospinal tract (upper motor neuron problems), *dementia*
S/S of PA alone	*achlorhydria, stomach cancer, autoantibodies against parietal cells and IF, correction of B_{12} absorption after giving IF*
PB findings in B_{12}/ folate deficiency	*pancytopenia* (intramarrow destruction of megaloblastic cells by macrophages), *macroovalocytes* (egg-shaped RBCs), *hypersegmented neutrophils* (>5 nuclear lobes)
lab findings in folate deficiency	*low serum folate* and *RBC folate* (better test), *high plasma homocysteine, increased urine FIGLu* (normally transfers carbons to FH_4), *high serum LDH* (destruction of RBCs), *slightly increased unconjugated bilirubin* (UCB; macrophage destruction of RBCs)
lab findings in PA	*low serum B_{12}, high plasma homocysteine, high urine methylmalonic acid* (most sensitive test), *high LDH, slightly increased UCB*
test used to localize B_{12} deficiency	**Schilling's test**: *absorption of radioactive B_{12} corrected with IF*: PA; *correction after a course of antibiotics*: bacterial overgrowth; *correction after pancreatic enzymes*: chronic pancreatitis; *no correction with the above*: rule out terminal ileal disease
treatment of folate and B_{12} deficiency	*folic acid for folate deficiency* and *intramuscular B_{12} for B_{12} deficiency* [Treatment with folate can correct the hematologic problems in B_{12} deficiency but not the neurologic problems.]

Table 12–3. MACROCYTIC ANEMIAS *Continued*

Question: Which of the following distinguishes PA from other causes of B$_{12}$ deficiency and folate deficiency? **SELECT 3**
  (A) Urine methylmalonic acid
  (B) Schilling's test
  (C) Plasma homocysteine
  (D) Antiparietal cell antibodies
  (E) Hypersegmented neutrophils
  (F) Neurologic exam
  (G) Achlorhydria

Answers: (B), (D), (G): Correction of the Schilling's test (choice B) with the addition of IF along with radioactive B$_{12}$ separates PA from other causes of B$_{12}$ deficiency and folate deficiency. Choices (D) and (G) also separate PA from the other types. The neurologic exam (choice F) is abnormal in B$_{12}$ deficiency and normal in folate deficiency. Methylmalonic acid (choice A) is increased in B$_{12}$ deficiency and FIGLu is increased in folate deficiency. Both deficiencies have hypersegmenting neutrophils (choice E) and an increase in homocysteine (choice C).

BCP = birth control pill, FH$_4$ = tetrahydrofolate, FIGLu = forminoglutamic acid, LDH = lactate dehydrogenase, PB = peripheral blood, RBC = red blood cell, S/S = signs and symptoms.

Table 12–4. NORMOCYTIC ANEMIAS

Most Common...	Answer and Explanation
initial effects of acute blood loss on the Hb concentration	*there are no effects since equal amounts of RBCs and plasma are lost* [Plasma is initially replaced and reveals the RBC deficit in a few hours to a few days. Isotonic saline reveals the deficit immediately.]
cause of acute blood loss	*GI bleed, most commonly from peptic ulcer disease* (e.g., duodenal ulcer)
known cause of aplastic anemia	*drugs* (e.g., chemotherapy, chloramphenicol) [Other causes: *infection* (NANB hepatitis), *chemicals* (benzene), *genetic* (Fanconi's anemia), *radiation, other anemias* (e.g., aplastic crises in HbSS, PNH). It is a stem cell disease with suppression of the trilineage myeloid stem cell.]
S/S in aplastic anemia	*bleeding* (thrombocytopenia), *fever* (infection secondary to neutropenia), *fatigue* (anemia)

Table continued on following page

Table 12–4. NORMOCYTIC ANEMIAS *Continued*

Most Common...	Answer and Explanation
lab findings in aplastic anemia	*normocytic anemia with corrected reticulocyte count <2%, pancytopenia, hypocellular bone marrow*
treatment for aplastic anemia	*bone marrow transplantation for patients <50 years of age* [Other modalities: *antithymocyte* and *lymphocyte globulins, cyclosporine, growth factors* (e.g., erythropoietin, CSF-GM and CSF-G, thrombopoietin)]
cause of anemia in renal disease	*deficiency of erythropoietin* [Recombinant therapy with erythropoietin is available.]
lab findings in renal disease	*normocytic anemia with corrected reticulocyte count <2%, burr cells* (undulating RBC membrane; correctable with dialysis), *prolonged bleeding time* (qualitative platelet defect)
anemia in malignancy	*ACD* [It is more commonly normocytic than microcytic.]
lab finding in hemolytic anemias	*corrected reticulocyte count >3%* (corrected for anemia and the presence or absence of marrow reticulocytes)
mechanisms of hemolysis in hemolytic anemias	**extravascular** (macrophage-induced) and *intravascular*
types of hemolytic anemias	**intrinsic** (membrane defect [congenital spherocytosis, PNH], abnormal Hb [sickle cell disease], deficient enzymes [G6PD deficiency]) or *extrinsic* (autoimmune, microangiopathic)
hemolytic anemias with predominantly extravascular hemolysis	*congenital spherocytosis, sickle cell disease, warm AIHA*
hemolytic anemias with predominantly intravascular hemolysis	*PNH, G6PD deficiency, microangiopathic hemolytic anemia, cold AIHA*
defect in congenital spherocytosis (AD)	*defect in spectrin in the RBC membrane* [The RBC has a reduced membrane, leading to formation of a sphere.]

Table 12–4. NORMOCYTIC ANEMIAS *Continued*

Most Common...	Answer and Explanation
clinical triad in congenital spherocytosis	*splenomegaly, anemia,* and *jaundice* (unconjugated hyperbilirubinemia) [Jet black calcium bilirubinate stones are commonly produced, leading to cholecystitis.]
test used to confirm congenital spherocytosis	*osmotic fragility of RBCs in various dilutions of saline* [There is increased osmotic fragility compared to normal RBCs.]
treatment of congenital spherocytosis	*splenectomy* [Pneumovax and Hib type b vaccines should be given prior to splenectomy. Spherocytes are still present after splenectomy, but they are not destroyed.]
defect in PNH	*acquired deficiency of decay accelerating factor* (DAF) [DAF normally degrades complement that deposits on RBCs, WBCs, and platelets during the night (complement attaches to cells owing to mild respiratory acidosis that occurs with sleep).]
clinical presentation of PNH	*episodic hemoglobinuria with pancytopenia*
screening and confirmatory test for PNH	*sugar water test* (screen; increases complement attachment to RBCs) and the *acidified serum test* (Ham's test), respectively
Hb disorder in blacks	*sickle cell trait and disease*
defect in sickle cell disease (AR)	*point mutation (adenine replaces thymidine), leading to a substitution of valine for glutamic acid at the sixth position of the β-globin chain*
cause of sickling of RBCs in HbSS	*increased amount of sickle Hb* [Other causes include *reduced O_2 tension, presence of other hemoglobins* (e.g., HbC), *dehydration.*]
Hb that inhibits sickling	*HbF* [Hydroxyurea therapy increases synthesis of HbF and reduces HbSS crises.]
PB RBC marker of a hemoglobinopathy	*target cells* [RBCs with excess membrane that forms a bulge in the center resembling a bull's-eye are always present in hemoglobinopathies.]

Table continued on following page

Table 12–4. NORMOCYTIC ANEMIAS *Continued*

Most Common...	Answer and Explanation
initial site for a vaso-occlusive crisis in HbSS	*hands and feet* (dactylitis) in a 6–9 month old black child [HbF prevents sickling prior to that time. Other sites for crises include the *brain* (strokes), *lungs* (acute chest syndrome), *liver, bone marrow* (aplastic crisis; low retic count), *spleen* (sequestration crisis; high retic count), *penis* (priapism).]
organism associated with an aplastic crisis in HbSS and congenital spherocytosis	*parvovirus* [It is a self-limited aplastic crisis.]
site of injury in sickle cell trait	*renal medulla* [Owing to the reduced O_2 tension, sickling may occur in peritubular capillaries, which leads to microhematuria, eventual loss of dilution/concentration, and the potential for renal papillary necrosis.]
PB finding in HbSS that indicates splenic dysfunction	*Howell-Jolly bodies* [These are nuclear remnants in RBCs that indicate splenic dysfunction, since macrophages would normally remove these from the cells. By 2–3 years of age, the spleen is nonfunctional. Splenomegaly persists into early adolescence, after which repeated infarctions cause it to be autosplenectomized.]
treatment of painful crises in HbSS	*hydration* (not blood transfusion), *analgesics,* and *oxygen*
crises in HbSS requiring blood transfusion	*acute chest syndrome* (fever, lung infiltrates, hypoxemia), *stroke, aplastic and sequestration crises*
screening tests to detect sickle cell trait	**sodium metabisulfite** (reduces O_2 tension; most sensitive test; sickle cells noted on a slide), *solubility test* (Sickledex; uses dithionite; high specificity but poor sensitivity)
confirmatory test for HbSA, HbSS, and other hemoglobinopathies	*Hb electrophoresis* (definitive test for all hemoglobinopathies) [HbSA has 60% HbA and 40% HbS (PB is normal), while HbSS has 90–95% HbS (PB has sickle cells), no HbA, and 5–10% HbF.]

Table 12–4. NORMOCYTIC ANEMIAS *Continued*

Most Common...	Answer and Explanation
prenatal method of detecting HbSS	*MSTII endonuclease testing* [Normally, the MSTII endonuclease enzyme cleaves the gene on the β-globin chain at the same mutation site involved in HbSA and HbSS. This divides a 1.35 kg segment into a 1.15 kb and a 0.2 kb segment. MSTII cannot cleave the 1.35 kb segment into these two fragments in the presence of a point mutation. In HbSA, there is (1) 1.35 kb segment (chromosome site with the point mutation), while the normal gene site is split into (1) 1.15 kb and (1) 0.2 kb segment. In HbSS, there are (2) 1.35 kb segments.]
COD in children with HbSS	*sepsis secondary to* Streptococcus pneumoniae, *and, less commonly,* Haemophilus influenzae [This underscores the importance of Pneumovax and Hib vaccination.]
defect in G6PD deficiency (SXR) causing hemolysis	*absence of GSH* [The production of GSH requires the enzyme G6PD. GSH normally neutralizes peroxide, which, if left unneutralized, denatures Hb to form Heinz bodies (identified with supravital stains) and also damages the RBC membrane.]
precipitating causes of hemolysis in G6PD deficiency	peroxide in RBCs is increased after **infections**, after taking certain *oxidizing drugs* (e.g., primaquine, dapsone), or after *eating fava beans* (Mediterranean variant)
defect in the black variant of G6PD versus the Mediterranean variant	*the black variant has defective G6PD only in the older RBCs, so hemolysis is not as severe, whereas the G6PD is defective and deficient in all RBCs in the Mediterranean variant, so hemolysis is more severe*
PB findings in G6PD deficiency	*bite cells* (macrophage removes part of the RBC membrane), *Heinz bodies* (only seen with supravital staining)
method of diagnosing G6PD deficiency in active hemolysis versus a nonhemolytic state	*in active hemolysis, Heinz bodies are present but enzyme studies are normal to increased, since only the RBCs containing enzyme remain behind. In the quiescent state, enzyme assays demonstrate low enzyme activity*

Table continued on following page

Table 12–4. NORMOCYTIC ANEMIAS *Continued*

Most Common...	Answer and Explanation
type of AIHA	**warm AIHA due to IgG antibodies in a patient with SLE**, followed by *drug-induced AIHA* [Cold AIHAs are due to IgM antibodies (primarily intravascular hemolysis; e.g., anti-i in infectious mononucleosis, anti-I in *Mycoplasma* infections).]
test used to identify an AIHA	**direct** and *indirect Coombs' test* [A direct Coombs detects IgG and/or C3 on the surface of RBCs, and the indirect Coombs identifies antibodies in the serum.]
S/S in AIHA	*fever, jaundice, generalized lymphadenopathy, and hepatosplenomegaly*
types of drug-induced AIHA	*penicillin* (IgG antibody against penicilloyl group on RBC membrane; type II hypersensitivity), *methyldopa* (autoantibody against an Rh factor; type II hypersensitivity), *quinidine* (immunocomplex destruction of RBC; type III hypersensitivity)
PB findings in AIHA	*spherocytes, shift cells* (marrow reticulocytes)
treatment of AIHAs	*avoid transfusion if possible*, **corticosteroids**, *splenectomy, alkylating agents*
cause of PCH	*a bithermal IgG antibody (called Donath-Landsteiner antibody)* [The antibody has anti-P specificity and along with complement attaches to the P antigen on RBCs in cold temperatures. The antibody detaches in warm (body) temperature, which leads to complement activation and intravascular hemolysis.]
diseases associated with PCH	*syphilis* [Other diseases: *infectious mononucleosis, mumps, and measles*]
cause of microangiopathic hemolytic anemia	*calcific aortic stenosis* [Other causes include *DIC, prosthetic heart valves, TTP, HUS, long-distance running.*]
PB finding in microangiopathic hemolytic anemia	*schistocytes* (fragmented RBCs)

Table 12–4. NORMOCYTIC ANEMIAS *Continued*

Question: Which of the following normocytic anemias have an increased corrected reticulocyte count? **SELECT 6**
(A) G6PD deficiency
(B) Sickle cell disease
(C) Chronic renal disease
(D) Congenital spherocytosis
(E) Aplastic anemia
(F) Warm AIHA
(G) Blood loss less than 1 week
(H) Anemia in a patient with aortic stenosis
(I) PNH

Answers: (A), (B), (D), (F), (H), (I): Only hemolytic anemias have an increased corrected retic count. Choices (C), (E), and (G) do not have an increased retic count.

ACD = anemia of chronic disease, AD = autosomal dominant, AIHA = autoimmune hemolytic anemia, AR = autosomal recessive, COD = cause of death, CSF-G = colony stimulating factor–granulocyte, CSF-GM = colony stimulating factor–granulocyte/macrophage, DIC = disseminated intravascular coagulation, G6PD = glucose 6-phosphate dehydrogenase, GI = gastrointestinal, GSH = glutathione, Hb = hemoglobin, HbSA = sickle cell trait, HbSS = sickle cell anemia, Hib = *Haemophilus influenzae* type b, HUS = hemolytic uremic syndrome, Ig = immunoglobulin, NANB = non-A, non-B, PB = peripheral blood, PCH = paroxysmal cold hemoglobinuria, PNH = paroxysmal nocturnal hemoglobinuria, RBC = red blood cell, SLE = systemic lupus erythematosus, S/S = signs and symptoms, SXR = sex-linked recessive, TTP = thrombotic thrombocytopenic purpura, WBC = white blood cell.

Table 12–5. WHITE BLOOD CELL DISORDERS

Most Common...	Answer and Explanation
cause of absolute neutrophilic leukocytosis [>7000 cells/µL]	*bacterial infection* (e.g., acute appendicitis, cellulitis) [Other causes: *decreased margination* (e.g., corticosteroids, catecholamines), *sterile inflammation* (e.g., AMI)]
PB findings of acute appendicitis	*absolute neutrophilic leukocytosis, toxic granulation* (prominence of azurophilic granules), and *left shift* (>10% band neutrophils)
cause of a leukemoid reaction [benign increase in WBCs >30,000 cells/µL]	*infection* (e.g., TB, whooping cough) or *malignancy* (e.g., renal adenocarcinoma) [The PB should not have myeloblasts or lymphoblasts present.]

Table continued on following page

Table 12–5. WHITE BLOOD CELL DISORDERS *Continued*

Most Common...	Answer and Explanation
cause of a leukoerythroblastic reaction [peripheralization of marrow elements]	*metastasis to bone* (e.g., breast cancer) with peripheralization of immature WBCs (e.g., myeloblasts) and RBCs (e.g., nucleated RBCs) [*Other causes: myelofibrosis, excess bone* (osteopetrosis), *multiple fractures, leukemia*]
cause of absolute neutropenia [<1500 cells/μL]	*decreased production due to drugs* (e.g., chemotherapy agents) [Other causes: *chemicals* (e.g., benzene), *increased margination* (e.g., normal finding in blacks, endotoxins), *infection* (e.g., typhoid), *destruction* (e.g., Felty's syndrome [autoimmune neutropenia + splenomegaly + rheumatoid arthritis])]
cause of absolute lymphocytosis [>8000 cells/μL in children; >4000 cells/μL in adults]	*viral infections* (e.g., HIV, infectious mononucleosis, infectious lymphocytosis) [Others: *bacterial* (e.g., *Bordetella pertussis*, TB), *Graves' disease, ALL* and *CLL, drugs* (e.g., phenytoin)]
cause of atypical lymphocytosis [antigenically stimulated lymphocytes]	*infectious mononucleosis* [Other causes: *viral hepatitis, CMV, toxoplasmosis, HIV, phenytoin*]
method of transmission of infectious mononucleosis	*kissing* (virus is in the saliva) [Others: *blood transfusion, sexually.* EBV attaches to CD_{21} receptors on B cells. T cells react against the infected B cells and become atypical lymphocytes.]
S/S of infectious mononucleosis	*exudative tonsillitis, cervical lymphadenopathy, generalized lymphadenopathy, rash with ampicillin, hepatosplenomegaly*
lab findings of infectious mononucleosis	*positive heterophile antibody test* (Monospot), *atypical lymphocytosis, elevated transaminases* (anicteric hepatitis), *increased anti-viral capsid antigen IgM* (most sensitive antibody)
cause of absolute lymphopenia [<3000 cells/μL in children, <1500 cells/μL in adults]	*viral infection* (initial phase) [Other causes: *drugs* (e.g., corticosteroids), *immunodeficiency syndromes* (e.g., AIDS, severe combined immunodeficiency)]

Table 12–5. WHITE BLOOD CELL DISORDERS *Continued*

Most Common...	Answer and Explanation
cause of eosinophilia [>700 cells/µL]	*type I hypersensitivity reactions* (e.g., drug reaction, hay fever, asthma) [Other causes: *invasive helminthic diseases* (no protozoal, not pinworm, not adult ascariasis), *Addison's disease, Hodgkin's disease, polyarteritis nodosa, MPD*]
cause of eosinopenia	*corticosteroids*
cause of basophilia [>110 cells/µL]	*MPDs* (e.g., PRV, CML) [Basophilia and eosinophilia are prominent in the MPDs.]
cause of monocytosis [>800 cells/µL]	*chronic inflammation* [Other causes: *autoimmune disease, malignancy*]
pathogenesis of the MPDs	*acquired, neoplastic stem cell disorders with unregulated proliferation of specific cell lines* [Myelofibrosis, leukemic transformation, and splenomegaly are characteristic findings.]
MPDs	*PRV* [Others: *CML, AMM, ET*]
cause of polycythemia	*relative polycythemia* (e.g., volume depletion) [There is a decrease in plasma volume, hemoconcentration of RBCs (reported as cells/µL), and a normal RBC mass (reported as mL/kg).]
pathogenesis of PRV	*clonal expansion of the trilineage myeloid stem cell* [There is an increased production of RBCs, WBCs (not lymphocytes), and platelets.]
clinical findings of PRV	*hypervolemia* (only MPD with an increased plasma volume), *hyperviscosity* (predisposes to thrombosis; most common cause of death), *hyperuricemia* (increased turnover of cells; gout), *histaminemia* (release of histamine from mast cells/basophils; plethoric face, headache, pruritus after bathing)
lab findings of PRV	*increased RBC mass* and *plasma volume, normal SaO$_2$* (inappropriate polycythemia; no physiologic stimulus for RBC production), *low erythropoietin* (O$_2$ content is increased), *thrombocytosis, leukocytosis, increased LAP score* (stain of neutrophils for alkaline phosphatase), *increased serum B$_{12}$* (increased WBC transcobalamin I)

Table continued on following page

Table 12–5. WHITE BLOOD CELL DISORDERS *Continued*

Most Common...	Answer and Explanation
treatment of PRV	*phlebotomy* [It decreases RBC mass and produces iron deficiency (decreases RBC production). Hydroxyurea is sometimes added.]
lab findings of polycythemias that are due to hypoxemia	*increased RBC mass, normal plasma volume, decreased SaO₂, increased erythropoietin* (appropriate polycythemia; stimulus for RBC production) [*Examples:* COPD, high altitude, cyanotic CHD]
lab findings of polycythemias that are due to a non-hypoxemic increase in erythropoietin	*increased RBC mass, normal plasma volume, normal SaO₂, increased erythropoietin* (inappropriate polycythemia; no hypoxemic stimulus for RBC production) [Examples: renal disorders (renal adenocarcinoma [includes von Hippel-Lindau disease], Wilms' tumor, cysts, hydronephrosis [uterine leiomyoma]), hepatocellular carcinoma]
lab findings of smoker's polycythemia	*RBC mass increased* (effect of carbon monoxide), *plasma volume decreased* (catecholamine effect), *SaO₂ variable, erythropoietin variable*
pathogenesis of CML	*neoplastic clonal expansion of the pluripotential stem cell prompted by a translocation of the* abl *oncogene from chromosome 9 to chromosome 22 with fusion with the break cluster region to form a fusion gene* (Philadelphia chromosome) *that enhances tyrosine kinase activity*
S/S of CML	*hypermetabolic state* (fever, weight loss, sweating), *hepatosplenomegaly* (metastasis), *generalized lymphadenopathy, chloromas* (soft tissue collections of neoplastic cells; orbit), *myeloblast or lymphoblast crisis after ~3 years*
lab findings of CML	*leukoerythroblastic smear* (50,000–150,000 cells/μL), *normocytic anemia, basophilia, thrombocytosis* (only leukemia with thrombocytosis), *myeloblasts* <10% in the bone marrow, *low LAP score* (neoplastic neutrophils do not stain for alkaline phosphatase), *Philadelphia chromosome* (t9;22)
treatment for CML	α-*interferon, busulfan, or hydroxyurea* [Bone marrow transplant is the only curative treatment.]

Table 12–5. WHITE BLOOD CELL DISORDERS *Continued*

Most Common...	Answer and Explanation
pathogenesis of AMM	*proliferation of neoplastic stem cells that begin in the marrow and move to the spleen, where hematopoiesis continues* [The marrow is fibrosed off by benign megakaryocytes secreting growth factors.]
S/S of AMM	*massive splenomegaly* (extramedullary hematopoiesis), *portal hypertension*
lab findings of AMM	*leukoerythroblastic smear, anemia, thrombocytosis, marrow fibrosis, tear drop RBCs in the PB, increased LAP, absent Philadelphia chromosome*
pathogenesis of ET	*clonal stem cell disorder primarily involving megakaryocytes*
S/S of ET	*bleeding* (usually GI; platelets are defective), *TIAs, splenomegaly*
lab findings of ET	*thrombocytosis* (>600,000 cells/μL), *iron deficiency anemia* (from bleeding), *neutrophilic leukocytosis, abnormal megakaryocytes in the marrow*
pathogenesis of myelodysplastic syndrome (MDS)	*clonal stem cell disorder with defects in maturation involving all hematopoietic cell lines* [Chromosomal abnormalities are common (e.g., 5q$^-$ and trisomy 8).]
clinical presentation of MDS	*elderly patient with severe anemia requiring constant transfusions; there is a tendency for progression into acute leukemia*
lab findings of MDS	*dimorphic RBC population* (micro-, macrocytic), *pancytopenia, increased myeloblasts and ringed sideroblasts in the marrow*
leukemia in the newborn-to–14 year old age bracket	*ALL*
leukemia in the 15 to 39 year old age bracket	*AML*
leukemia in the 40 to 60 year old age bracket	*AML and CML*

Table continued on following page

Table 12–5. WHITE BLOOD CELL DISORDERS *Continued*

Most Common...	Answer and Explanation
leukemia in the >60 year old age bracket	*CLL* [CLL is also the most common cause of generalized lymphadenopathy in a patient over 60 years old.]
method of distinguishing acute from chronic leukemia	*a blast count in the bone marrow that is >30%* (e.g., myeloblasts, lymphoblasts, monoblasts, erythroblasts) *signals acute leukemia; chronic leukemias have less than 30% blasts in the marrow and more evidence of differentiation in the PB*
causes of leukemia	*chromosomal abnormalities, radiation, alkylating agents, benzene, immunodeficiency syndromes, viruses* (HTLV-1)
S/S of leukemia	*fever, hepatosplenomegaly, generalized lymphadenopathy, bleeding, bone pain*
initial step in a leukemia work-up	*bone marrow aspirate and biopsy* [The diagnosis of leukemia can only be made on a bone marrow aspirate.]
ancillary lab findings in leukemia	*hyperuricemia* (increased cell turnover), *increased LDH* (nonspecific tumor marker)
stains used in diagnosing AML	*specific esterase, Sudan black B, peroxidase*
stain used in diagnosing ALL	*PAS* (chunks of PAS-positive material are noted in the cytoplasm)
stain used in diagnosing HCL	*TRAP stain*
stain used in diagnosing monocytic leukemias	*nonspecific esterase*
type of immunotyping for B and T cell leukemias	*flow cytometry with identification of B and T cell markers, common ALL antigen* (CALLA), *tdT* (terminal deoxynucleotidyl transferase; very early B cell marker, T cell marker, and marker of blasts of myeloid lineage)
type of ALL	*CALLA-positive, tdT-positive ALL* [It is a pre-B leukemia.]
sites for residual blasts in ALL	*CNS, testes, bone marrow*

Table 12–5. WHITE BLOOD CELL DISORDERS *Continued*

Most Common...	Answer and Explanation
treatment regimen in ALL	*remission/induction* (prednisone, vincristine, asparaginase), *consolidation* (same drugs at lower doses), *maintenance* (6-mercaptopurine, methotrexate)
cell type of CLL	*virgin B cells* [They are unable to produce plasma cells, hence the presence of hypogammaglobulinemia.]
complication associated with CLL	*hypogammaglobulinemia* (infections are the most common COD; neoplastic B cells cannot produce plasma cells) [Other complications: *AIHA warm and cold, second malignancies*]
cause of adult T cell leukemia	*HTLV-1 retrovirus* [It is more common in Japan than in the United States.]
complications associated with adult T cell leukemia	*hypercalcemia due to lytic bone lesions, skin infiltration* (feature of T cell malignancies in general)
cause of HCL	*stem cell disorder involving B cells* [The lymphocytes have projections off the cytoplasm. The splenic red pulp is the primary site for neoplastic proliferation.]
acute nonlymphocytic leukemia	*FAB classification M2* (acute myelogenous leukemia with maturation)
cytoplasmic abnormality in AML	*Auer rods* [They are found only in acute leukemia arising from neutrophils (missing in monocytic leukemias and CML).]
leukemia associated with DIC	*FAB classification: M3* (acute progranulocytic leukemia) [The blasts are hypergranular. A t(15;17) is characteristic. High doses of retinoic acid can produce remissions.]
leukemia associated with gum infiltration	*FAB classification: M5* (acute monocytic leukemia)
leukemia with bizarre, multinucleated erythroblasts	*FAB classification: M6* (DiGuglielmo's disease) [The blasts are also PAS positive.]
COD in leukemia	**infections** (usually gram-negative), *bleeding*

Table continued on following page

268 MOST COMMONS IN PATHOLOGY AND LABORATORY MEDICINE

Table 12–5. WHITE BLOOD CELL DISORDERS *Continued*

Question: Which of the following distinguish PRV from all other causes of polycythemia? **SELECT 2**
(A) RBC mass
(B) SaO₂
(C) RBC count
(D) Plasma volume
(E) Erythropoietin concentration

Answers: (D), (E): PRV is the only polycythemia with an increased plasma volume and a low erythropoietin, the latter owing to the high O₂ content, which suppresses erythropoietin.

AIDS = acquired immunodeficiency syndrome, AIHA = autoimmune hemolytic anemia, ALL = acute lymphoblastic leukemia, AMI = acute myocardial infarction, AML = acute myelogenous leukemia, AMM = agnogenic myeloid metaplasia, CHD = congenital heart disease, CLL = chronic lymphocytic leukemia, CML = chronic myelogenous leukemia, CMV = cytomegalovirus, CNS = central nervous system, COD = cause of death, COPD = chronic obstructive pulmonary disease, DIC = disseminated intravascular coagulation, EBV = Epstein-Barr virus, ET = essential thrombocythemia, FAB = French-American-British, GI = gastrointestinal, HCL = hairy cell leukemia, HIV = human immunodeficiency virus, HTLV = human T cell leukemia virus, Ig = immunoglobulin, LAP = leukocyte alkaline phosphatase, LDH = lactate dehydrogenase, MPD = myeloproliferative disease, PAS = periodic acid–Schiff, PB = peripheral blood, PRV = polycythemia rubra vera, RBC = red blood cell, SaO₂ = arterial oxygen saturation, S/S = signs and symptoms, TB = tuberculosis, TIA = transient ischemic attack, TRAP = tartrate-resistant acid phosphatase, WBC = white blood cell.

Table 12–6. LYMPH NODE DISORDERS

Most Common...	Answer and Explanation
location for B cells in a lymph node and spleen	*germinal follicles, mantle zone around T cells in the periarteriolar lymphocyte sheath,* respectively
location for T cells in a lymph node and spleen	*paracortex, periarteriolar lymphocyte sheath in the white pulp,* respectively
location for histiocytes in a lymph node and spleen	*sinuses, cords of Billroth in the red pulp,* respectively

Table 12–6. LYMPH NODE DISORDERS *Continued*

Most Common...	Answer and Explanation
roles of IL-2, IL-4, and IL-5 in B cell differentiation in a lymph node	*IL-2 activates B cells, IL-4 stimulates B cell growth and enhances isotype switching from synthesis of IgM to IgG, and IL-5 stimulates B cell differentiation* [All of these interleukins are secreted by CD₄ helper T cells.]
proliferative change in an enlarged painful lymph node	*reactive hyperplasia* [The reactive germinal centers are clearly demarcated from the surrounding paracortex and contain lymphocytes with various shapes and sizes.]
malignancy associated with Virchow's node	*stomach adenocarcinoma* [Virchow's nodes are left supraclavicular nodes that drain the abdominal cavity; therefore, other abdominal malignancies may also metastasize to these nodes (e.g., pancreas, colon).]
malignancies causing para-aortic lymph node enlargement	*primary malignant lymphomas, metastatic testicular cancers*
causes of hilar lymph node enlargement	*primary lung cancer* (most common initial site of metastasis), *sarcoidosis, TB, systemic fungal infections*
causes of generalized non-tender lymphadenopathy	*acute and chronic leukemias* [Other causes include *non-Hodgkin's malignant lymphoma.*]
causes of generalized tender lymphadenopathy	*infections* (e.g., HIV, IM, CMV, secondary syphilis) [Other causes include *drugs* (e.g., phenytoin), *autoimmune disease* (e.g., SLE, RA).]
benign lymph node disorder most often confused with metastatic malignant melanoma	*dermatopathic lymphadenopathy* [The lymph nodes drain skin lesions with excessive squamous proliferation (e.g., chronic dermatitis, psoriasis), thereby increasing macrophage phagocytosis of melanin pigment.]
cause of cat-scratch disease	*Bartonella henselae* [It is primarily identified with silver stains. Granulomatous microabscesses are present in the lymph nodes.]

Table continued on following page

Table 12–6. LYMPH NODE DISORDERS *Continued*

Most Common...	Answer and Explanation
benign reactive lymph node hyperplasia most often confused with Hodgkin's disease	*lymph nodes in IM* [The infected B cells transform into plasmacytoid immunoblasts that resemble Reed-Sternberg cells.]
drug producing reactive lymph node hyperplasia and atypical lympho-cytosis in the PB	*phenytoin* [Fever, generalized lymphadenopathy, skin rash, and eosinophilia are commonly present as well.]
benign lymph node change in nodes draining a breast cancer	*sinus histiocytosis* [In breast cancer, it is a favorable prognostic sign.]
type of malignant lymphoma	**non-Hodgkin's malignant lymphoma (NHL)** followed by *Hodgkin's disease* (HD)
extranodal site for a primary malignant lymphoma	*stomach* [The majority arise in the mucosa-associated lymphoid tissue. *Helicobacter pylori* is one of the causes of a low-grade B cell lymphoma in this area.]
primary site for HIV-induced malignant lymphoma	*central nervous system* [AIDS is the most common cause for the increase in primary CNS lymphomas in the United States.]
malignancy of lymph nodes	*metastasis* (e.g., breast cancer, primary lung cancer)
organ metastasized to	*lymph nodes* [Since carcinomas are more common than sarcomas and generally drain to regional lymph nodes, lymph nodes have this dubious reputation.]
initial site in a lymph node for metastasis	*subcapsular sinus*
CD antigen marker for malignant lymphomas	*CD45* [It identifies ~90% of malignant lymphomas.]
translocations associated with malignant lymphoma	*t(8;14) in Burkitt's lymphoma, t(14;18) in B cell follicular lymphomas*

Table 12–6. LYMPH NODE DISORDERS *Continued*

Most Common...	Answer and Explanation
cause for the increase in NHL in the United States	*increase in HIV-positive patients* [Other causes: *immunosuppressive therapy* (alkylating agents), *congenital immunodeficiencies* (e.g., Wiskott-Aldrich syndrome), *autoimmune disease* (e.g., Sjögren's syndrome), *EBV infections*]
location for Burkitt's lymphoma	*equatorial Africa* [There is a strong relationship with EBV and involvement of the jaw.]
classification scheme for NHL that utilizes pattern and size of the cells	*Rappaport classification* [Patterns are nodular or diffuse and the size is based on comparison with endothelial cells; smaller cells are called lymphocytic and larger cells are called histiocytic. Nodular is more favorable than diffuse and lymphocytic more favorable than histiocytic.]
classification scheme based on marker studies	*Lukes-Collins classification* [It is more accurate than the Rappaport system but is more expensive and more complicated.]
classification scheme for NHL used in the Working Formulation	*NHL is subdivided into grade* (low, intermediate, high) to facilitate treatment of the patient [An example of a low-grade NHL is a B cell follicular center cell lymphoma of the small cleaved type, which is the overall most common NHL. Examples of high-grade NHLs are Burkitt's lymphoma and immunoblastic lymphomas.]
B cell NHL due to inactivation of a gene involved with apoptosis (programmed cell death)	*follicular center cell lymphoma: small cleaved type* [Translocation of the B cell immunoglobulin heavy chain gene site located on chromosome 14 to a location in proximity to the *bcl*-2 oncogene site on chromosome 18 causes overexpression of the *bcl*-2 gene protein product. This product inactivates the apoptosis gene responsible for programmed cell death of the B cell, so the cells do not die.]
B cell NHL confused with CLL involving lymph nodes	*small lymphocyte lymphocytic lymphoma* [It involves the bone marrow and has a leukemic phase, hence its confusion with CLL.]
NHL in children	*Burkitt's lymphoma* (small non-cleaved lymphocytic lymphoma) [It is a high-grade B cell lymphoma.]

Table continued on following page

Table 12–6. LYMPH NODE DISORDERS *Continued*

Most Common...	Answer and Explanation
site for Burkitt's lymphoma	*abdominal cavity* [In boys, it is most often in the small intestine; in girls, the pelvic organs. The African type is more common in the jaws and has the greater relationship with EBV.]
microscopic appearance of Burkitt's lymphoma	*"starry sky" appearance* [The round B lymphocytes are the dark of night and the stars are macrophages with tingible bodies (apoptotic B cells).]
NHL due to immunosuppression	*B cell immunoblastic lymphoma* [It is a high-grade lymphoma.]
T cell malignant lymphoma with skin and PB involvement	*mycosis fungoides* [The neoplastic T cells (CD₄ T helper cells) involve the skin, lymph nodes, and other organs. It is called *Sezary syndrome* when the neoplastic cells (characteristic nuclear cleft) enter the PB. Collections of neoplastic cells in the epidermis are called Pautrier's microabscesses.]
T cell malignant lymphoma in children that has a leukemic phase resembling ALL	*lymphoblastic lymphoma* [It is a high-grade tumor that commonly involves the anterior mediastinum and PB, the latter site resembling ALL.]
diseases encompassed by the term histiocytosis X	*eosinophilic granuloma* (benign), *Hand-Schuller-Christian disease* (malignant), and *Letterer-Siwe disease* (malignant) [Histiocytes are CD₁ positive.]
S/S of an eosinophilic granuloma	*unifocal lytic lesion in bone in an adolescent or adult* [Bone pain and pathologic fractures may occur. Histiocytes have a coffee bean shape.]
clinical triad associated with Hand-Schuller-Christian disease	*diabetes insipidus* (hypothalamic involvement), *lytic lesions in the skull*, and *exophthalmos* (retro-orbital infiltration) [It usually affects children.]
S/S of Letterer-Siwe disease	*diffuse eczematous rash, multifocal cystic lesions, organ infiltration in an infant or young child* [It is the most aggressive histiocytosis X.]

Table 12–6. LYMPH NODE DISORDERS *Continued*

Most Common...	Answer and Explanation
features distinguishing HD from NHL	*HD is more likely to involve younger people; is more often associated with fever; is less likely to involve Waldeyer's ring* (tonsils, adenoids), *skin,* and *GI tract*; and *is more likely to have localized rather than generalized lymphadenopathy*
subtypes of HD in order of increasing number of RS cells, decreasing survival, and increasing age	*lymphocyte predominant* (LP; male dominant), *nodular sclerosing* (NS; female dominant; most common type), *mixed cellularity* (MC; male dominant), *lymphocyte depletion* (LD; male dominant). [RS cells, the neoplastic cell (B or T cell) in HD, must be present to diagnose HD. RS cells are single cells with two or more nuclei or nuclear lobes with a large red nucleolus surrounded by a clear halo ("owl-eye" appearance).]
RS cell variants	*L and H variant* ("popcorn" cell; LP HD), *lacunar cell* (multilobulated nucleus; NS HD), *mononuclear variants* (single rather than a double nucleus; MC HD), *sarcomatous type* (LD HD)
HD subtype with mediastinal involvement	*NS HD* [Broad bands of birefringent collagen separate nodular areas containing spaces (lacunae) with lacunar cells.]
factors determining the prognosis of HD	the **clinical stage** and *type of HD* (LP best; LD worst)
stage when HD initially presents itself	*stage IIA* [Stage IIA refers to the involvement of two or more lymph node regions on the same side of the diaphragm. Large case letter A indicates absence of fever, night sweats, and weight loss (B indicates the presence of symptoms).]
complication of therapy of HD	*second malignancies* (e.g., acute nonlymphocytic leukemia, B cell NHL) [These are more often related to the alkylating agents than to the radiation.]

Table continued on following page

Table 12–6. LYMPH NODE DISORDERS *Continued*

Question: Which of the following lymph node disorders has the best prognosis?
(A) Burkitt's lymphoma
(B) Letterer-Siwe disease
(C) Immunoblastic lymphoma
(D) B cell follicular center cell lymphoma
(E) Lymphocyte predominant HD

Answer: (E): LP HD (90% 5-year survival) has the best prognosis of all the types of lymphoma listed, most of which represent high-grade malignancies, except for (D), which is low grade.

AIDS = acquired immunodeficiency syndrome, ALL = acute lymphoblastic leukemia, CLL = chronic lymphocytic lymphoma, CMV = cytomegalovirus, CNS = central nervous system, EBV = Epstein-Barr virus, GI = gastrointestinal, HD = Hodgkin's disease, HIV = human immunodeficiency virus, Ig = immunoglobulin, IL = interleukin, IM = infectious mononucleosis, NHL = non-Hodgkin's lymphoma, PB = peripheral blood, RA = rheumatoid arthritis, RS = Reed Sternberg, SLE = systemic lupus erythematosus, S/S = signs and symptoms, TB = tuberculosis.

Table 12–7. PLASMA CELL DISORDERS, AMYLOIDOSIS, MAST CELL DISORDERS, AND DISORDERS OF THE SPLEEN

Most Common...	Answer and Explanation
monoclonal gammopathy (MG)	*MGUS* (56%) [It most commonly occurs in the elderly. ~25% may develop MM or a related disorder over the next 20 years.]
primary malignancy of bone	*MM* [It accounts for ~20% of all cases of MG. The median age is ~60 years, and it is more common in women than men.]
urine finding in MM	*BJ protein* [It represents the presence of light chains in urine. It is best detected by urine electrophoresis. BJ protein has a negative dipstick reaction for protein (only detects albumin) but it is strongly positive with sulfosalicylic acid (SSA detects albumin and **globulins**).]

Table 12–7. PLASMA CELL DISORDERS, AMYLOIDOSIS, MAST CELL DISORDERS, AND DISORDERS OF THE SPLEEN *Continued*

Most Common...	Answer and Explanation
S/S of MM	*anemia, multifocal lytic lesions* (pathologic fractures; release of osteoclast activating factor by plasma cells), *bone pain, renal failure* (nephrocalcinosis, BJ protein casts, amyloidosis [derived from light chains]), *recurrent infections* (most common cause of death) [Alkylating agents are the mainstay of therapy.]
lab findings of MM	*IgG* (IgA, light chains less common) *monoclonal spike, sheets of malignant plasma cells* (>10%) *in the marrow, BJ proteinuria, hypercalcemia* (25%), *rouleaux, increased ESR, prolonged bleeding time* (qualitative platelet defect)
MG associated with hyperviscosity	*Waldenstrom's macroglobulinemia with increased IgM* [Unlike MM, there are no lytic areas and lymphadenopathy is more likely present.]
heavy chain disease	*α-heavy chain disease* [It most commonly presents as a small bowel lymphoma with malabsorption or localized disease in the upper respiratory tract. *γ-Heavy chain* disease presents like a malignant lymphoma. *μ-Heavy chain* disease presents like CLL. The MG protein is part of the heavy chain without light chains. BJ proteinuria is uncommon.]
stain and EM appearance of amyloid	*after Congo red staining, it has an apple-green birefringence under polarized light; EM reveals linear, non-branching fibrils with hollow cores on cross section*
types of protein converted into amyloid	*light chains* (e.g., primary amyloidosis; multiple myeloma) [Other proteins include *serum-associated amyloid* (SAA; secondary or reactive amyloidosis), *β-amyloid* (Alzheimer's disease; coded by chromosome 21; Down syndrome relationship), *β$_2$-microglobulin* (hemodialysis related; joints and bones), *prealbumin* (senile amyloidosis), *calcitonin* (medullary carcinoma of the thyroid).]

Table continued on following page

**Table 12–7. PLASMA CELL DISORDERS, AMYLOIDOSIS,
MAST CELL DISORDERS, AND DISORDERS
OF THE SPLEEN** *Continued*

Most Common...	Answer and Explanation
sites of amyloid deposition	*spleen* (light chain deposits in white pulp [sago spleen], SAA deposits in red pulp [lardaceous spleen]), *liver* (increased serum alkaline phosphatase), *tongue* (macroglossia), *kidneys* (nephrotic syndrome), *neurons* (Alzheimer's disease), *nerves* (peripheral neuropathy), *heart* (restrictive cardiomyopathy, low voltage ECG, conduction defects), *adrenals* (Addison's disease)
method of diagnosing amyloidosis	*rectal or gingival mucosal biopsy* [Other methods include *omental fat pad biopsy, biopsy of organ involved, SPE* (positive in light chain types of amyloidosis).]
causes of massive splenomegaly (>1000 g)	**MPD** (CML, PRV, AMM), *CLL*
benign tumor of the spleen	*hemangioma*
malignancy of the spleen	*metastatic malignant lymphoma*
cause of hypersplenism [exaggeration of normal function]	*portal hypertension secondary to cirrhosis* [Hypersplenism may trap RBCs, WBCs, and platelets, leading to cytopenias.]
findings in Felty's syndrome	*splenomegaly, rheumatoid arthritis, autoimmune neutropenia*
cause of autosplenectomy	*sickle cell disease*

Table 12–7. PLASMA CELL DISORDERS, AMYLOIDOSIS, MAST CELL DISORDERS, AND DISORDERS OF THE SPLEEN *Continued*

Most Common...	Answer and Explanation
cause of a ruptured spleen	*trauma*
infectious cause of hemolytic anemia and splenomegaly worldwide	*malaria*
autoimmune disease associated with "onion skinning" of the penicilliary arterioles	*SLE* ["Onion skinning" refers to hyperplastic arteriolosclerosis.]
cause of congestive splenomegaly	*portal hypertension secondary to cirrhosis* [The spleen is often encased by fibrotic material with the appearance of icing on a cake ("sugar-coated spleen"). Gamna Gandy bodies (calcium and iron concretions) are present in collagen. Hypersplenism is commonly present.]
source of embolization in splenic infarction	*left heart* [Pale infarcts are the rule except with splenic vein thrombosis, which produces a hemorrhagic infarction. Friction rubs may be present.]
association with congenital asplenia	*malformations of the heart* (~80%)
hematologic abnormalities with splenectomy	*target cells, Howell-Jolly bodies* (nuclear remnants), *reticulocytosis, thrombocytosis*
leukemia with only red pulp infiltration	HCL [Most other leukemias involve both the red and white pulp.]

Table continued on following page

Table 12-7. PLASMA CELL DISORDERS, AMYLOIDOSIS, MAST CELL DISORDERS, AND DISORDERS OF THE SPLEEN *Continued*

Question: A 65-year-old woman with a pathologic fracture, anemia, and elevated BUN and creatinine levels would most likely have which of the following?
(A) MGUS
(B) Secondary amyloidosis
(C) An IgM monoclonal spike
(D) Malignant plasma cells in the bone marrow
(E) α-Heavy chain disease

Answer: (D): A patient with a pathologic fracture, anemia, and renal disease most likely has MM. MM is most often due to an increase in IgG originating from malignant plasma cells in the marrow. Primary amyloidosis is associated with MM rather than secondary amyloidosis (choice B). Waldenstrom's macroglobulinemia due to an IgM MG is an age-related finding and would not be expected to include bone disease not associated with pathologic fractures (choice C). MGUS is an age-related finding and would not be expected to include bone disease and anemia (choice A). α-Heavy chain disease involves the small bowel or upper respiratory tract (choice E).

AMM = agnogenic myeloid metaplasia, BJ = Bence-Jones, BUN = blood urea nitrogen, CLL = chronic lymphocytic lymphoma, CML = chronic myelogenous leukemia, ECG = electrocardiogram, EM = electron microscopy, ESR = erythrocyte sedimentation rate, HCL = hairy cell leukemia, Ig = immunoglobulin, MGUS = monoclonal gammopathy of undetermined significance, MM = multiple myeloma, MPD = myeloproliferative disease, PRV = polycythemia rubra vera, RBC = red blood cell, SLE = systemic lupus erythematosus, SPE = serum protein electrophoresis, S/S = signs and symptoms, WBC = white blood cell.

Table 12-8. BLOOD BANKING

Most Common...	Answer and Explanation
ABO blood group	*blood group O* [The O gene is inactive, so neither A nor B antigens are present. O cells have H antigen (fucose attached to the terminal end of a glycolipid) on their surface.]
ABO blood group with *N*-acetylgalactosamine attached to H antigen	*blood group A*

Table 12–8. BLOOD BANKING *Continued*

Most Common...	Answer and Explanation
ABO blood group with galactose attached to H antigen	*blood group B* [AB people have either A or B sugars attached to H antigen.]
ABO blood group that are universal recipients	*blood group AB* [They have no isohemagglutinins (anti-A or anti-B) in their plasma to attack A or B antigens on other RBCs.]
ABO blood group that can only be transfused with blood group O	*blood group O* [O patients have anti-A IgM, anti-B IgM, and anti-A,B IgG; therefore, they can only receive blood negative for A or B antigens.]
ABO blood group designated the universal donor	*blood group O* [Anti-A IgM from B patients and anti-B IgM from A patients cannot destroy O RBCs, since they lack A and B antigens.]
ABO blood group involved in ABO incompatibility in newborns	*blood group O* [O mothers have anti-A,B IgG (normal antibody; it is not from a previous sensitization), which can cross the placenta and attach to fetal RBCs with A or B antigen leading to their extravascular destruction.]
ABO blood groups with an increased incidence of duodenal ulcer and gastric cancer	*blood group O and blood group A*, respectively
source of IgG in the cord blood of newborns	*maternally derived IgG* [Newborns begin synthesizing IgG in a few months.]
Rh antigen	*D antigen* (85% of the population is positive; designated Rh-positive) [*Other Rh antigens:* C, c, E, e (there is no d antigen)]
antibody in clinical medicine	*anti-D antibodies* [They are IgG antibodies.]
antigen that is a receptor for *Plasmodium vivax*	*Duffy antigen* [Blacks commonly lack this antigen, so they are protected from contracting *P. vivax* malaria.]

Table continued on following page

Table 12–8. BLOOD BANKING *Continued*

Most Common...	Answer and Explanation
cold (IgM) antibodies of clinical significance	*anti-I* (hemolytic anemia in *Mycoplasma pneumoniae* infections) and *anti-i* (hemolytic anemia in infectious mononucleosis) antibodies [Anti-P antibodies are also cold-reacting, even though they are IgG (antibody noted in PCH).]
naturally occurring antibody	*anti-Lewis IgM antibodies* [They are weak antibodies and have no clinical significance.]
tests performed on donor blood in the blood bank	*ABO, Rh, ABS* (indirect Coombs'), *RPR or VDRL, HBsAg, anti-HCV antibodies, anti-HIV-1 and HIV-2 antibodies*
infection transmitted by blood transfusion	*CMV* [It is present in lymphocytes. CMV-negative blood must be transfused into newborns, immunocompromised patients, patients with T cell immunodeficiencies. There is a 1 in 676,000 chance of contracting HIV infection per unit of blood and a 1 in 200,000 chance of contracting HBV per unit of blood.]
cause of post-transfusion hepatitis	*HCV* (90%) [There is a 1 in 3300 chance of contracting HCV per unit of blood.]
preservative used in the blood bank	*CPDA-1* [It represents **c**itrate (anticoagulant; binds calcium), **p**hosphate (maintain 2,3 BPG; levels 100% for 1 week), **d**extrose (fuel for RBCs), **a**denine (substrate for ATP). The shelf life is 35 days.]
tests performed on a patient who is going to be transfused with blood	*ABO, Rh, ABS* (look for atypical antibodies), *direct Coombs'* (look for antibodies on the patient's RBCs), *major cross-match* (patient serum against donor RBCs; the goal is not to have any antibodies that will attack donor antigens)
method of preventing GVH and CMV infection in the recipient of a blood transfusion	*irradiation* [It kills donor lymphocytes that could cause GVH and kills lymphocytes containing CMV.]
risks when transfusing blood	*development of antibodies against foreign antigens* [Other risks include *transmitting infection* (e.g., CMV, HCV), *transfusion reactions* (see below), *volume overload, GVH reaction*.]

Table 12–8. BLOOD BANKING *Continued*

Most Common...	Answer and Explanation
indication for transfusing packed RBCs	*symptomatic anemia that cannot be adequately corrected by medical therapy* [Whole blood transfusions are reserved for those who have lost massive amounts of whole blood.]
antigens located on platelets	*ABO, HLA, PL$_{Al}$* [Rh antigens are not present.]
indication for transfusing platelet concentrates	*symptomatic thrombocytopenia* (bleeding) [Other indications: *count <50,000 cells/μL and major surgery is going to be performed, counts <20,000 cells/μL, qualitative bleeding disorder* (e.g., patient on aspirin who has significant bleeding)]
indication for infusion of FFP	*multiple coagulation deficiencies* (e.g., cirrhosis, DIC, overanticoagulated with warfarin)
components in cryoprecipitate	*factor VIII* (VIII:Ag, VIII:C, VIII:vWF), *fibrinogen, factor XIII*
indication for ISG	*prevention of HAV in a patient exposed to an active HAV infection* [Other indications: *B cell immunodeficiencies* (e.g., Bruton's agammaglobulinemia, CLL), *temporary prevention of hemolysis or thrombocytopenia in AIHA and autoimmune thrombocytopenia* (IgG blocks macrophage Fc receptors for IgG), *treatment of Kawasaki's disease*]
transfusion reaction	*febrile reaction* [The patient has anti-HLA antibodies against donor leukocyte HLA antigens (type II hypersensitivity). Micropore filters (filter out the leukocytes) or washing the RBCs prior to infusion prevents further reactions.]
transfusion reaction associated with urticaria or anaphylactic reactions	*allergic reactions* [The patient has IgE antibodies against plasma proteins or IgA (IgA deficiency patient with anti-IgA antibodies) in the donor unit (type I hypersensitivity).]

Table continued on following page

Table 12–8. BLOOD BANKING *Continued*

Most Common...	Answer and Explanation
type of hemolytic transfusion reaction	*previously undetected antibodies in the recipient against a donor antigen* (extravascular hemolysis; type II hypersensitivity) [An ABO mismatch (e.g., blood group A recipient receives B blood) is less common and the result of human error (e.g., not checking the patient bracelet number with the number on the unit). It is an intravascular hemolytic anemia.]
S/S of a hemolytic transfusion reaction	*fever, drop in Hb and Hct, hypotension, oliguria, jaundice, bleeding* (secondary to DIC)
type of HDN	*ABO incompatibility between an O mother and a blood group A or B baby* [Maternal anti-A,B IgG antibodies cross into the fetal circulation and attach to fetal A or B cells. They are extravascularly removed by macrophages in the fetal spleen (fetus develops a mild anemia; type II hypersensitivity). The UCB produced by this hemolysis is removed by the mother's liver.]
cause of jaundice in the newborn in the first 24 hours	*ABO incompatibility* [After delivery, the newborn's liver is unable to handle the increased UCB load.]
lab findings on newborn cord blood in ABO incompatibility	*weakly positive direct Coombs'* (maternal anti-A,B on the surface of fetal A or B cells), *anti-A,B IgG in the serum* (maternal origin), *mild anemia, spherocytes* (macrophage damage to RBCs)
cause of Rh HDN	*anti-D antibodies that developed in an Rh-negative woman from a previous pregnancy* [The pathophysiology of the anemia and hyperbilirubinemia are similar to those described for ABO incompatibility.]

Table 12–8. BLOOD BANKING *Continued*

Most Common...	Answer and Explanation
differences distinguishing Rh HDN from ABO HDN	*anemia is more severe in Rh HDN; Rh-negative mother can be any bloodtype; the fetus is not affected in the first Rh-incompatible pregnancy but subsequent pregnancies involving Rh-positive fetuses have an increased risk for HDN; Rh HDN can be prevented with RhIG;* and *spherocytes are not present in newborn blood* [ABO incompatibility protects against Rh sensitization, since O mothers have anti-A and anti-B IgM antibodies that would immediately destroy A or B Rh-positive fetal cells spilling into the maternal circulation during delivery of the baby (fetal-maternal bleed).]
complications of HDN	*anemia in the newborn, which may be severe enough to result in hydrops fetalis* (heart failure secondary to severe anemia), *unconjugated hyperbilirubinemia with a risk for kernicterus* (free, unbound UCB [fetal albumin binding sites are fully saturated, hence UCB is unbound] enters the CNS and produces permanent neurologic damage)
method of antenatal protection for Rh sensitization	*injection of RhIG at 28 weeks in anti-D negative women* [RhIG is pooled, purified IgG human anti-D (very little crosses the placenta). A booster dose is given if the baby is Rh-positive at delivery.]
postnatal method of protecting Rh-negative, anti-D negative women (who have not received RhIG) with an Rh-positive child	*maternal blood is taken and a Kleihauer-Betke test* (or similar test) *is performed to identify fetal RBCs in her circulation* (fetal-maternal bleed) [The number of vials of RhIG that are given to the mother is based on the amount of fetal RBCs in her blood. The anti-D in RhIG somehow protects the mother from developing an antibody response against the Rh-positive fetal cells. RhIG is usually given within 3 days of delivery. RhIG is not given to women who already have anti-D antibodies.]

Table continued on following page

Table 12–8. BLOOD BANKING *Continued*

Most Common...	Answer and Explanation
method of following women who are anti-D positive during pregnancy	*repeated amniocenteses and spectrophotometer detection of bilirubin pigment (absorbance wavelength of 450 nm) in AF* [The presence of bilirubin pigment means the baby has HDN. The ΔOD (optical density) 450 (measurement from the baseline to the top of the spike) is then plotted on a Liley graph to determine the severity of hemolysis and the need for delivery and/or exchange transfusion.]
method of lowering UCB levels in newborns	*placing the baby under UVB light* [It oxidizes UCB in the skin to a harmless, water-soluble dipyrrole.]
reasons for performing an exchange transfusion in a baby with HDN	*correct anemia, remove UCB, remove free antibodies, remove RBCs coated by antibodies*
blood exchanged in ABO incompatibility	*group O packed RBCs (same Rh type as the baby's) with AB plasma*
blood exchanged in Rh HDN	*group O Rh-negative packed RBCs with AB plasma*

Table 12–8. BLOOD BANKING *Continued*

Question: Which of the following components have no risk for transmitting infection to the patient? **SELECT 2**
- (A) FFP
- (B) Cryoprecipitate
- (C) RhIG
- (D) Packed RBCs
- (E) ISG
- (F) Platelet concentrates
- (G) Whole blood

Answers: (C), (E): Neither ISG nor RhIG can transmit infections owing to the manufacturing techniques used in their preparation. However, all the other products can transmit disease.

ABS = antibody screen, AF = amniotic fluid, AIHA = autoimmune hemolytic anemia, ATP = adenosine triphosphate, BPG = bisphosphoglycerate, CLL = chronic lymphocytic lymphoma, CMV = cytomegalovirus, CNS = central nervous system, DIC = disseminated intravascular coagulation, FFP = fresh frozen plasma, GVH = graft versus host, HAV = hepatitis A virus, Hb = hemoglobin, HBsAg = hepatitis B surface antigen, HBV = hepatitis B virus, Hct = hematocrit, HCV = hepatitis C virus, HDN = hemolytic disease of the newborn, HIV = human immunodeficiency virus, HLA = human leukocyte antigen, Ig = immunoglobulin, ISG = immune serum globulin, PCH = paroxysmal cold hemoglobinuria, RBC = red blood cell, RPR = rapid plasma reagin, S/S = signs and symptoms, UCB = unconjugated bilirubin, UVB = ultraviolet B, VDRL = Venereal Disease Research Laboratories, VIII:Ag = VIII antigen, VIII:C = VIII coagulant, VIII:vWF = VIII von Willebrand's factor.

CHAPTER

13

GASTROINTESTINAL PATHOLOGY

CONTENTS

Table 13–1. UPPER AND LOWER GASTROINTESTINAL BLEEDING

Most Common...	Answer and Explanation
causes of hematemesis [vomiting blood]	**duodenal ulcer** followed in descending order by *gastric ulcer, esophageal varices*
causes of melenemesis [vomiting coffee ground–like material]	**duodenal ulcer** followed by *gastric ulcer* [Acid in the stomach converts Hb into the black pigment hematin.]
cause of melena [black, tarry stools]	*duodenal ulcer* [The majority of causes of melena are proximal to the ligament of Treitz (junction of the duodenum with the jejunum). It requires 50–100 mL of blood to produce melena.]
cause of hematochezia [passage of bright red blood in the stool]	**diverticulosis** followed by *angiodysplasia* [Diverticulitis does not produce bleeding because of scarring of the vessels. Most causes of hematochezia are below the ligament of Treitz.]
causes of chronic lower GI bleeding	**internal hemorrhoids** and *colorectal cancer*
causes of iron deficiency due to a GI bleed	**duodenal ulcer**, *colorectal cancer*

Table continued on following page

287

Table 13–1. UPPER AND LOWER GASTROINTESTINAL BLEEDING *Continued*

Most Common...	Answer and Explanation
lab test used to identify blood in the stool	*Hemoccult slide test* [The test uses guaiac to detect peroxidase activity in Hb. Newer tests have antibodies against Hb or detect heme in the stool.]
causes of a false-positive Hemoccult slide test result	**myoglobin in meat,** *nonheme peroxidases in vegetables* (e.g., horseradish, cruciferous vegetables)
test used to distinguish fetal blood from maternal blood in the stool of a newborn	*Apt test* [Bloody stools due to intrinsic bleeding contain fetal Hb (resistant to alkali denaturation), while those due to swallowing of maternal blood contain adult Hb (denatured by alkali).]
recommendation for screening for colorectal cancer in a low-risk patient (no family history of colon cancer)	*annual stool guaiac beginning at age 50 with a flexible sigmoidoscopy every 3–5 years.* [Intermediate-risk patients (family member with colon cancer after age 50) should begin the above at age 40. High-risk patients (family member with colon cancer before age 50) should have colonoscopic examinations.]

Question: The first step in the work-up of a patient with melena is which of the following?
  (A) Colonoscopy
  (B) Flexible sigmoidoscopy
  (C) Barium enema
  (D) Upper GI endoscopy
  (E) CEA screening test

Answer: (D): Melena is most commonly due to a lesion above the ligament of Treitz, so upper GI endoscopy looking for PUD is the first step in the work-up. CEA testing is no longer used as a screen for colorectal cancer. The other tests are for working up lower GI bleeds.

CEA = carcinoembryonic antigen, GI = gastrointestinal, Hb = hemoglobin, PUD = peptic ulcer disease.

Table 13–2. ABDOMINAL PAIN

Most Common . . .	Answer and Explanation
order to follow in evaluating the abdomen	*inspection, auscultation, percussion, and palpation*

Table 13–2. ABDOMINAL PAIN *Continued*

Most Common...	Answer and Explanation
causes of pain in hollow viscera	*stretching of the wall, inflammation, ischemia or distention, forceful contractions*
causes of pain of solid viscera	*stretching or inflammation of the capsule (e.g., hepatomegaly)*
types of abdominal pain	*visceral, parietal, referred pain*
nerve fibers responsible for visceral pain	*unmyelinated afferent C fibers, which localize the pain* (dull, slow in onset) *to the midline closest to the viscera*
nerve fibers responsible for parietal pain	*both C fibers and myelinated A δ fibers, the latter localizing the pain (acute, sharp) to the exact location of peritoneal irritation* (pus, blood, bile, pancreatic secretions)
route of pain migration in acute appendicitis	*initially periumbilical (C fibers; inflamed appendix), then moves to McBurney's point in the RLQ* (A fibers; localized peritonitis)
site of referred pain in acute cholecystitis	*right scapular area*
site of referred pain in a perforated peptic ulcer with air under the diaphragm	*right shoulder via irritation of the phrenic nerve, since the diaphragm is higher on the right than the left and is more likely to collect air*
cause of colicky pain [pain followed by pain-free interval]	*obstruction of a viscus that has peristalsis* (e.g., obstruction due to bowel adhesions) [Other types of pain are steady.]
sequence of pain and vomiting in a surgical abdomen	*pain occurs first and is then followed by nausea/vomiting*
cause of obstipation [absence of stooling and flatus]	*obstruction, which produces both constipation (no bowel movements) and obstipation*
causes of hyperperistalsis [increased bowel sounds]	**diarrhea** and *early obstruction*

Table continued on following page

Table 13–2. ABDOMINAL PAIN *Continued*

Most Common...	Answer and Explanation
cause of adynamic and dynamic ileus [absent bowel sounds]	*intestinal obstruction due to inhibition of bowel motility* (e.g., peritonitis) *and mechanical intestinal obstruction* (e.g., adhesions), *respectively*

Question: Intermittent, colicky pain would most likely be present in which of the following? **SELECT 2**
  (A) PUD
  (B) Crohn's disease
  (C) Ulcerative colitis
  (D) Acute appendicitis
  (E) Peritonitis
  (F) A small bowel obstruction
  (G) Acute pancreatitis

Answers: (B), (F): Crohn's disease involving the terminal ileum produces narrowing of the lumen and signs of obstruction, therefore the pain is colicky rather than steady. Bowel obstruction is the classic example of colicky pain. All the other choices have a steady pain.

PUD = peptic ulcer disease, RLQ = right lower quadrant.

Table 13–3. ORAL CAVITY DISORDERS

Most Common...	Answer and Explanation
congenital disorder in the oral cavity	*cleft lip with or without an associated cleft palate* (50% of cases) [Cleft lips are usually located on the upper lip, are usually unilateral, and are more common in males. They are examples of multifactorial inheritance and are due to failure of fusion of the facial processes.]
cause of herpangina and hand-foot-mouth disease in children	*Coxsackie A* [Herpangina is associated with fever, pharyngitis, and palatal ulcers/vesicles surrounded by erythema. Hand-foot-mouth disease has vesicular lesions in these locations.]
cause of gingivostomatitis in children	*Herpes simplex type I* [Painful vesicles occur in the oral cavity. Primary disease has systemic signs (fever, lymphadenopathy), while recurrent disease does not.]
causes of exudative tonsillitis	**viruses** (e.g., EBV, coxsackievirus) *account for >50% of cases* [Group A *Streptococcus pyogenes* accounts for only 20–35% of cases. It is not possible to distinguish bacterial from

Table 13–3. ORAL CAVITY DISORDERS *Continued*

Most Common...	Answer and Explanation
Continued	viral tonsillitis by clinical exam. Documentation by culture or direct antigen detection for streptococcal infection is recommended before using antibiotics.]
causes of oral candidiasis	**newborn passing through an infected birth canal** and *immunocompromised patient* (most common fungal infection in AIDS)
initial step in evaluating a white lesion (leukoplakia) in the mouth	*determine whether the white material scrapes off* [Milk scrapes off entirely. Candida scrapes off and leaves a bloody base (KOH reveals pseudohyphae and yeasts). True leukoplakia (see below) does not scrape off and biopsy is recommended.]
cause of leukoplakia on the lateral border of the tongue in an HIV-positive patient	*hairy leukoplakia secondary to EBV* [It is one of the early infections predating the onset of AIDS.]
cause of Hutchinson's and mulberry teeth	*congenital syphilis* [The former are peg-shaped upper incisors, and the latter are molar teeth resembling mulberries.]
cause of lost teeth in patients <35 years old	*dental caries*
predisposing causes of dental caries	*sucrose, Streptococcus mutans* (acts on sucrose to produce dextran [enhances plaque formation] and acid [erodes enamel]), *reduced salivation* (e.g., Sjögren's syndrome)
mechanism of fluoride in preventing dental caries	*changes hydroxyapatite in enamel into fluorapatite,* and *it is bactericidal*
cause of a submandibular sinus draining pus and yellow granules	*Actinomyces israelii* [It is a gram-positive, anaerobic, filamentous bacterium (best identified in the yellow, sulfur granules). It usually occurs in patients with dental abscesses.]
bullous lesion located in the oral cavity	*pemphigus vulgaris* [It is due to IgG antibodies directed against intercellular attachments between keratinocytes. Pemphigus produces suprabasilar vesicles (basal cells look like tombstones) with acantholytic cells (free squamous cells) in the fluid.]

Table continued on following page

Table 13–3. ORAL CAVITY DISORDERS *Continued*

Most Common...	Answer and Explanation
diseases associated with aphthous ulcers [painful ulcerations]	**early symptomatic phase of AIDS,** *Reiter's syndrome* (HLA-B27, positive arthritis, urethritis, conjunctivitis), *Crohn's disease, Behçet's syndrome* (genital ulcerations, conjunctivitis, uveitis)
syndrome associated with mucosal pigmentation	*Peutz-Jeghers* syndrome [It is an AD polyposis syndrome.]
endocrine disorder associated with mucosal pigmentation	*Addison's disease* [Hypocortisolism leads to an increase in ACTH, which stimulates melanin synthesis.]
heavy metal pigmentation of the gums	*lead poisoning*
antibiotic causing tooth discoloration	*tetracycline*
cause of chalky discoloration of the teeth	*excess fluoride* (fluorosis)
cause of macroglossia	**primary hypothyroidism** [Other causes: *amyloidosis, acromegaly.*]
cause of leukoplakia [white patch] or erythroleukoplakia [red and white patch]	*tobacco smoking or chewing* [Leukoplakia does not rub off and should be biopsied to rule out squamous dysplasia or cancer.]
cause of Wickham's stria [net-like leukoplakia] in the mouth	*lichen planus*
benign odontogenic tumor	*ameloblastoma* [The tumor derives from enamel organ epithelium or dentigerous cysts. It has a soap bubble appearance in the mandible on x-ray.]
cancers and their locations in the oral cavity	*squamous cell carcinoma* involving the **lateral border of the tongue,** *lower lip,* and *ventral aspect of the tongue*

Table 13–3. ORAL CAVITY DISORDERS *Continued*

Most Common...	Answer and Explanation
predisposing causes of squamous cancer	**smoking** and *alcohol* [They have an additive effect, which further increases the risk for cancer.]
cancer associated with smokeless tobacco	*verrucous carcinoma* [It is a variant of squamous cancer. The cancer most commonly develops in the mandibular sulcus and rarely metastasizes.]
cancer of the upper lip	*basal cell carcinoma* [It is sunlight-induced.]
infection of the salivary glands	*mumps* [Mumps is a paramyxovirus infection. It produces bilateral parotitis and may be associated with unilateral orchitis (adolescents), oophoritis, and pancreatitis.]
extrasalivary complication of mumps	*meningoencephalitis* [The CSF has a mixed infiltrate of cells, increased protein, and low glucose. The disease is self-limited.]
site for salivary gland tumors	*parotid glands* [This is true whether the tumor is benign or malignant. Most parotid tumors are benign, whereas a greater percentage of minor salivary gland tumors are malignant.]
overall benign salivary gland tumor in both major and minor salivary glands	*mixed tumor* (pleomorphic adenoma) [The tumors are most commonly located in the parotid. They have an incomplete capsule and commonly recur. Rarely, they may develop into carcinoma.]
malignant tumor in both the major and minor salivary glands	*mucoepidermoid carcinoma* [This cancer is most commonly located in the parotid.]
benign salivary gland tumor that is exclusively located in the parotid	*papillary cystadenoma lymphomatosum* (Warthin's tumor, adenolymphoma) [The tumor arises from the parotid duct subjacent to a lymph node, hence the heavy benign lymphoid infiltrate.]

Table continued on following page

Table 13-3. ORAL CAVITY DISORDERS *Continued*

Question: Tobacco products are most closely related to the etiology of which of the following? **SELECT 2**
   (A) Hairy leukoplakia
   (B) Wickham's stria
   (C) Mucosal pigmentation
   (D) Ulcerative lesion on the upper lip
   (E) White patch in the mandibular sulcus
   (F) Ulcerative lesion on the lower lip

Answers: (E), (F): Leukoplakia in the mandibular sulcus is most likely associated with smokeless tobacco and could be a precursor for verrucous carcinoma. The lower lip is a common location for squamous cancer. Choice A is associated with EBV, choice B with lichen planus, choice C with Peutz-Jeghers or other pigment disorders, and choice D with a basal cell carcinoma.

AD = autosomal dominant, AIDS = acquired immunodeficiency syndrome, CSF = cerebrospinal fluid, EBV = Epstein-Barr virus, HIV = human immunodeficiency virus, HLA = human leukocyte antigen, Ig = immunoglobulin, KOH = potassium hydrocide.

Table 13-4. ESOPHAGEAL DISORDERS

Most Common...	Answer and Explanation
manifestation of esophageal disease	*heartburn* (burning sensation in the retrosternal area)
cause of dysphagia for solids but not liquids	*obstructive lesions in the esophagus* (e.g., esophageal web, esophageal cancer, lye stricture)
cause of dysphagia for solids and liquids	*motility disorders* (e.g., PSS, CREST syndrome, achalasia, previous stroke)
cause of odynophagia [painful swallowing]	*inflammation* (e.g., **infectious esophagitis,** GERD)
congenital esophageal disorder	*TE fistula* [In most cases, a TE fistula has a proximal esophagus that ends blindly and a distal esophagus arising from the trachea (stomach is distended with air).]
esophageal disorder associated with maternal polyhydramnios	*TE fistula* [Fetuses swallow amniotic fluid, and a block in the proximal esophagus leads to polyhydramnios.]
cause of an esophageal web	*chronic iron deficiency* [Chronic iron deficiency is the cause of the Plummer-Vinson syndrome, which, in addition to iron defi-

Table 13–4. ESOPHAGEAL DISORDERS *Continued*

Most Common...	Answer and Explanation
continued	ciency, consists of an esophageal web, achlor-hydria, and glossitis.]
esophageal diverticulum	*Zenker's diverticulum* [This diverticulum is located in the upper esophagus and is caused by a defect in the cricopharyngeus muscle leading to an outpouching consisting of mucosa, submucosa, and part of the muscularis (false diverticulum or pulsion diverticulum). Halitosis and diverticulitis may occur.]
systemic collagen vascular disease involving the esophagus	*PSS* [The smooth muscle in the lower esophagus is replaced with collagen, leading to aperistalsis, proximal esophageal dilatation, and a relaxed LES. The CREST syndrome, a localized variant of PSS, has similar problems.]
neuromuscular disorder of the esophagus	*achalasia* [Achalasia is characterized by an absence of ganglion cells in the myenteric plexus of the LES (loss of the vasodilator, vasointestinal peptide) leading to sustained contraction of the LES, aperistalsis and dilatation of the proximal esophagus. Esophageal manometry (pressure readings) is diagnostic.]
infectious disease producing achalasia	*Chagas' disease due to* Trypanosoma cruzi [The disease also destroys ganglion cells in the rectum, producing Hirschsprung's disease.]
hiatal hernia	*sliding hiatal hernia* [It is due to the herniation of the proximal stomach through a widened diaphragmatic hiatus. Reflux esophagitis (GERD) occurs at night.]
cause of heartburn	*GERD* [GERD is due to relaxation of the LES and reflux of acid and bile into the distal esophagus.]
predisposing causes of GERD	*sliding hiatal hernia, PUD, factors lowering the LES* (e.g., smoking, alcohol, caffeine, fatty foods)
complications associated with GERD	**esophageal ulceration leading to glandular metaplasia** (Barrett's esophagus) [Other complications include an *increased risk for adenocarcinoma, nocturnal cough* (acid reflux into airways), *nocturnal asthma* (acid reflux into airways).]

Table continued on following page

Table 13–4. ESOPHAGEAL DISORDERS *Continued*

Most Common...	Answer and Explanation
lab test used to diagnose GERD	*pH electrode left in the distal esophagus overnight*
cause of infectious esophagitis in AIDS	**Candida** [Other causes include: *CMV* and *HSV*]
causes of corrosive esophagitis	**ingestion of lye** (strong alkali; causes liquefactive necrosis) and *acid* (causes coagulation necrosis) *with subsequent stricture formation*
cause of esophageal varices	*portal hypertension secondary to alcoholic cirrhosis* [The left gastric (coronary) vein (branch of the portal vein) is the dilated vessel in the submucosa in esophageal varices. Rupture is the most common cause of death in cirrhosis.]
cause of a tear or rupture of the distal esophagus/proximal stomach	*severe vomiting (retching) in an alcoholic or patient with bulimia nervosa* [A tear is called Mallory-Weiss syndrome, and a rupture, Boerhaave's syndrome.]
benign tumor of the entire GI tract, including esophagus	*leiomyoma*
malignant tumor of the esophagus	*squamous carcinoma, most often located in the mid-esophagus* [It first spreads locally to regional nodes and then to distant sites (**liver,** lung).]
predisposing cause for squamous carcinoma	**smoking and alcohol** [Other causes include *nitrosamines, lye strictures, Plummer-Vinson syndrome.* Alcohol and smoking have an additive effect on producing cancer. It is common in Northern China and Iran.]
clinical presentation of esophageal cancer	*weight loss and dysphagia for solids*
cause of adenocarcinoma of the distal esophagus	*Barrett's esophagus due to GERD*
diaphragmatic hernia presenting at birth	*Bochdalek hernia* (pleuroperitoneal) [In this hernia, the visceral contents extend through the defect in the posterolateral diaphragm into the left chest cavity.]

Table 13–4. ESOPHAGEAL DISORDERS *Continued*

Question: A 57-year-old smoker and alcoholic presents with weight loss and dysphagia for solids but not liquids. The most likely diagnosis is which of the following?
(A) Esophageal adenocarcinoma
(B) Esophageal varices
(C) Achalasia
(D) PSS
(E) Squamous carcinoma of the esophagus

Answer: (E): Smoking and alcohol have an additive effect on producing squamous cancers in the oral cavity, larynx, and esophagus. Adenocarcinomas (A) are more likely with a long history of GERD, leading to a Barrett's esophagus. Choices B, C, and D are not associated with smoking or alcohol.

AIDS = acquired immunodeficiency syndrome, CMV = cytomegalovirus, CREST = calcinosis, Raynaud's phenomenon, esophageal dysfunction, sclerodactyly, telangiectasia, GERD = gastroesophageal reflux disease, GI = gastrointestinal, HSV = herpes simplex virus, LES = lower esophageal sphincter, PSS = progressive systemic sclerosis, PUD = peptic ulcer disease, TE = tracheoesophageal.

Table 13–5. STOMACH DISORDERS

Most Common...	Answer and Explanation
cause of hypergastrinemia	**patient on an H_2 blocker** [Acid has a negative feedback on the release of gastrin from the G cells in the antrum. *Other causes* of hypergastrinemia include gastric distention, PA, ZE syndrome.]
cause of an increased BAO and MAO in a gastric analysis	*duodenal ulcer disease* [A basal acid output (BAO) is collected over a 1-hour period on an empty stomach. The maximal acid output (MAO) is collected over 1 hour after pentagastrin stimulation. Gastric ulcers have a normal or slightly low BAO and MAO. ZE syndrome has an extremely high BAO and MAO.]
serious complication of achlorhydria	*adenocarcinoma of the stomach*
cause of projectile vomiting of bile-stained fluid at birth	*duodenal atresia* [The atretic bowel is distal to the entrance of bile, so the vomitus is bile stained. A "double-bubble" sign is present on an abdominal radiograph. It is a cause of polyhydramnios in the mother and is associated with Down syndrome.]

Table continued on following page

Table 13–5. STOMACH DISORDERS *Continued*

Most Common...	Answer and Explanation
cause of projectile vomiting of non-bile–stained fluid 2–4 weeks after birth	*congenital pyloric stenosis* [CPS is a male-dominant disorder transmitted by multifactorial inheritance. Visible peristalsis and a palpable knot are present on physical exam of the abdomen.]
cause of acute erosive gastritis	**NSAIDs** [*Other causes include* CMV (AIDS patients), smoking, alcohol, burns (Curling's ulcers), CNS injury (Cushing's ulcers), uremia.]
cause of type A (body and fundus) chronic atrophic gastritis	**PA** [Autoimmune destruction of parietal cells in the body and fundus leads to chronic atrophic gastritis, achlorhydria, hypergastrinemia, G cell hyperplasia (potential for a carcinoid tumor), and an increased risk for adenocarcinoma.]
cause of type B (antrum) chronic atrophic gastritis	*Helicobacter pylori* [The organism is a gram-negative, curved rod that produces urease. It is transmitted by the fecal-oral route and is found in the mucus layer lining the antrum. Urease converts urea into ammonia, which destroys the bicarbonate-rich mucus layer, leading to gastritis and PUD.]
test used to identify *H. pylori*	*Clo-test* [The test detects urease in a gastric biopsy obtained by endoscopy. Serologic tests are also very sensitive.]
disease caused by *H. pylori*	**duodenal ulcer** [Other diseases include *gastric ulcer, type B chronic atrophic gastritis, gastric adenocarcinoma, low-grade B cell malignant lymphoma*.]
cause of type AB (environmental) chronic atrophic gastritis	*H. pylori in concert with vitamin C deficiency* from diets lacking fruits and vegetables [Vitamin C normally prevents nitrosamination. Nitrosamines are also implicated in gastritis and increased risk for adenocarcinoma.]
cause of chemical gastritis	*NSAIDs* [Superficial erosions with bleeding may occur.]
cause of protein-losing enteropathy	*Menetrier's disease* [It is characterized by giant rugal folds and glands that secrete an excessive amount of protein-rich mucus.]
cause of PUD	*H. pylori* [The mechanisms involve the generation of ammonia by the action of urease on urea and factors produced by the bacteria

Table 13–5. STOMACH DISORDERS *Continued*

Most Common...	Answer and Explanation
continued	that inhibit bicarbonate secretion. Disruption of the bicarbonate-rich mucus barrier (maintained by prostaglandin E) leading to acid injury are operative in both gastric and duodenal ulcers.]
arteries responsible for bleeds in gastric and duodenal ulcers	*left gastric artery and gastroduodenal artery,* respectively
differences that distinguish duodenal ulcers from gastric ulcers	*most common PUD; more commonly associated with H. pylori; greater male-to-female ratio; more likely to bleed and perforate; most often located on the anterior portion of the first part of the duodenum; blood group O relationship; greater BAO and MAO; MEN I relationship; never malignant; more likely to wake the patient up at night*
differences that distinguish gastric ulcers from duodenal ulcers	*most often on the lesser curvature of the antrum* (type B chronic atrophic gastritis); *low risk for cancer developing in the ulcer; pain after eating that is aggravated by food but improved with antacids; BAO and MAO normal to decreased*
treatment of *H. pylori*	*combination of tetracycline, metronidazole, bismuth subsalicylate*
aggravating causes for PUD	*alcohol, renal failure*
complication of PUD	*bleeding* (duodenal > gastric ulcers)
cause of ZE syndrome	malignant pancreatic islet cell tumor secreting excessive gastrin
S/S of ZE syndrome	*solitary ulcers in the usual locations; occasionally multiple ulcers in unusual places* (e.g., jejunum), *malabsorption* (excessive acid inhibits digestion of foods in the small intestine)
screening and confirmatory test for ZE syndrome	*screening: BAO* (markedly increased) and *MAO* (maximally increased; BAO/MAO >0.60 *Confirmatory: intravenous secretin test* (paradoxical increase in already high serum gastrin levels)

Table continued on following page

Table 13–5. **STOMACH DISORDERS** *Continued*

Most Common...	Answer and Explanation
location for pancreatic heterotopic rests (choristoma)	*wall of the stomach*
polyp	**hyperplastic polyp** (most common type; hamartomatous; rarely malignant) [Other types: *adenomatous polyp* (neoplastic; potential for malignant transformation), *Peutz-Jeghers polyp* (AD; hamartomatous; rarely malignant).]
benign soft tissue tumor	*leiomyoma* (most common location is the stomach) [They may bleed.]
malignancy	**intestinal type of adenocarcinoma** (*H. pylori*–related; decreasing incidence) [Other type: *diffuse type* (not *H. pylori*–related; increasing incidence).]
cause of gastric adenocarcinoma	***H. pylori*** [*Other factors:* nitrosamines, smoked foods, blood group A, all types of chronic atrophic gastritis.]
location of gastric adenocarcinoma	**lesser curvature of pyloroantrum** (50%; same site as gastric ulcers) [Other sites: *cardia* (25%; rapidly increasing), *body and fundus* (25%).]
gastric cancer with signet ring cells (mucus pushes nucleus to periphery)	*diffuse type* (linitis plastica, or "leather bottle" stomach) [Barium studies reveal no peristalsis.]
S/S of gastric cancer	**weight loss** [Other S/S: *epigastric pain, early satiety, vomiting.*]
site of metastasis of gastric cancer	**regional lymph nodes** [Other sites: *liver, lung, ovaries* (Krukenberg tumor; bilateral; signet ring cells), *Virchow's left supraclavicular node, umbilicus* (Sister Mary Joseph sign).]
paraneoplastic syndromes associated with gastric cancer	*acanthosis nigricans* (dark, papillomatous plaques in intertriginous areas), *Leser-Trélat sign* (multiple outcroppings of seborrheic keratoses)

Table 13–5. STOMACH DISORDERS *Continued*

Most Common...	Answer and Explanation
extranodal site for malignant lymphoma	*stomach* [It is usually a high-grade, B-cell immunoblastic lymphoma. Low-grade B-cell lymphomas are *H. pylori*–related.]

Question: Which of the following differentiate duodenal from gastric ulcers? **SELECT 4**
  (A) Greater tendency for perforation
  (B) MEN I association
  (C) Low risk for cancer
  (D) Blood group A
  (E) Low BAO and MAO
  (F) Greater *H. pylori* association
  (G) Greater tendency to bleed

Answers: (A), (B), (F), (G): Choices (C), (D), and (E) are more common with gastric ulcers. Duodenal ulcers are usually associated with blood group O, have high BAO and MAO, and are never malignant.

AD = autosomal dominant, AIDS = acquired immunodeficiency syndrome, CMV = cytomegalovirus, CNS = central nervous system, CPS = congenital pyloric stenosis, H$_2$ = histamine, MEN = multiple endocrine neoplasia, NSAID = nonsteroidal anti-inflammatory drug, PA = pernicious anemia, PUD = peptic ulcer disease, S/S = signs and symptoms, ZE = Zollinger-Ellison.

Table 13–6. SMALL BOWEL DISORDERS INCLUDING MALABSORPTION AND DIARRHEAL CONDITIONS

Most Common...	Answer and Explanation
cause of malabsorption	**small bowel disease** (necessary for absorption) [Other causes: *pancreatic disease* (necessary for breakdown of lipids, proteins, and fats), *bile salt deficiency* (necessary for lipid absorption).]
clinical finding suggesting malabsorption	*steatorrhea* [The term refers to excess undigested (pancreatic problem) or malabsorbed fats in the stool.]
cause of pancreatic insufficiency	*chronic pancreatitis secondary to alcoholism*
cause of bile salt deficiency	**liver disease** (e.g., cirrhosis) [Other causes: *cholestasis* (intra- or extrahepatic), *drugs* (e.g., cholestyramine), *bacterial overgrowth, terminal ileal disease* (e.g., Crohn's disease).]

Table continued on following page

Table 13–6. SMALL BOWEL DISORDERS INCLUDING MALABSORPTION AND DIARRHEAL CONDITIONS *Continued*

Most Common...	Answer and Explanation
screening test for malabsorption	**quantitative stool for fat** (gold standard) [A *qualitative stool for fat* using fat stains, if positive, does not require a quantitative study. *Serum carotene* levels lack sensitivity.]
screening test for small bowel disease	*D-xylose* [It is a five-carbon sugar that does not require pancreatic amylases for absorption. It is decreased in the serum/urine in small bowel disease.]
screening test for bile salt deficiency	*radioactive bile breath test* [The presence of bacteria breaks down ingested radioactive glycocholate into radioactive CO_2, which is reabsorbed and measured in the breath.]
screening tests for pancreatic insufficiency	*CT scan of the pancreas* (look for dystrophic calcifications), *bentiromide test* (checks for the ability of chymotrypsin to cleave and absorb PABA from bentiromide), *ERCP* (enzyme measurements, radiography)
small bowel disease causing malabsorption	*celiac disease, an autoimmune disease with antibodies against gliadin* (alcohol extract of gluten in wheat) [There are HLA-B8, -Dr3, and -DQ2 associations. Anti-gliadin antibodies are the best screen.]
G/M findings in celiac disease	*atrophy of the villi in the jejunum and distal ileum with hyperplasia and chronic inflammation of the intestinal crypts* [Villi reappear after gluten-free diets.]
skin disease associated with celiac disease	*dermatitis herpetiformis* (vesicular skin disease)
cause of Whipple's disease	*Tropheryma whippeli* [The bacteria is a defective rod that can be identified only with EM.]
G/M findings in Whipple's disease	*villous atrophy and foamy macrophages in the lamina propria* (blocks lymphatic reabsorption of chylomicrons)
S/S of Whipple's disease	*polyarthritis, fever, generalized lymphadenopathy, skin pigmentation, and steatorrhea in a man* [Antibiotics are curative.]

Table 13-6. SMALL BOWEL DISORDERS INCLUDING MALABSORPTION AND DIARRHEAL CONDITIONS *Continued*

Most Common...	Answer and Explanation
infectious disease simulating Whipple's disease	*disseminated MAI in a patient with AIDS* [It is a common cause of diarrhea in AIDS patients.]
complications in malabsorption	*fat-soluble vitamin deficiencies* (vitamin A: nyctalopia; vitamin D: hypocalcemia; vitamin E: ataxia, hemolytic anemia; vitamin K: hemorrhagic diathesis), *hypoalbuminemia, combined anemias* (iron, folate, and B_{12} deficiencies), *failure to thrive*
type of diarrhea	**osmotic** [Other types: *secretory, invasive*].
cause of osmotic diarrhea [loss of a hypotonic stool]	**lactase deficiency** [Other causes: *certain laxatives.* The bowel mucosa is normal. The fluids lost are hypotonic in relation to plasma. Lactase deficiency is common in blacks and Asians.]
cause of secretory diarrhea [toxin-induced stimulus of cAMP]	**traveler's diarrhea** (e.g., enterotoxigenic *Escherichia coli*) [Other causes: *cholera* (*Vibrio cholerae*; "rice water" stools). The bowel mucosa is normal. The fluids lost are isotonic in relation to plasma.]
cause of invasive diarrhea	***Campylobacter jejuni*** [Other causes: *Shigella sonnei, Salmonella typhimurium, Escherichia coli* (enteroinvasive and enterohemorrhagic strains).]
test used to distinguish the types of diarrhea	**fecal smear for leukocytes** [Presence of leukocytes indicates an invasive diarrhea (e.g., shigellosis) versus an osmotic or secretory diarrhea. *Stool cultures* are also useful.]
gold standard test for lactase deficiency	*hydrogen breath test* after giving the patient lactose [Colonic bacteria convert undigested lactose into hydrogen gas (cause of explosive diarrhea) and fatty acids, the latter having osmotic activity.]
cause of diarrhea in children	*rotavirus* [The infection usually occurs in winter months. The Rotazyme test on stool may be used for the diagnosis. Norwalk virus is a common cause in adults.]

Table continued on following page

Table 13–6. SMALL BOWEL DISORDERS INCLUDING MALABSORPTION AND DIARRHEAL CONDITIONS *Continued*

Most Common...	Answer and Explanation
bacteria producing food poisoning secondary to formation of a preformed toxin	***Staphylococcus aureus*** [Other causes: *Bacillus cereus* (gram-positive rod; contaminated fried rice), *Clostridium botulinum* (adults; gram-positive rod).]
bacteria producing food poisoning after colonizing the bowel	*Salmonella enteritidis* (animal reservoirs; e.g., turtles, iguanas), *Clostridium perfringens, Clostridium botulinum* (infants; contaminated honey)
infectious diarrhea associated with sinus bradycardia, neutropenia, and splenomegaly	*Salmonella typhi* [It is the cause of typhoid fever (human reservoir). The blood (septicemic phase) is the best fluid to culture during the first week of infection. The organism invades Peyer's patches. A chronic carrier state (gallbladder most common site) may occur. Ampicillin and surgery are used to treat the chronic carrier state.]
diarrhea associated with pseudomembranous inflammation	***Clostridium difficile*** (gram-positive rod; ampicillin most common offending drug; toxin assay of stool best test; metronidazole best treatment) [Other causes: *Shigella species* (gram-negative rod; no animal reservoir), *Campylobacter jejuni* (gram-negative curved rod; poultry relationship), *enterohemorrhagic E. coli.*]
strain of *E. coli* associated with HUS	*enterohemorrhagic strain* (O157:H7 serotype) [This bacterium often contaminates improperly cooked beef.]
cause of intestinal TB in the United States	*Mycobacterium tuberculosis* [The disease is secondary to swallowing the organisms from a primary location in the lungs. The organisms infect Peyer's patches and commonly cause intestinal strictures with obstruction. *Mycobacterium bovis* is more common in Third World countries where milk is unpasteurized.]
protozoal cause of diarrhea in the United States	*Giardia lamblia* [The infection occurs from ingestion of cysts in contaminated water. Metronidazole is the treatment of choice.]

Table 13–6. SMALL BOWEL DISORDERS INCLUDING MALABSORPTION AND DIARRHEAL CONDITIONS *Continued*

Most Common...	Answer and Explanation
organisms detected with the Enterotest (string test)	*Cryptosporidium parvum, G. lamblia,* and *Strongyloides stercoralis* [A string with one end attached to the cheek is swallowed and allowed to remain in the duodenum for a few hours. It is retrieved and the material is examined. A *stool for ova and parasites* is the gold standard test for parasitic GI disorders.]
organisms producing diarrhea in AIDS	*Microsporidia species, Cryptosporidium parvum* (oocysts, partially acid-fast), *CMV, MAI, Shigella species, Entamoeba histolytica*
diverticular disease of the small bowel	*Meckel's diverticulum* (persistence of the vitelline duct) [The diverticulum contains all layers of the bowel (true diverticulum) Bleeding is the most common complication.]
diverticular disease causing malabsorption and B_{12} deficiency	*duodenal diverticula* (pulsion type) [Diverticula are sites for bacterial overgrowth and subsequent bile salt and B_{12} deficiencies.]
site and presentation of an intussusception	the *terminal ileum telescopes into the cecum, leading to obstruction* (colicky pain) and *infarction* (bloody diarrhea) [Intussusceptions are most common in children. Prominence of Peyer's patches is the nidus for intussusception. In adults, the nidus is more likely to be a polyp or cancer.]
GI site for transmural infarctions	*small bowel, owing to a single blood supply* (superior mesenteric artery)
cause of a small bowel infarction	**thrombosis of the SMA** [Other causes: embolism to the SMA (atrial fibrillation in the left atrium), SMV thrombosis (PRV), nonocclusive (digitalis).]
S/S of a small bowel infarction	*sudden onset of pain, bloody diarrhea, hypotension, and adynamic ileus* [Neutrophilic leukocytosis and hyperamylasemia (bowel origin) are commonly present.]

Table continued on following page

Table 13–6. SMALL BOWEL DISORDERS INCLUDING MALABSORPTION AND DIARRHEAL CONDITIONS *Continued*

Most Common...	Answer and Explanation
cause of small bowel obstruction	**adhesions from previous surgery** [Entrapment of small bowel in an *indirect hernia sac* is the second most common cause. *Potassium chloride* may produce jejunal strictures.]
radiographic finding in bowel obstruction	*air-fluid levels with a step-ladder effect*
type of hernia	*indirect inguinal hernia* [This hernia is due to protrusion of a new peritoneal process into the inguinal canal (bowel directly hits the finger). It is lateral to the triangle of Hesselbach (rectus abdominis: medial border; inguinal ligament: inferior border; superficial epigastric artery: lateral border).]
type of hernia extending through the center of the triangle of Hesselbach	*direct inguinal hernia*
hernia in patients with ascites	*umbilical hernia*
hernia with the highest rate of incarceration	*femoral hernia* below the inguinal ligament
cause of gallstone ileus	*a fistulous communication of the gallbladder with the small bowel and passage of the stone into the bowel with obstruction at the ileocecal valve* [There is air in the biliary tree.]
cause of meconium ileus	*cystic fibrosis* [Inspissated meconium leads to obstruction.]
malignant tumor of the small bowel	**carcinoid tumor** (terminal ileum) [Other tumors: *adenocarcinoma* (duodenum), *malignant lymphoma* (terminal ileum).]
site for a carcinoid tumor	*tip of the appendix* [Tumors are usually <2 cm, hence they rarely metastasize. They have a bright yellow color.]

Table 13–6. SMALL BOWEL DISORDERS INCLUDING MALABSORPTION AND DIARRHEAL CONDITIONS *Continued*

Most Common...	Answer and Explanation
site for a carcinoid tumor leading to a carcinoid syndrome [flushing, diarrhea, right heart valvular lesions]	*terminal ileum* [Tumors >2 cm have the greatest potential for metastasis to the liver, which is true for small bowel carcinoids. Metastatic nodules in the liver bypass liver conversion of serotonin into 5-HIAA by entering directly into the hepatic vein. Circulating serotonin and bradykinin produce the carcinoid syndrome. 5-HIAA levels in urine are markedly elevated.]
location for Peutz-Jeghers polyps	*small bowel*

Question: A patient with long-standing steatorrhea has a positive test for anti-gliadin antibodies. You would expect the patient to have which of the following? **SELECT 3**
(A) Hypocalcemia
(B) Normal PT
(C) Hypoalbuminemia
(D) Normal D-xylose test
(E) Anemia
(F) Positive stool for fecal leukocytes

Answers: (A), (C), (E): The patient has celiac disease and would be expected to have fat-soluble vitamin deficiencies (choice A: hypocalcemia from hypovitaminosis D; choice B: prolonged PT from vitamin K deficiency), hypoalbuminemia (choice C), combined anemia (iron/folate)[B_{12} deficiencies] (choice E), decreased D-xylose absorption (choice D), and a normal fecal leukocyte smear (choice F).

AIDS = acquired immunodeficiency syndrome, cAMP = cyclic adenosine monophosphate, CMV = cytomegalovirus, CT = computed tomographic, EM = electron microscopy, ERCP = endoscopic retrograde cholangiopancreatography, GI = gastrointestinal, G/M = gross and microscopic, 5-HIAA = 5-hydroxyindoleacetic acid, HLA = human leukocyte antigen, HUS = hemolytic-uremic syndrome, MAI = *Mycobacterium avium-intracellulare,* PABA = para-aminobenzoic acid, PRV = polycythemia rubra vera, PT = prothrombin time, SMA = superior mesenteric artery, SMV = superior mesenteric vein, S/S = signs and symptoms, TB = tuberculosis.

Table 13–7. LARGE BOWEL, APPENDIX DISORDERS

Most Common...	Answer and Explanation
cause of Hirschsprung's disease	*absent ganglion cells in the submucosal and myenteric plexuses in the rectum cause aperistalsis beyond the rectum and proximal bowel dilatation* [There is an absence of stool in the rectal ampulla.]
site for diverticula in the GI tract	*sigmoid colon* (pulsion type)
cause of diverticulosis in the colon	*low-fiber diet with increased constipation*
complication of diverticulosis	**diverticulitis** [Other complications include *hematochezia* (diverticular sac is next to an artery) *perforation, fistula formation.*]
causes of fistulas in the GI tract	**diverticulosis** and *Crohn's disease*
causes of hematochezia	**diverticulosis** and *angiodysplasia*
cause and site of ischemic colitis	*atherosclerosis of the SMA and/or IMA with ischemia located at the splenic flexure where the SMA overlaps with the IMA* ("watershed infarctions") [Ischemic ulcers present with pain and bloody diarrhea. Repair by fibrosis may lead to ischemic strictures with obstruction. Transmural infarctions are rare.]
sites of angiodysplasia	*cecum and right colon in elderly patients* [Submucosal blood vessels are dilated and bleed. Colonoscopy and angiography confirm the diagnosis.]
associations with angiodysplasia	**calcific aortic stenosis** and *von Willebrand's disease*
site of a volvulus	*sigmoid colon*, particularly in elderly patients [The bowel twists around the mesenteric root, leading to obstruction and infarction.]
inflammatory bowel diseases (IBD)	**ulcerative colitis** (UC) and *Crohn's disease* (CD)
location of UC and CD	*rectum* and *terminal ileum*, respectively [UC begins in the rectum (friable, bloody mucosa) and may involve the entire colon in continu-

Table 13–7. LARGE BOWEL, APPENDIX DISORDERS
Continued

Most Common...	Answer and Explanation
continued	ity. CD involves the terminal ileum alone (30%), colon alone (20%), or combined (50%).]
G/M findings in UC	*inflammatory pseudopolyps, mucosal/sub-mucosal inflammation, neutrophilic crypt abscesses*
G/M findings in CD	**transmural inflammation** (skip areas) [Other findings include *subserosal lymphoid infiltrates, skip lesions* (lesions are not in continuity), *noncaseating granulomas* (60%), *cobblestoning, strictures, fistulas, aphthous ulcers* (early finding).]
S/S of UC	*LLQ cramping pain with diarrhea containing blood* and *mucus*
S/S of CD	**RLQ colicky pain with diarrhea and bleeding** (if the colon is involved), *anal fistulas and fissures*
radiographic findings in UC	*toxic megacolon* (bowel distended >6 cm), *"lead pipe" appearance*
radiographic finding in CD	*"string sign" in the terminal ileum from narrow lumen*
extraintestinal findings noted in UC rather than CD	*PSC, HLA-B27 positive ankylosing spondylitis*
renal finding noted in CD rather than UC	*renal stones* (oxalate)
risk factors for adenocarcinoma in UC	*pancolitis and duration of disease >10 years* [This underscores the importance of annual colonoscopy exams.]
intrinsic colonic motility disorder	*irritable bowel syndrome* [It is a female-dominant disease with alternating bouts of diarrhea and constipation. Sigmoidoscopy is normal.]
cause of melanosis coli	*laxative abuse* [Laxatives containing phenanthrene pigments are phagocytosed by colonic macrophages in the lamina propria, giving the mucosa a black color.]

Table continued on following page

Table 13–7. LARGE BOWEL, APPENDIX DISORDERS
Continued

Most Common...	Answer and Explanation
overall site for GI polyps	*colorectal area*
polyp in the GI tract	*hyperplastic polyp* [It is a hamartomatous polyp with no malignant potential. Histologically, it has a "saw tooth" appearance.]
rectal polyp in children	*juveile polyp* [It is a solitary hamartomatous polyp that presents with rectal bleeding.]
syndromes associated with juvenile polyps	*juvenile polyposis* (AD or **nonhereditary**) with a small risk for malignancy and *Cronkhite-Canada syndrome* (nonhereditary; polyps + ectodermal abnormalities of the nails; small cancer risk)
polyposis associated with ovarian tumors	*Peutz-Jeghers polyp* (AD) [It may be associated with sex cord stromal tumors with annular tubules.]
premalignant dysplastic polyp of the colon	*adenoma:* **tubular** (stalked polyp) [Other types: *tubulovillous, villous types* (sessile polyp with finger-like projections). The majority are located in the rectosigmoid colon.]
risk factors for malignancy in adenomas	*size of a tubular adenoma* (>2 cm) and *amount of villous component* (villi look like those in the small intestine, mucus-secreting component) [Villous adenomas are sessile and have the greatest malignant potential; tubular adenomas have the least.]
clinical/lab findings of a villous adenoma	*excessive mucus coating the stool, hypoalbuminemia, hypokalemia*
polyposis syndrome	*familial polyposis* (AD) [Polyps are not present at birth.]
pathogenesis of familial polyposis	*inactivation of the APC suppressor gene on chromosome 5* [Activation of a *ras* oncogene and inactivation of the p53 suppressor gene are also operative in malignant transformation from an adenoma to cancer.]
polyposis syndrome with benign bone and soft tissue tumors	*Gardner's syndrome* (AD) [It is associated with benign osteomas and desmoid tumors (fibromatosis) of the abdominal sheath.]

Table 13–7. LARGE BOWEL, APPENDIX DISORDERS
Continued

Most Common...	Answer and Explanation
polyposis syndrome with malignant brain tumors	*Turcot's syndrome* (AR) [It is the only AR polyposis syndrome.]
site for colorectal cancer	**rectosigmoid** (60%), *cecum/ascending colon* (25%)
risk factor for colorectal cancer	**age** [Other risk factors: *low fiber/high saturated fat diet, smoking, polyposis syndrome, hereditary non-polyposis syndrome* (Lynch syndrome), *past history of polyps in the patient or family member.*]
S/S of colorectal cancer	*left-sided cancers obstruct* (annular, "napkin-ring" appearance) and *right-sided cancers bleed* (polypoid)
staging system for colorectal cancer	*Aster-Collins modified Duke's staging system*
site for metastasis of colon cancer	**regional lymph nodes,** *liver, lungs* [Metastasis or recurrence causes an increase in CEA.]
disorder of the appendix	*acute appendicitis*
cause of appendicitis	*fecalith obstructing the proximal lumen leading to ischemia, mucosal injury, and bacterial invasion of the wall*
complication of appendicitis	**periappendiceal abscess** [Other complications: *perforation, pylephlebitis* (infection of portal vein), *subphrenic abscess.*]
S/S of acute appendicitis	**fever,** *periumbilical pain* → *nausea/vomiting* → *shift of pain to RLQ* → *rebound tenderness at McBurney's point* (localized peritonitis) [*Rovsing's sign:* pain in RLQ on palpation of LLQ; *psoas sign:* pain on extension of right thigh; *obturator sign:* pain on internal rotation of right thigh.]
lab findings of acute appendicitis	neutrophilic leukocytosis, left shift
tumor of the appendix	*carcinoid tumor*

Table continued on following page

Table 13–7. LARGE BOWEL, APPENDIX DISORDERS
Continued

Most Common...	Answer and Explanation
cause and S/S of internal hemorrhoids	*straining at stool, painless bleeding*, respectively [Internal hemorrhoids derive from the superior hemorrhoidal vein. Pregnancy and portal hypertension are other causes.]
S/S of external hemorrhoids	*bleeding, painful thrombosis*
anal cancer	*epidermoid carcinoma* [It is increased in homosexual men and has an HPV-16, -18 association.]
cancer located at the squamocolumnar junction	*transitional cell* (basaloid, cloacogenic) *carcinoma*

Question: Which of the following are more often associated with UC than CD? **SELECT 6**
- (A) Transmural inflammation
- (B) Adenocarcinoma
- (C) "String sign"
- (D) Crypt abscesses
- (E) Noncaseating granulomas
- (F) Toxic megacolon
- (G) Fistula formation
- (H) Rectal involvement
- (I) PSC
- (J) Renal stones
- (K) HLA-B27–positive ankylosing spondylitis
- (L) Skip areas

Answers: (B), (D), (F), (H), (I), (K): CD is more often transmural (A) and UC mucosal/submucosal; CD is associated with the "string" sign (C) due to luminal obstruction; CD is more likely to have granulomas (E), fistula formation (G), renal stones (J), and skip areas (L).

AD = autosomal dominant, AR = autosomal recessive, CEA = carcinoembryonic antigen, GI = gastrointestinal, G/M = gross and microscopic, HLA = human leukocyte antigen, HPV = human papilloma virus, IBD = inflammatory bowel disease, IMA = inferior mesenteric artery, LLQ = left lower quadrant, PSC = primary sclerosing cholangitis, RLQ = right lower quadrant, SMA = superior mesenteric artery, S/S = signs and symptoms.

CHAPTER

14

HEPATOBILIARY AND PANCREATIC PATHOLOGY

CONTENTS

Table 14–1. LIVER FUNCTION TESTING

Most Common...	Answer and Explanation
indices of liver cell necrosis	*transaminases AST and ALT* [ALT is more specific for liver disease than AST.]
transaminase pattern in viral hepatitis	*ALT is higher than AST* [ALT is the last transaminase to return to normal.]
transaminase pattern in alcohol-related liver disease	*AST is higher than ALT* [Alcohol is a mitochondrial poison. AST is located in mitochondria, hence its preferential increase over ALT.]
indices of cholestasis [obstruction to bile flow]	*ALP and GGT* [Cholestasis may be intra- or **extrahepatic.** The enzymes are synthesized by bile duct epithelium rather than released from necrotic tissue.]
liver enzyme increased by drugs enhancing the cytochrome P450 system	*GGT* [**Alcohol** and barbiturates produce hyperplasia of the SER housing the cytochrome system. GGT is synthesized whenever the system undergoes hyperplasia.]
method of determining the origin of ALP (e.g., liver versus bone)	*measurement of GGT* [If the ALP and GGT are increased, ALP is most likely of liver origin. If GGT is normal, ALP is most likely from another source (e.g., bone placenta).]
index of liver excretion	*total bilirubin with fractionation into CB and UCB* [Fractionation is expressed as CB% (CB = CB/TB × 100).]

Table continued on following page

313

Table 14–1. LIVER FUNCTION TESTING *Continued*

Most Common...	Answer and Explanation
bilirubin patterns for jaundice	*CB < 20%:* primarily UCB (e.g., extravascular hemolysis, decreased uptake or conjugation of UCB) *CB 20–50%:* mixed UCB and CB (e.g., hepatitis, cirrhosis) **CB > 50%:** intra- and extrahepatic cholestasis (e.g., stone in CBD)
urine bilirubin (UB) and urobilinogen (UBG) findings in jaundice	<table><tr><td></td><td>UB</td><td>Urine UBG</td></tr><tr><td>*CB <20%:*</td><td>negative</td><td>increased</td></tr><tr><td>*CB 20–50%:*</td><td>increased</td><td>increased</td></tr><tr><td>*CB >50%:*</td><td>increased</td><td>absent</td></tr></table>
indices of severity of liver disease	**PT** and *serum albumin* [The PT is increased (decreased synthesis of coagulation factors) and albumin is decreased (decreased synthesis).]
autoantibodies	*anti-mitochondrial* (primary biliary cirrhosis) and *anti–smooth muscle* (autoimmune hepatitis)
tumor markers	*AAT and AFP for hepatocellular carcinoma, CEA for metastatic disease to liver*
lab findings in viral hepatitis (arrows indicate magnitude)	*ALT (↑ ↑ ↑), AST (↑ ↑), ALP (↑), GGT (↑), TB (↑), CB 20–50%*
lab findings in obstructive jaundice	*ALT (↑ ↑), AST (↑), ALP (↑ ↑ ↑), GGT (↑ ↑ ↑), TB (↑ ↑), CB >50%*
lab findings in alcoholic hepatitis	*AST (↑ ↑), ALT (↑), ALP (↑ ↑), GGT (↑ ↑ ↑), TB (↑), CB 20–50%*
lab findings in focal metastatic disease to liver	*ALP (↑), GGT (↑), and LDH (↑), normal TB and transaminases* [Focal disease does not produce enough necrosis to elevate transaminases or enough bile duct compression to produce cholestasis. ALP and GGT are synthesized owing to compression of tumor nodules on bile duct epithelium. LDH is a nonspecific tumor marker.]

Table 14–1. LIVER FUNCTION TESTING *Continued*

Question: Which of the following tests are most useful in separating alcoholic hepatitis from viral hepatitis? **SELECT 2**
- (A) ALT
- (B) AST
- (C) CB%
- (D) UCB
- (E) UB
- (F) UBG
- (G) GGT

Answers: (B), (G): In alcoholic hepatitis, AST > ALT, and GGT is markedly elevated owing to enhancement of the cytochrome system. All the other choices have similar results.

AAT = α_1-antitrypsin, AFP = alpha-fetoprotein, ALP = alkaline phosphatase, ALT = alanine transaminase, AST = aspartate transaminase, CB = conjugated bilirubin, CBD = common bile duct, CEA = carcinoembryonic antigen, GGT = γ-glutamyl transferase, LDH = lactate dehydrogenase, PT = prothrombin time, SER = smooth endoplasmic reticulum, TB = total bilirubin, UCB = unconjugated bilirubin

Table 14–2. OVERVIEW, JAUNDICE

Most Common...	Answer and Explanation
functions of the liver	*gluconeogenesis; ketone body synthesis; synthesis of VLDL; synthesis of bile salts/acids; biotransformation of drugs, hormones, and toxins; protein synthesis* (e.g., albumin, coagulation factors), *urea synthesis*
disorder involving the portal vein	**PH** [Other disorders include *pylephlebitis* (inflammation; acute appendicitis most common cause), *schistosomiasis* (*Schistosoma mansoni*; eggs produce fibrosis ["pipestem cirrhosis"] and PH).]
disorder involving intrahepatic bile ducts	**primary biliary cirrhosis** [Other disorders: *ascending cholangitis, intrahepatic biliary atresia.*]
disorder involving the limiting plate [demarcation separating portal triad from parenchyma]	*chronic active (aggressive) hepatitis* [Inflammation of the triads in CAH leads to disruption of the plate, which is called piecemeal necrosis.]

Table continued on following page

Table 14–2. OVERVIEW, JAUNDICE *Continued*

Most Common...	Answer and Explanation
disorders involving zone 1 [zone next to the triad]	*necrosis associated with yellow phosphorus poisoning, eclampsia* [Zone 1 receives most of the oxygenated blood as the hepatic artery and portal vein empty blood into the sinusoids.]
disorder involving zone 2 [mid-zonal region]	*hepatitis associated with yellow fever*
disorder involving zone 3 [zone around the THV]	**right heart failure** ("nutmeg liver") [Other disorders: *tissue hypoxia secondary to shock* (fatty change), *alcohol-related liver disease* (fibrosis around the THV, fatty change). Zone 3 has the least amount of oxygen.]
cause of pruritus in liver disease	*bile salt deposition in the skin*
cause of dark colored urine and acholic ("clay colored") stools	*obstructive liver disease* [Dark colored urine is due to excess CB (water soluble) and the acholic stools to absence of urobilin pigment (see below).]
cause of pitting edema of the legs and ascites	*cirrhosis of the liver with portal hypertension* (ascites) and *hypoalbuminemia* (ascites and pitting edema)
S/S of hyperestrinism secondary to cirrhosis	*gynecomastia, spider angiomas, palmar erythema, secondary female sex characteristics* (male cirrhotic)
S/S of PH in cirrhosis	**ascites,** *caput medusae, hemorrhoids*
initial site of visible jaundice	*sclera* [The sclera has increased elastic tissue, which has an increased affinity for UCB or CB. TB must be >2.5 mg/dL.]
site for synthesis of UCB	*bone marrow with macrophage destruction of senescent RBCs* [UCB (lipid soluble) is the end-product of Hb breakdown. UCB binds with albumin in the blood.]
fate of UCB	*uptake and conjugation of UCB into water soluble CB in the hepatocyte*
fate of CB	*secreted into bile canaliculi → enters CBD → stored and concentrated in GB → converted in the terminal ileum and colon by bacteria into UCB* (β-glucuronidases; some UCB is re-*

Table 14–2. OVERVIEW, JAUNDICE *Continued*

Most Common...	Answer and Explanation
continued	absorbed), which is *further reduced to urobilinogen* (colorless) → *UBG oxidized to urobilin* (normal color of stool and urine) *or partially reabsorbed* (90% to the liver, 10% to the urine)
cause of jaundice in the United States	*HAV*
genetic cause of jaundice	*Gilbert's syndrome* (second overall most common cause of jaundice) [It is a problem with uptake and conjugation of UCB (CB <20%). A liver biopsy is totally normal.]
method of diagnosing Gilbert's syndrome	*fast the patient and note doubling of the TB over the baseline value* [The syndrome has no clinical significance.]
genetic cause of conjugating enzyme deficiency	*Crigler-Najjar syndrome* [Type I has a total enzyme lack and is incompatible with life, while type II is a milder disease (phenobarbital is used to enhance conjugation of UCB). The CB is <20%.]
genetic causes of a defect in the canalicular transport system	*Dubin-Johnson syndrome* and *Rotor's syndrome* [The former is associated with a black liver (non-melanin pigment) and the latter is not. The CB is >50%.]
acquired causes of a CB <20%	*extravascular hemolytic anemia* (e.g., congenital spherocytosis, ABO incompatibility), *impaired uptake of UCB* (e.g., cirrhosis, hepatitis), *impaired conjugation UCB* (e.g., physiologic jaundice of NB [jaundice peaks at 3 days; also increased production of UCB], breast milk jaundice [fatty acids in milk inhibit conjugating enzymes; also, breast milk has β-glucuronidases, hence increasing UCB absorption from the bowel]
cause of jaundice in the first 24 hours after birth	*ABO incompatibility* (O mother with an A or B baby)
acquired causes of a CB 20–50%	**viral hepatitis,** *alcoholic hepatitis*
acquired cause of a CB >50%	**extrahepatic obstruction** (e.g., **stone in CBD** [Other causes include *carcinoma of the head of the pancreas, intrahepatic obstruction* (usually drug-induced).]

Table continued on following page

Table 14–2. OVERVIEW, JAUNDICE *Continued*

Most Common...	Answer and Explanation
cause of dark urine in viral hepatitis	*increase in urobilin* (from increased UBG) and *CB in the urine* [The inflamed liver has a problem in uptake of UCB for conjugation, a problem with liver cell necrosis and release of CB into the blood, and a problem in uptake of UBG recycled from the bowel, so most of it ends up in the urine.]
cause of dark urine in extravascular hemolysis	*an increase in production of UBG from the increase in UCB, so more UBG enters the urine and more urobilin is produced* [Albumin-bound and lipid-soluble UCB cannot enter the urine.]
cause of kernicterus in newborns	*Rh incompatibility due to anti-D* [Excessive amounts of unbound UCB from extravascular hemolysis of fetal RBCs enter the brain through the poorly developed blood-brain barrier.]

Question: Which of the following are primarily unconjugated hyperbilirubinemias? **SELECT 4**
  (A) Gilbert's syndrome
  (B) Stone in CBD
  (C) Crigler-Najjar syndrome
  (D) Dubin-Johnson syndrome
  (E) Primary biliary cirrhosis
  (F) ABO incompatibility
  (G) Physiologic jaundice of the newborn

Answers: (A), (C), (F), (G): All the other choices are primarily conjugated hyperbilirubinemias.

CAH = chronic active hepatitis, CB = conjugated bilirubin, CBD = common bile duct, GB = gallbladder, HAV = hepatitis A, Hb = hemoglobin, NB = newborn, PH = portal hypertension, RBC = red blood cell, S/S = signs and symptoms, TB = total bilirubin, THV = terminal hepatic venule, UCB = unconjugated bilirubin, UBG = urobilinogen, VLDL = very low density lipoprotein.

Table 14–3. LIVER INFECTIONS

Most Common...	Answer and Explanation
types of viral hepatitis in descending order of incidence	**HAV,** *HBV, HCV, HDV,* and *HEV*
types of viral hepatitis transmitted by fecal-oral route	**HAV** and *HEV* [The other types are primarily transmitted parenterally.]
viral hepatitis with the greatest risk for chronic disease	*HCV* (40–60%)
types of viral hepatitis without a chronic state	**HAV** and *HEV*
cause of traveler's hepatitis	*HAV*
viral cause of fulminant hepatitis	*HBV*
types of viral hepatitis with a serum sickness–like prodrome	**HBV** and *HCV* [Patients may present with urticaria, vasculitis (polyarteritis nodosa relationship), polyarthritis, glomerulonephritis. It is a type III immunocomplex disease.]
hepatitis requiring HBsAg	*HDV* [It is an incomplete RNA virus.]
hepatitis transmitted by coinfection and superinfection	*HDV* [Coinfection means that both HBV and HDV are transmitted in the same needle, while superinfection means that HDV is transmitted at a later date (more serious infection).]
hepatitis in child day care centers	*HAV*
cause of post-transfusion hepatitis	*HCV*
beneficial effects of HBV immunization	**prevents HBV,** *HDV,* and *hepatocellular carcinoma* secondary to HBV-related postnecrotic cirrhosis (true tumor vaccine)
hepatitis that worsens in pregnancy	*HEV* [The patients develop fulminant hepatitis.]

Table continued on following page

Table 14–3. LIVER INFECTIONS *Continued*

Most Common...	Answer and Explanation
types of viral hepatitis in which the antibody indicates infection, not protection	*HCV, HDV* [Anti-HAV IgG, anti-HBs, and anti-HEV-IgG are protective antibodies.]
marker of active HAV, HBV, HCV, HDV, and HEV	*anti-HAV-IgM, HBsAg, anti-HCV, anti-HDV,* and *anti-HEV-IgM,* respectively
markers of infectivity in HBV	**HBV-DNA** and *HBeAg*
sequence of antigens and antibodies in HBV	*HBsAg* (not infective) → *HBeAg and HBV-DNA* (infective) → *anti-HBc-IgM* → *loss of HBeAg and HBV-DNA* → *loss of HBsAg* (not infective) → *persistence of anti-HBc-IgM in the window period when anti-HBs is not present* → *anti-HBs* (protective antibody), *anti-HBc-IgG, anti-HBe*
indicator of chronic HBV	*persistence of HBsAg >6 months* ["Healthy carriers" only have HBsAg (low risk of infectivity), while infective carriers (high risk of infectivity) have HBsAg, HBeAg, and HBV DNA.]
serologic marker of someone who has received recombinant HBV vaccine	*anti-HBs* [Presence of anti-HBs and anti-HBc-IgG indicates that the patient had HBV and has recovered.]
clinical phases of viral hepatitis	*prodromal phase, icteric phase, recovery phase* [The prodromal phase is flu-like. Most viral hepatitis is anicteric. When icteric, the urine is darker and stools lighter (mild cholestasis phase). The recovery phase lasts for a few months.]
G/M findings of acute viral hepatitis	*hepatomegaly with ballooning degeneration* (swelling of hepatocytes), *acidophilic bodies* (apoptosis of hepatocytes), *hyperplasia of Kupffer's cells, patchy lymphocytic infiltrate, liver cell regeneration, inflammation of the portal triads* [Fatty change is noted only in HCV hepatitis.]
microscopic findings in chronic hepatitis	*CPH*: mild inflammation of the portal triads; hepatocytes with a "ground glass" appearance have HBsAg

Table 14–3. LIVER INFECTIONS *Continued*

Most Common...	Answer and Explanation
continued	*CAH*: piecemeal necrosis, liver cell necrosis, fibrosis between triads, triads and THV, or THV to THV.
cause of "ring granulomas" in the liver	*Q fever due to Coxiella burnetii*
S/S of ascending cholangitis	*Charcot's triad of fever, jaundice, and RUQ pain* [It is due to an infection (usually *E. coli*) of an obstructed CBD (stone or stricture) that ascends into the triads.]
cause of liver abscesses in the United States	*ascending cholangitis* [Parasitic diseases are more likely in Third World countries.]
cause of infectious and noninfectious granulomatous hepatitis	*TB and sarcoidosis,* respectively
cause of hepar lobatum	*granulomatous hepatitis due to Treponema pallidum* (tertiary syphilis), *which causes diffuse fibrosis and gumma formation*
cause of an "anchovy-paste" liver abscess	*Entamoeba histolytica* [Amebiasis starts in the cecum with excystation and burrowing of the trophozoites (contain ingested RBCs) into the bowel wall ("flask-shaped" ulcers). Some organisms may penetrate the portal vein tributaries and enter the right lobe of liver, where they digest the parenchyma (looks like anchovy paste). From this location, ameba can enter the right lung cavity and disseminate. Metronidazole is the treatment of choice.]
cause of "sheep herder's" disease	*Echinococcus granulosus* or *multilocularis* (cestode tapeworm) [The dog is the definitive host (has the adult worms with the eggs), while the sheep herder is the intermediate host (carries the larval form). Ingested eggs develop into larva, which penetrate the bowel wall and liver to form hydatid cysts containing scolices. Rupture of a cyst can produce anaphylactic shock. Albendazole and surgery are treatment options.]

Table continued on following page

Table 14–3. LIVER INFECTIONS *Continued*

Most Common...	Answer and Explanation
cause of "pipe stem" cirrhosis leading to PH	*Schistosoma mansoni* (trematode) [Cercaria penetrate the skin and find their way into the mesenteric veins and the portal vein, where they form adults. Adults lay eggs, which produce a hypersensitivity reaction leading to fibrosis and PH. Praziquantel is the treatment of choice.]
parasitic cause of cholangiocarcinoma	*Clonorchis sinensis* (Chinese liver fluke) [Humans ingest the encysted metacercaria larvae in uncooked fish sauce. The larvae enter the bile ducts, where adults develop. Praziquantel is the treatment of choice.]

Question: What is the most likely cause of a sudden onset of fulminant hepatitis in an intravenous drug abuser with previously stable chronic HBV?
 (A) Acetaminophen
 (B) HAV
 (C) HCV
 (D) HDV
 (E) Hepatocellular carcinoma

Answer: (D): The patient most likely developed a superinfection with HDV. Since HDV is cytolytic, every cell infected by the virus is immediately destroyed, hence the fulminant hepatitis. Acetaminophen is the most common drug producing fulminant hepatitis. The other viruses do not produce this type of scenario.

anti-HBc = anti-hepatitis B core antibody, anti-HBe = anti-hepatitis B e antibody, anti-HBs = anti-hepatitis B surface antibody, CAH = chronic active hepatitis, CBD = common bile duct, CPH = chronic persistent hepatitis, G/M = gross and microscopic, HAV = hepatitis A, HBeAg = hepatitis Be antigen, HBsAg = hepatitis B surface antigen, HBV = hepatitis B, HCV = hepatitis C, HDV = hepatitis D, HEV = hepatitis E, Ig = immunoglobulin, PH = portal hypertension, RBC = red blood cell, RUQ = right upper quadrant, S/S = signs and symptoms, TB = tuberculosis, THV = terminal hepatic venule.

Table 14–4. MISCELLANEOUS LIVER DISORDERS, PERITONEAL DISORDERS

Most Common...	Answer and Explanation
cause of liver congestion	*right heart failure* [There is a backup of venous blood into the THV producing the classic "nutmeg" liver. Chronic congestion may produce cardiac cirrhosis.]

Table 14–4. MISCELLANEOUS LIVER DISORDERS, PERITONEAL DISORDERS *Continued*

Most Common...	Answer and Explanation
cause of hepatic vein thrombosis (Budd-Chiari syndrome)	**polycythemia rubra vera** [Other causes include *oral contraceptives, paroxysmal nocturnal hemoglobinuria* (release of TXA_2 from platelets). The liver becomes enlarged and painful; PH develops with ascites.]
cause of portal vein thrombosis	*pylephlebitis secondary to acute appendicitis* [Areas of red-blue discoloration occur in the liver owing to a combination of venous congestion and liver cell atrophy (this condition is misnamed as "infarcts" of Zahn).]
cause of peliosis hepatis [RBCs accumulate in space of Disse]	*anabolic steroids*
types of alcohol-related disease	**fatty change,** *alcoholic hepatitis,* and *cirrhosis*
risk factors for alcohol-related liver disease	**amount and duration of alcohol** [Other factors include *female sex, coexisting HCV,* and *certain genetic tendencies.*]
pathway for alcohol metabolism	alcohol $\xrightarrow{\text{alcohol dehydrogenase}}$ acetaldehyde $+ NADH_2 \xrightarrow{\text{aldehyde dehydrogenase}}$ acetate $+ NADH_2 \longrightarrow$ acetyl Co-A
lab findings related to the increase in NADH in alcohol metabolism	*conversion of pyruvate to lactate* (lactic acidosis), *increase in DHAP leading to an increase in G-3P and synthesis of VLDL, fasting hypoglycemia* (pyruvate is in the form of lactate), *hyperuricemia* (lactic acid competes with uric acid for renal excretion)
lab findings secondary to the increase in acetyl CoA in alcohol metabolism	*conversion into fatty acids* (substrate for VLDL synthesis), *conversion into ketone bodies, particularly β-OHB, since AcAc is converted into β-OHB by the increase in NADH* [Alcoholics have both lactic and β-OHB ketoacidosis.]
cause of fibrosis related to alcohol	*acetaldehyde binds with lysine residues in proteins to form an acetaldehyde-protein complex.* [This complex stimulates myofibroblasts and Ito cells (normally a storage cell for retinoic acid) to produce collagen around the THV (perivenular fibrosis, a prominent

Table continued on following page

Table 14–4. MISCELLANEOUS LIVER DISORDERS, PERITONEAL DISORDERS *Continued*

Most Common...	Answer and Explanation
continued	finding in alcohol-related liver damage). Collagen also replaces necrotic hepatocytes located around islands of regenerating hepatocytes (regenerative nodules of cirrhosis).]
reversible and irreversible types of alcohol-related liver disease	*reversible:* fatty change (begins in zone 3; see Chapter 2), alcoholic hepatitis *irreversible*: cirrhosis
histologic finding in alcoholic hepatitis	**fatty change** [Other findings: *Mallory bodies* (altered prekeratin intermediate filaments), *neutrophilic infiltrate, intrahepatic cholestasis.*]
S/S of alcoholic hepatitis	*painful hepatomegaly, jaundice, fever, ascites,* and *hepatic encephalopathy* (in severe cases)
histologic findings in alcoholic cirrhosis	*regenerative nodules* (regenerating hepatocytes without sinusoids or portal triads) *surrounded by fibrosis*
clinical and lab findings of autoimmune hepatitis	*clinical*: hepatosplenomegaly, jaundice *lab*: positive ANA, positive anti–smooth muscle antibody
primary bile acids and salts	*bile acids*: cholic and chenodeoxycholic acids [They are synthesized from cholesterol.] *bile salts: glycocholic* and *taurochenodeoxycholic acids*
secondary bile salts	*deoxycholic* and *lithocholic acids* [These are deconjugated products of primary bile salts.]
cause of intrahepatic cholestasis	**drugs** (e.g., oral contraceptives) [Other causes include *viral hepatitis* (early cholestatic phase), *PBC, genetic* (Dubin-Johnson), *biliary atresia, alcoholic hepatitis.*]
cause of extrahepatic cholestasis	**stone in the CBD** [Other causes include *carcinoma of the head of pancreas, PSC.*]
G/M features of intra- and extrahepatic cholestasis	*gross*: enlarged, green liver *intra-*: bile plugs in the canaliculi around zone 3 *extra-*: bile lakes and infarcts from rupture of bile ducts

Table 14–4. MISCELLANEOUS LIVER DISORDERS, PERITONEAL DISORDERS *Continued*

Most Common...	Answer and Explanation
S/S of cholestasis	**jaundice,** *pruritus* (bile salts), *skin xanthomas* (CH deposition; CH is eliminated in bile), *hepatomegaly, secondary biliary cirrhosis, acholic stools* (absent urobilin), *dark urine* (CB; no UBG)
lab findings of cholestasis	*marked elevation of ALP and GGT, mild to moderate increase in ALT and AST, CB > 50%, hypercholesterolemia* (lipoprotein X [high in free CH and low in esterified CH]; characteristic of obstructive jaundice)
disease associated with PSC	*ulcerative colitis* (UC) [PSC is a multifocal, obliterative fibrosis of large bile ducts leading to strictures, obstruction, and secondary biliary cirrhosis. ERCP is confirmatory.]
cause of destruction of bile duct radicals in the portal triads	*PBC* [It is an autoimmune disease in middle-aged women.]
microscopic findings of PBC	*granulomatous inflammation with destruction of the portal triad bile duct radicles, with eventual replacement by fibrosis* (cirrhosis)
S/S of PBC	*early presentation with* **pruritus** *and markedly elevated ALP without evidence of jaundice* (late finding) [Signs of PH develop later. It is often associated with other autoimmune diseases (e.g., rheumatoid arthritis).]
lab findings of PBC	*increased ALP and GGT, presence of antimitochondrial antibodies* (90%), *increased IgM, hypercholesterolemia*
drugs associated with hepatitis (acute and chronic)	*isoniazid, halothane* (fever after 1 week and then jaundice), *methyldopa, salicylates*
drugs associated with intrahepatic cholestasis	**estrogen derivatives** [Others drugs include *anabolic steroids, erythromycin estolate, amoxicillin, chlorpromazine, thiazides.*]
drugs associated with fatty change	*amiodarone, corticosteroids, tetracycline* (microvesicular type)
drug associated with fibrosis	*methotrexate*

Table continued on following page

Table 14–4. MISCELLANEOUS LIVER DISORDERS, PERITONEAL DISORDERS *Continued*

Most Common...	Answer and Explanation
drugs/chemicals associated with liver tumors	*liver cell adenoma*: oral contraceptives *nodular hyperplasia*: azathioprine *hepatocellular carcinoma* (HCC): oral contraceptives *angiosarcoma*: vinyl chloride, arsenic, Thorotrast
drugs associated with granulomatous hepatitis	*allopurinol, sulfonamides*
chemicals associated with liver necrosis	*yellow phosphorus* (zone 1), *carbon tetrachloride* (CCl$_3$ · free radical, zone 3), *Amanita poisoning* (zone 3)
genetic cause of iron overload	*hemochromatosis* (AR) [It has an HLA-A3 relationship, males are involved more than females, and the abnormal gene is on chromosome 6. There is an unrestricted absorption of iron from the small bowel. Recent studies indicate that it is one of the most common genetic diseases in the United States.]
target organ involved in hemochromatosis	**liver** (cirrhosis; HCC most common cause of death) [Other organs involved: *heart* (restrictive cardiomyopathy), *pancreas* (DM, malabsorption), *hypothalamus* (DI), *joints* (osteoarthritis), *skin* (hyperpigmentation), and *gonads* (hypogonadism).]
lab findings in hemochromatosis	*high serum iron, low TIBC* (screening test), *high percent saturation, high serum ferritin* (screening test)
acquired cause of iron overload	*hemosiderosis* (multiple blood transfusions, drinking well water, alcoholics)
treatment for iron overload	*phlebotomy* [The goal is to have a low serum ferritin level.]
cause of Wilson's disease (AR)	*defect of copper excretion in bile leading to chronic liver disease, low ceruloplasmin levels* (decreased synthesis), and *deposition of free copper into the lenticular nuclei degeneration* (spasticity, dementia, choreoathetosis) and *Descemet's membrane in the eye* (Kayser-Fleischer ring)

Table 14–4. MISCELLANEOUS LIVER DISORDERS, PERITONEAL DISORDERS *Continued*

Most Common...	Answer and Explanation
lab findings in Wilson's disease	*decreased total copper* (due to decrease in ceruloplasmin and amount of copper bound to that protein) and *increased free copper levels*
treatment for Wilson's disease	*penicillamine* [It is a copper chelating agent.]
glycogen storage disease involving the liver	*von Gierke's disease* (AR) [It is due to a deficiency of the gluconeogenic enzyme glucose 6-phosphatase. Patients have hypoglycemia and hepatorenomegaly.]
target organs involved in AAT deficiency (AR)	*liver* (cholestatic hepatitis, cirrhosis, carcinoma; PAS positive globules of AAT in the liver) and *lungs* (panacinar emphysema of the lower lobes)
liver disease in pregnancy	**viral hepatitis** [Other diseases: *benign intrahepatic cholestasis* (estrogen-induced), *acute fatty liver* (abnormality in β-oxidation of fatty acids; must deliver the baby), *preeclampsia/eclampsia* (periportal necrosis, HELLP syndrome [**h**emolytic anemia, **el**evated transaminases, **l**ow **p**latelets]).]
cause of neonatal cholestasis	**neonatal hepatitis** (multinucleated giant cells; cholestatic hepatitis) [Other causes include *biliary atresia* (extrahepatic more common than intrahepatic), *infection* (e.g., CMV), *CF, AAT deficiency.*]
causes of Reye's syndrome in children	*influenza or chickenpox with ingestion of aspirin* [Its pathogenesis may involve an alteration in the β-oxidation of fatty acids.]
target organs in Reye's syndrome	*brain* (cerebral edema; convulsions, coma; encephalopathy is the most common cause of death) and *liver* (microvesicular steatosis; megamitochondria on EM)
lab findings in Reye's syndrome	**increased transaminases**, *increased ammonia* (alteration in the urea cycle), *hypoglycemia, jaundice* (uncommon)
primary malignant tumor in children	*hepatoblastoma* (increased AFP; contains both epithelial and mesenchymal components)

Table continued on following page

Table 14–4. MISCELLANEOUS LIVER DISORDERS, PERITONEAL DISORDERS *Continued*

Most Common...	Answer and Explanation
morphologic types of cirrhosis	*micronodular* (nodules <3 mm; alcohol, PBC, hemochromatosis), *macronodular* (nodules >3 mm; viral, AAT, Wilson's), **mixed pattern**
cause of cirrhosis	**alcohol-related liver disease** [Other causes include *postnecrotic cirrhosis* (**HBV**, HCV), *hemochromatosis, PBC, Wilson's disease, AAT deficiency.*]
COD in cirrhosis	**ruptured esophageal varices,** *hepatocellular failure*
causes of hepatocellular failure	*fulminant hepatic failure* (FHF; acute liver failure with encephalopathy within 8 weeks of hepatic dysfunction) and *cirrhosis* (differs from FHF in that it is associated with PH)
cause of FHF	*drugs* (acetaminophen most common) and *viral infections* (HBV most common)
disorders associated with hepatocellular failure	*coagulation defects* (bleeding; PT increases while the transaminases decrease from massive loss of hepatocytes), *encephalopathy* (somnolence, asterixis [flapping tremor]), *hepatorenal syndrome* (renal failure without microscopic alterations), *dysfunctional urea cycle* (low BUN, high ammonia), *hyperestrinism* (inability to metabolize estrogen and 17-KS [aromatized to estrogen]), *chronic respiratory alkalosis* (toxic byproducts stimulate the respiratory center), *hypoglycemia* (defective gluconeogenesis, low glycogen stores), *ascites* (see below)
cause of ascites in cirrhosis	**PH** (increased hydrostatic pressure) [Other causes include *hypoalbuminemia* (decreased oncotic pressure), *secondary aldosteronism* (inability to metabolize aldosterone; stimulation of the RAA system; salt and water retention).]
cause of PH	**cirrhosis** [Other causes include *portal vein thrombosis* (prehepatic), *Budd-Chiari syndrome* (post-hepatic), *right heart failure* (post-hepatic).]
cause of PH in cirrhosis	*obstruction to portal vein blood flow due to intrasinusoidal obstruction by fibrosis and regenerative nodules, intrahepatic anastomoses between the hepatic arterial and venous systems*

Table 14–4. MISCELLANEOUS LIVER DISORDERS, PERITONEAL DISORDERS *Continued*

Most Common...	Answer and Explanation
cause of a liver mass with a central stellate-shaped scar	*focal nodular hyperplasia* (no identifiable cause)
benign tumor of the liver	*cavernous hemangioma*
benign tumor of liver associated with birth control pills or anabolic steroids	*liver cell adenoma* [It may rupture during pregnancy.]
malignancy of the liver	*metastasis* (primary sites: **lung,** colorectum, pancreas, stomach, breast)
primary malignancy of the liver	*HCC*
causes of HCC	*postnecrotic cirrhosis* secondary to **HBV** (enhanced with aflatoxins) or *HCV, hemochromatosis, alcohol*
G/M findings of HCC	*gross*: nodular mass(es) in a background of cirrhosis *microscopic*: vessel invasion, neoplastic hepatocytes with bile
S/S of HCC	*fever, hepatomegaly, abdominal pain, weight loss, bloody ascitic fluid*
lab finding of HCC	**increased AFP** [Other findings include AAT, ALP, polycythemia (ectopic erythropoietin), hypoglycemia (ectopic insulin-like factor).]
cause of angiosarcoma	*vinyl chloride, arsenic, Thorotrast*
bile duct site for primary cancer	*adenocarcinoma of the ampulla of Vater*
causes of cholangiocarcinoma	*PSC, Clonorchis sinensis*
causes of acute peritonitis	*ruptured viscus* (e.g., duodenal ulcer, diverticulum, appendix), *ruptured cyst* (e.g., benign follicular cyst), *ischemic bowel, spontaneous* (ascites in alcoholic cirrhosis with *Eschericha coli* most common cause; ascites in a child with nephrotic syndrome with *Streptococcus pneumoniae* as the most common cause)

Table continued on following page

330 MOST COMMONS IN PATHOLOGY AND LABORATORY MEDICINE

Table 14–4. MISCELLANEOUS LIVER DISORDERS, PERITONEAL DISORDERS *Continued*

Question: Which of the following would be expected findings in a man with alcoholic cirrhosis? **SELECT 3**
(A) High serum BUN
(B) High serum ammonia
(C) Hyperglycemia
(D) Gynecomastia
(E) Impotence
(F) Bloody ascitic fluid
(G) Hypernatremia

Answers: (B), (D), (E): Dysfunction of the urea cycle causes an increase in ammonia (B) and decrease in urea (A). Hypoglycemia (C; decreased glycogen and gluconeogenesis) and hyponatremia (G; kidney reabsorption of more water than salt) are commonly present. Bloody ascitic fluid (F) is a feature of HCC. Impotence (E) is due to hyperestrinism (D) with increased production of sex hormone–binding globulin, which binds free testosterone and the effect of alcohol on reducing testosterone synthesis by the Leydig cells.

AAT = α₁-antitrypsin, AcAc = acetoacetate, AFP = alpha-fetoprotein, ALP = alkaline phosphatase, ALT = alanine transaminase, ANA = antinuclear antibodies, AR = autosomal recessive, AST = aspartate transaminase, BUN = blood urea nitrogen, CB = conjugated bilirubin, CBD = common bile duct, CF = cystic fibrosis, CH = cholesterol, CMV = cytomegalovirus, CoA = coenzyme A, COD = cause of death, DHAP = dihydroxyacetone phosphate, DI = diabetes insipidus, DM = diabetes mellitus, EM = electron microscopy, ERCP = endoscopic retrograde cholangiopancreatography, FHF = fulminant hepatic failure, G-3P = glycerol 3-phosphate, GGT = γ-glutamyl transferase, G/M = gross and microscopic, HBV = hepatitis B, HCV = hepatitis C, HLA = human leukocyte antigen, IgM = immunoglobulin M, 17-KS-17-ketosteroids, NADH₂ = nicotinamide adenine dinucleotide (reduced form), β-OHB = β-hydroxybutyrate, PAS = periodic acid-Schiff, PBC = primary biliary cirrhosis, PH = portal hypertension, PSC = primary sclerosing cholangitis, PT = prothrombin time, RAA = renin-angiotensin-aldosterone, RBC = red blood cell, S/S = signs and symptoms, THV = terminal hepatic venule, TIBC = total iron binding capacity, TXA₂ = thromboxane A₂, UBG = urobilinogen, VLDL = very low density lipoprotein.

Table 14–5. GALLBLADDER AND PANCREATIC DISORDERS

Most Common...	Answer and Explanation
causes of stone formation	*an* **increase of CH** *or a decrease in bile salts in bile*
types of stones	**CH** *and pigment stones*
risk factors for stone formation	*obese female, ethnicity* (e.g., black, Native American), *DM, cirrhosis, chronic extravascular hemolysis* (e.g., sickle cell disease)

Table 14–5. GALLBLADDER AND PANCREATIC
DISORDERS *Continued*

Most Common...	Answer and Explanation
cause of black pigment stones	*extravascular hemolytic anemia* (e.g., sickle cell disease, congenital spherocytosis)
complication associated with stones	**cholecystitis** (acute and chronic) [Other complications include *CBD obstruction, GB cancer.*]
cause of acute cholecystitis	*stone impacted in the cystic duct* [*Escherichia coli* is the most common pathogen. The majority of cases resolve in 3–7 days when the stone falls out of the duct.]
test used to identify stones in the cystic duct	*radionuclide scan*
test used to identify stones in the GB	*ultrasonography* (gold standard test)
S/S of acute cholecystitis	*fever, RUQ pain 15–30 minutes after eating, radiation of pain to the right scapula, Murphy's sign* (pain when the GB hits the examiner's finger on patient inspiration)
cause of chronic cholecystitis	*stones in the GB with repeated attacks of minor inflammation*
G/M of a strawberry GB (cholesterolosis)	*presence of CH-laden macrophages in the lamina propria* giving the mucosa a yellow-strawberry appearance
cause of hydrops of the GB	*obstruction of the cystic duct* [This leads to mucous distention of the GB.]
causes of GB cancer	**stones** and a *porcelain GB* (dystrophically calcified GB) [It is the most common primary cancer of the biliary tract.]
defect in cystic fibrosis (CF; AR disease)	*defective gene on chromosome 7 that codes for CF transmembrane regulator* (CFTR) [CFTR normally controls the transport of chloride ions through certain epithelial cells.]
DNA defect in CF	*deletion of three nucleotide bases on chromosome 7 that normally codes for phenylalanine leads to a defective CFTR*

Table continued on following page

Table 14–5. GALLBLADDER AND PANCREATIC DISORDERS *Continued*

Most Common...	Answer and Explanation
abnormality in the sweat glands and respiratory epithelium in CF	*sweat glands*: neither chloride nor sodium ions can be reabsorbed out of the lumen (basis of the sweat test) *respiratory epithelium*: chloride cannot be secreted into the lumen while sodium and water are reabsorbed out of the lumen, leading to thick secretions [Similar changes occur in the pancreatic epithelial cells.]
S/S of CF	**recurrent pulmonary infections** and *malabsorption* (duct obstruction with subsequent exocrine gland atrophy) [Others include: DM (late), secondary biliary cirrhosis, meconium ileus in newborns (impacted meconium), secondary biliary cirrhosis (thick bile secretions), bronchiectasis (CF most common cause), nasal polyps, cor pulmonale, atresia of vas deferens (males are sterile), woman may bear children (problems with fertility).]
lab test to confirm CF	**sweat chloride test** (>60 mEq/L is diagnostic) [Children have a salty taste when kissed. There is an increase in serum immunoreactive trypsin in newborns due to obstructed pancreatic ducts.]
COD in CF	*progressive respiratory failure*
causes of acute pancreatitis	**stone impacted in distal end of the CBD** and **alcoholism** [Other causes include *trauma* (most common in children), *infection* (e.g., mumps, CMV in AIDS), *drugs* (azathioprine, estrogen, pentamidine), *hypertriglyceridemia, hypercalcemia.*]
initiating events responsible for acute pancreatitis	*zymogen activation* (intra-acinar autoactivation of trypsinogen to form trypsin, which activates other enzymes, complement, and the kinin system) and *increased duct permeability* (due to obstruction with increased pressure leading to gland fibrosis and atrophy, not necrosis)
G/M findings in acute pancreatitis	*gross*: edematous, focally hemorrhagic pancreas with chalky areas representing enzymatic fat necrosis *microscopic*: liquefactive necrosis, neutrophil infiltrate, saponified adipose

Table 14–5. GALLBLADDER AND PANCREATIC DISORDERS *Continued*

Most Common...	Answer and Explanation
S/S of acute pancreatitis	**severe, boring, midepigastric pain with radiation into the back** [Other S/S include *fever, Grey-Turner sign* (flank hemorrhage), *Cullen's sign* (periumbilical hemorrhage).]
lab finding in acute pancreatitis	**elevated serum amylase** (returns to normal in 3–5 days owing to increased clearance by the kidneys; FP from bowel infarction, ruptured ectopic pregnancy, mumps) [Other findings include *elevated serum lipase, neutrophilic leukocytosis, hypocalcemia* (used up in enzymatic fat necrosis; poor sign).]
radiographic findings in acute pancreatitis	*sentinel loop* (localized ileus) *near duodenum or transverse colon, left-sided pleural effusion* (10%; contains amylase) [CT is the best imaging technique for pancreatic disease.]
complication of acute pancreatitis	**pancreatic necrosis** [Other complications include *pseudocyst* (persistence of hyperamylasemia beyond 1 week), *pancreatic abscess* (fever, leukocytosis), *ARDS, hypovolemic shock* (third space loss of fluids), *DIC.*]
cause of chronic pancreatitis	*alcoholism* [CF is the most common cause in children. Obstruction (calcified concretions) with duct dilatation produces a "chain of lakes" appearance with radiographic dyes.]
clinical triad of chronic pancreatitis	*pancreatic calcifications* (CT is the best study), *steatorrhea,* and *DM*
pancreatic cancer	**adenocarcinoma,** *islet cell tumors* (see Chapter 17).
causes of pancreatic carcinoma	**smoking,** *chronic pancreatitis* [Point mutations of the p53 suppressor gene and *ras* oncogene have been strongly implicated.]
pancreatic sites for cancer	**head of the pancreas,** *body,* and *tail*
S/S in carcinoma of the head of pancreas	**epigastric pain** [Other S/S include *jaundice* (CB >50%), *acholic stools, weight loss, palpable GB* (Courvoisier's sign), *Trousseau's superficial thrombophlebitis.* It has a poor prognosis.]

Table continued on following page

Table 14–5. GALLBLADDER AND PANCREATIC
DISORDERS *Continued*

Most Common...	Answer and Explanation
lab findings in pancreatic cancer	*elevated CA19-9* (gold standard tumor marker) [Enzymes are not commonly elevated.]

Question: Gallstones are involved in the pathogenesis of which of the following disorders? **SELECT 4**
- (A) Cholecystitis
- (B) UCB hyperbilirubinemia
- (C) Cholesterolosis
- (D) Acute pancreatitis
- (E) GB cancer
- (F) Primary sclerosing cholangitis
- (G) Ascending cholangitis
- (H) Pancreatic adenocarcinoma
- (I) Chronic pancreatitis

Answers: (A), (D), (E), (G): Hyperbilirubinemia (B) is due to an increase in GB. Cholesterolosis (C) had no relation to stones and is not clinically symptomatic. PSC (F) is associated with ulcerative colitis and not stones. There is no relation of pancreatic carcinoma (H) or chronic pancreatitis with stones (I).

AIDS = acquired immunodeficiency syndrome, AR = autosomal recessive, ARDS = adult respiratory distress syndrome, CB = conjugated bilirubin, CBD = common bile duct, CF = cystic fibrosis, CH = cholesterol, CMV = cytomegalovirus, COD = cause of death, CT = computed tomography, DIC = disseminated intravascular coagulation, DM = diabetes mellitus, FP = false positive, GB = gallbladder, G/M = gross and microscopic, PSC = primary sclerosing cholangitis, RUQ = right upper quadrant, S/S = signs and symptoms, UCB = unconjugated bilirubin.

CHAPTER
15

KIDNEY, LOWER URINARY TRACT, MALE REPRODUCTIVE PATHOLOGY

CONTENTS

Table 15–1. OVERVIEW, RENAL FUNCTION TESTS

Most Common...	Answer and Explanation
S/S of kidney disease	**proteinuria** (usually a kidney problem) [Other S/S include *pain* (flank pain), *hematuria* (source from kidney, ureters, bladder, prostate, urethra), *oliguria* (prerenal, renal, postrenal).]
S/S of lower urinary tract disease	**dysuria** (painful urination; usually infection) [Other S/S include *increased frequency of urination* (usually infection).]
S/S of male genital disease	*testicular pain* (e.g., orchitis, epididymitis), *testicular mass* (most commonly cancer), *erectile dysfunction* (e.g., stress, testosterone deficiency)
kidney site for tissue hypoxia	*renal medulla* [Normally, it only receives 10% of the total renal blood flow.]
manifestation of tubular damage	**loss of concentrating ability** and *dilution*
contributor to synthesis of the GBM	*visceral epithelial cells* (podocytes)
type of capillary in the glomerulus	*capillary lined by fenestrated endothelial cells for ease in filtration*
components of the GBM	*type IV collagen* and *GAGs* [Heparin is the main GAG and is responsible for the negative charge of the GBM).]

Table continued on following page

335

Table 15–1. OVERVIEW, RENAL FUNCTION TESTS *Continued*

Most Common...	Answer and Explanation
function of mesangial cells	**support** [Other functions include *phagocytosis, release of inflammatory mediators, regulation of intraglomerular blood flow via AT II.* They are modified smooth muscle cells.]
cause of glomerular diseases	*immunocomplex deposition* (type III hypersensitivity; e.g., post-streptococcal GN)
cause of tubular diseases	*ischemia* (e.g., acute tubular necrosis)
cause of interstitial nephritis (tubulointerstitial disease)	**infection** (e.g., pyelonephritis), *drugs* (e.g., methicillin)
cause of vascular disease	**small vessel disease of DM** and *hypertension* (hyaline arteriolosclerosis), *renal artery atherosclerosis* (e.g., renovascular hypertension)
tests for renal function	**urinalysis** (UA), *serum BUN, serum creatinine, BUN:creatinine ratio, CCr, UOsm, FENa*
source of urea	*end-product of amino acid and pyrimidine metabolism*
cause of an increased serum BUN	*decreased GFR* (e.g., CHF, shock, hypovolemia), which leads to an increased proximal reabsorption of urea *(prerenal azotemia)* [The *BUN:creatinine ratio increases from a normal of 10:1 to >15:1.* Creatinine increases slightly due to a reduction in GFR.]
source of creatinine	*creatine in muscle* [This underscores why creatinine is a measure of muscle mass.]
cause of an elevated creatinine	*prerenal azotemia* (decreased GFR) [Creatinine is a poor screen for renal disease, since >50% of renal mass must be destroyed before it increases.]
clearance substance used in clinical medicine	*creatinine* [The creatinine clearance formula is: $CCr = UOsm \times V/POsm$, where V = volume of a 24-hr urine collection in mL/min.]
cause of a decreased CCr	*increasing age* [It is an age-dependent finding. Pathologic causes include chronic renal failure secondary to glomerulonephritis and other disorders.]

Table 15–1. OVERVIEW, RENAL FUNCTION TESTS *Continued*

Most Common...	Answer and Explanation
cause of an increased CCr	**pregnancy and early diabetic nephropathy** [The increase in plasma volume in pregnancy increases the GFR and, subsequently, the CCr. Hyperfiltration is a characteristic feature of early DM.]
effect of a decreased GFR on the BUN:creatinine ratio	*increases the normal 10:1 ratio to >15:1* [A decrease in the GFR increases the proximal reabsorption of urea but not creatinine, since it is not reabsorbed. There is a disproportionate increase in urea and only a slight increase in creatinine due to the slower GFR.]
effect of renal failure on the serum BUN:creatinine ratio	*maintenance of the 10:1 ratio* [Both the serum BUN and creatinine are equally affected by intrinsic renal disease, so both increase at the same rate and maintain the normal 10:1 ratio (e.g., serum BUN 80 mg/dL and creatinine 8 mg/dL; this is called *renal azotemia* [uremia]).]
effect of postrenal obstruction on the serum BUN:creatinine ratio	*>15:1 ratio* [This is due to back diffusion of urea in urine into the blood secondary to obstruction behind the kidney (e.g., ureters, bladder, urethra; e.g., serum BUN 80 mg/dL and creatinine 2 mg/dL; this is called *postrenal azotemia*).]
use of UOsm	*to evaluate the concentrating* (usually >800 mOsm/kg) and *diluting capacity of the kidneys* (commonly <100 mOsm/kg)
use of the FENa [fractional excretion of sodium]	*work-up of oliguria* (urine flow <400 mL/day) [FENa = UNa × PCr/PNa × UCr × 100. Values <1 indicate intact tubular function; those >1 indicate tubular dysfunction.]
cause of a dark yellow urine	**concentrated urine** [Other causes include *coloring from vitamins, CB, increased UBG.*]
cause of a red urine	**hematuria** (Hb) [Other causes include *myoglobin, drugs* (phenazopyridine), *porphyrias.*]
cause of a black urine	*alkaptonuria* (AR) [Homogentisic acid must be oxidized on exposure to air before it turns black.]
urine dipstick components	*specific gravity, pH, protein, glucose, ketones, bilirubin, UBG, leukocyte esterase, nitrites*

Table continued on following page

Table 15–1. OVERVIEW, RENAL FUNCTION TESTS *Continued*

Most Common...	Answer and Explanation
cause of isosthenuria [fixed specific gravity]	*chronic renal failure with complete loss of concentration and dilution*
dipstick urine pH findings in meat eaters and vegans	*acid pH* (inorganic/organic acids from meat) and *alkaline pH* (citrates converted into bicarbonate), respectively
uses of urine pH	*alter pH to prevent renal stones* (e.g., alkalinize urine in uric acid stones), *alter pH to excrete drugs* (e.g., alkalinize to excrete salicylates), *diagnose renal tubular acidosis* (urine pH >5.5)
cause of an alkaline urine smelling like ammonia	*urease-producing bacterial infection* (e.g., *Proteus* species) [Urease breaks urea down into ammonia.]
cause of a positive dipstick for protein	**primary renal disease** (the most common initial finding) [Dipstick protein only detects albumin (not globulins). Positive dipstick proteins are confirmed with SSA, which detects both albumin and globulins (e.g., Bence-Jones protein [light chains]).]
cause of a negative dipstick protein and strongly positive SSA	*Bence-Jones proteinuria in multiple myeloma* [Both the dipstick and SSA reading should be the same if only albumin is present. A disproportionate increase in SSA indicates globulins are present.]
test used to detect microalbuminuria (<30 mg albumin/ day)	*microalbumin dipsticks* [These dipsticks are sensitive to 1.5–8 mg/dL, unlike the standard dipsticks, which only detect as low as 30 mg/dL. Microalbuminuria is the first sign of diabetic nephropathy.]
cause of a positive dipstick for glucose	**DM** [Other causes include *normal pregnancy* (low renal threshold for glucose), *benign glucosuria* (low threshold), proximal renal tubular acidosis. The test is specific for glucose.]
use of Clinitest	*it detects urine-reducing substances* (e.g., glucose, galactose, lactose, ascorbic acid, fructose, but not sucrose, since it is not a reducing sugar)
cause of a positive dipstick for ketones	**volume depletion** [Other causes include *DKA, normal pregnancy, ketogenic diets.* Nitroprusside only reacts with acetone and AcAc, not β-OHB.]

Table 15–1. OVERVIEW, RENAL FUNCTION TESTS *Continued*

Most Common...	Answer and Explanation
cause of a positive dipstick for bilirubin	**viral hepatitis with excretion of CB** [CB is also present in *obstructive jaundice* but not in jaundice due to UCB.]
cause of an increased dipstick reaction for UBG	**viral hepatitis** [In viral hepatitis, the UBG normally recycled back to the liver (entero-hepatic circulation) is redirected to the kidneys. UBG is also increased in *extravascular hemolysis* and is absent in obstructive jaundice. Urobilin, the oxidation product of UBG, gives the normal color to urine (and stool).]
causes of a positive dipstick for blood	**hematuria** (e.g., **cystitis,** renal adenocarcinoma, bladder cancer), *myoglobinuria* (dipstick reagents are positive for myoglobin or Hb; a serum creatine kinase is useful in this differentiation)
cause of a positive dipstick for leukocyte esterase	**cystitis with neutrophils in the urine** (neutrophils contain esterase) [*Sterile pyuria* refers to neutrophils with a negative standard urine culture (e.g., urethritis due to *Chlamydia trachomatis*, renal TB).]
cause of a positive dipstick for nitrites	*cystitis secondary to a nitrate reducer, most commonly Escherichia coli*
cause of dysmorphic [abnormally shaped] RBCs in the urine	*glomerulonephritis* [They are best seen with a phase contrast microscope. Dysmorphic RBCs indicate a glomerular origin for the hematuria.]
causes of WBCs in the urine	**infection (cystitis,** pyelonephritis, urethritis), *drug-induced interstitial nephritis.*
cause of oval fat bodies [epithelial cells or macrophages with lipid] and free lipid in the urine	*nephrotic syndrome* (proteinuria >3.5 g/24 hours) [If polarization of the urine reveals *Maltese crosses* in the oval fat bodies, casts, or free lipid in the urine, it indicates CH rather than TG is present.]
cause of eosinophiluria	*drug-induced interstitial nephritis*
cause of hemosiderinuria	*chronic intravascular hemolytic anemia* (e.g., microangiopathic hemolytic anemia in a patient with aortic stenosis)

Table continued on following page

Table 15–1. OVERVIEW, RENAL FUNCTION TESTS *Continued*

Most Common...	Answer and Explanation
location of urine cast formation	*diseases originating in the kidneys* (e.g., GN, pyelonephritis) [Casts are molds of tubular lumens and contain cellular elements, etc. that are involved in the disease process.]
cast in the urine	*hyaline casts* (acellular, clear casts) composed of Tamm-Horsfall protein [They usually have no clinical significance, unless they are present in great numbers.]
casts associated with the nephritic syndrome [inflammatory types of GN]	**RBC casts,** *WBC casts* to a lesser extent
casts associated with the nephrotic syndrome	*fatty casts with Maltese crosses*
cast associated with acute pyelonephritis	*WBC cast*
cast associated with acute tubular necrosis	*renal tubular cast*
casts in chronic renal disease	*broad casts* and *waxy casts*
progression of degeneration of a cellular cast in a renal tubule	*cellular cast* (e.g., WBC cast) → *coarsely granular cast* → *finely granular cast* → *waxy cast* (usually after 3 months, which is why it is an indicator of chronic renal disease)
clinically important crystals in an acid urine	*uric acid* (gout, idiopathic) and *calcium oxalate* (looks like the back of an envelope; calcium oxalate stone former, Crohn's disease, ethylene glycol poisoning [ethylene glycol is converted into oxalic acid, which binds with calcium])
clinically important crystal in an alkaline urine	*triple phosphate* (looks like a coffin lid) in patients with urease-producing organisms (e.g., *Proteus* species)
inborn error of metabolism with a pathognomonic urine crystal	*cystinuria with a hexagonal crystal*

Table 15–1. OVERVIEW, RENAL FUNCTION TESTS *Continued*

Most Common...	Answer and Explanation
benign cause of proteinuria	*postural (orthostatic) proteinuria* [Proteinuria occurs with standing and disappears after lying down.]
pathologic cause of proteinuria	*loss of GBM negative charge or size barrier* (e.g., GN) [The strong negative charge and the size of proteins are most important in restricting proteins from entering the urine.]

Question: A urine specimen from a 25-year-old man with dysuria reveals a positive dipstick for leukocyte esterase (negative nitrite), a sediment with numerous WBCs, no visible bacteria, and a negative routine culture. Possible causes include which of the following? **SE-LECT 2**

    (A) *E. coli*
    (B) TB
    (C) *Proteus* species
    (D) *Chlamydia*
    (E) Improper collection

Answers: (B), (D): This is a sterile pyuria, which may be due to TB or *Chlamydia*, usually the latter. Choices (A) and (C) would have a positive culture and positive nitrite. Choice (E) is not likely because the patient is symptomatic.

AcAc = acetoacetic acid, AR = autosomal recessive, AT II = angiotensin II, β-OHB = β-hydroxybutyric acid, BUN = blood urea nitrogen, CB = conjugated bilirubin, CCr = creatinine clearance, CH = cholesterol, CHF = congestive heart failure, DKA = diabetic ketoacidosis, DM = diabetes mellitus, GAG = glycosaminoglycans, GBM = glomerular basement membrane, GFR = glomerular filtration rate, GN = glomerulonephritis, Hb = hemoglobin, PCr = plasma creatinine, PNa = plasma sodium, POsm = plasma osmolality, RBC = red blood cell, S/S = signs and symptoms, SSA = sulfosalicylic acid, TB = tuberculosis, TG = triglyceride, UBG = urobilinogen, UCr = urine creatinine, UNa = urine sodium, UOsm = urine osmolality, WBC = white blood cell.

Table 15–2. CYSTIC AND GLOMERULAR DISORDERS

Most Common...	Answer and Explanation
cause of a palpable flank mass in a newborn	*cystic disease of the kidney(s)*
cystic disease in children	*renal dysplasia* [It refers to abnormal development of one or both kidneys.]

Table continued on following page

Table 15–2. CYSTIC AND GLOMERULAR DISORDERS *Continued*

Most Common...	Answer and Explanation
genetic cystic disease in children	*autosomal recessive polycystic kidney disease* [It involves both kidneys and is associated with cysts in other sites (e.g., liver).]
type of cyst in adults	*acquired retention cysts* [These are derived from tubular obstruction.]
genetic adult cystic disease	*adult polycystic kidney disease* (APKD), an AD disease. [Cysts are not present at birth.]
complications associated with APKD	**hypertension** [Other complications include *intracranial berry aneurysms, cysts in other sites, renal failure.*]
cell type causing crescents in a glomerulus	*proliferation of parietal cells in Bowman's capsule* [It is associated with RPGN.]
cause of a linear IF pattern in the glomerulus	*Goodpasture's syndrome* [Anti-GBM antibodies (against α_3 type IV collagen) line up on the endothelial side of the membrane, producing a smooth IF pattern.]
cause of a granular ("lumpy-bumpy") IF pattern in the glomerulus	*IC deposition* [IC deposition is dependent on charge, size, and solubility, hence it has a more granular pattern of distribution.]
GN where IF is diagnostic of the disease	*IgA nephropathy* (Berger's disease) [IgA must be identified to confirm the diagnosis.]
type of glomerular disease with fusion of the podocytes	*nephrotic syndrome* (e.g., minimal change disease)
antigens involved in IC types of GN	**DNA** (SLE GN), *bacterial products* (group A streptococcus GN), *HBV* (membranous GN), *HCV* (membranoproliferative GN), *CEA* (membranous GN)
EM manifestation of IC deposits	*densities in a subendothelial, intramembranous, subepithelial,* or *mesangial distribution*
S/S and lab findings of the nephritic syndrome	*oliguria, hypertension, periorbital edema, hematuria, proteinuria* (not in nephrotic range), *RBC casts, WBCs in the sediment*

Table 15–2. CYSTIC AND GLOMERULAR DISORDERS *Continued*

Most Common...	Answer and Explanation
S/S and lab findings of the nephrotic syndrome	*generalized pitting edema,* infections (*Streptococcus pneumoniae* due to hypogammaglobulinemia), *thrombosis* (loss of AT III in the urine), *proteinuria* (>3.5 g/24 hrs), *fatty casts, oval fat bodies, hypoproteinemia, hypercholesterolemia*
GN	*IgA nephropathy* [It presents with gross (children) or asymptomatic microscopic (adults) hematuria, often following an upper respiratory infection, and is primarily nephritic.]
pathologic and lab findings of post-strep GN	*diffuse proliferative GN (nephritic) after group A strep infection* (usually skin), *granular IF, subepithelial deposits, low C3* (alternative pathway activation) [Good prognosis in children]
pathologic and lab findings of SLE GN	*diffuse proliferative GN most common* (type IV; nephritic or nephrotic), *granular IF, subendothelial deposits, low C3* (classical pathway activation), *anti-ds DNA, poor prognosis*
genetic GN with nerve deafness	*Alport's syndrome* (SXD; primarily nephritic) [It commonly occurs in members of the Church of Latter Day Saints. There is a defect in α_5 type IV collagen.]
GN in Goodpasture's syndrome	*RPGN* (primarily nephritic; male dominant) [Goodpasture's syndrome has anti-BM antibodies against pulmonary capillaries and GBM (begins in the lungs with hemoptysis and ends with renal failure due to RPGN).]
nephrotic syndrome in children	*minimal change disease* (nil disease, lipoid nephrosis) [It is a cellular immune reaction with a loss of negative charge (polyanions) in the GBM.]
S/S and pathologic findings in minimal change disease	*normotensive, pitting edema, respond well to steroids, normal glomeruli on H&E staining, fusion of the podocytes on EM* [It often follows an upper respiratory infection and may complicate Hodgkin's disease or patients with an atopic history.]
nephrotic syndrome in adults	*diffuse membranous GN* [It is an IC disease with subepithelial deposits (epimembranous spikes are visible with stains).]

Table continued on following page

Table 15–2. CYSTIC AND GLOMERULAR DISORDERS *Continued*

Most Common...	Answer and Explanation
causes of membranous GN	**idiopathic,** *drugs* (captopril), *infections* (**HBV,** malaria), *malignancy* (colon cancer)
GN in AIDS and IV drug abuse	*FSG* (primarily nephrotic) [FSG is associated with hypertension and a poor prognosis.]
GN in patients with HCV	*type I MPGN* (primarily nephrotic) [It is an IC disease with subendothelial deposits, "tram tracking" (mesangium splits the GBM), and low C3 levels.]
GN associated with autoantibodies against C3 convertase	*type II MPGN* (primarily nephrotic) [It is associated with a C3 nephritic factor that stabilizes C3 convertase leading to sustained activation of C3 (low). In addition, there are dense deposits ("dense deposit disease") throughout the GBM.]
systemic disease secondarily affecting the glomerulus	*DM* (type I DM > type II DM)
initial lab findings in DM nephropathy	*microalbuminuria* [It is due to increased intraglomerular pressure (increased GFR) and increased permeability of the glomerular capillaries. Proteinuria may be in the nephrotic range later in the disease.]
G/M changes in DM nephropathy	*large kidneys with afferent and efferent hyaline arteriolosclerosis and nodular densities in the mesangium* (resemble Christmas balls; called Kimmelstiel-Wilson disease, or nodular glomerulosclerosis)
treatment for early DM nephropathy	*angiotensin-converting enzyme inhibitors* (e.g., captopril) [ACE inhibitors reduce the effect of AT II on increasing intraglomerular pressure.]
type of renal disease in amyloidosis	*nephrotic syndrome* [It is most common with secondary or reactive amyloidosis.]
glomerular disease with pre-eclampsia/ eclampsia	*hypertension with heavy proteinuria, pitting edema,* and *swelling of the endothelial cells in the glomerulus* (endotheliosis)
causes of chronic GN in descending order of incidence	**RPGN,** *FSG, type I MPGN*

Table 15–2. CYSTIC AND GLOMERULAR DISORDERS *Continued*

Question: Which of the following characterize various types of GN that primarily present as the nephritic syndrome? **SELECT 3**
(A) Fusion of podocytes
(B) Anti-GBM antibodies
(C) Apple green birefringence
(D) Fatty casts
(E) RBC casts
(F) Hypertension
(G) C3 nephritic factor
(H) Epimembranous spikes
(I) Tram tracks
(J) Hyaline arteriolosclerosis

Answers: (B), (E), (F): Anti-GBM antibodies (B) connote Goodpasture's syndrome. RBC casts (E) predominate in the nephritic syndrome, and hypertension (F) is primarily noted in nephritic types of GN. Hypertension is also noted in the nephrotic syndrome (except in primary glomerular diseases producing the nephrotic syndrome. Fusion of the podocytes (A) is noted in minimal change disease). Apple green birefringence (C; amyloid) is involved in amyloid kidneys (nephrotic). Fatty casts (D) are the key cast of the nephrotic syndrome. C3 nephritic factor (G; type II MPGN), epimembranous spikes (H; membranous GN), tram tracks (I; type I MPGN), and hyaline arteriolosclerosis (J; KW disease) are most commonly nephrotic.

ACE = angiotensin-converting enzyme, AD = autosomal dominant, AIDS = acquired immunodeficiency syndrome, anti-BM = anti-basement membrane, anti-ds DNA = anti-double stranded DNA, AT II = antithrombin II, AT III = antithrombin III, CEA = carcinoembryonic antigen, DM = diabetes mellitus, EM = electron microscopy, FSG = focal segmental glomerulosclerosis, GBM = glomerular basement membrane, GFR = glomerular filtration rate, G/M = gross and microscopic, GN = glomerulonephritis, HBV = hepatitis B virus, HCV = hepatitis C virus, H&E = hematoxylin and eosin, IC = immunocomplex, IF = immunofluorescent/immunofluorescence, Ig = immunoglobulin, IV = intravenous, KW = Kimmelstiel-Wilson, MPGN = membranoproliferative glomerulonephritis, RBC = red blood cell, RPGN = rapidly progressive crescentic glomerulonephritis, SLE = systemic lupus erythematosus, S/S = signs and symptoms, SXD = sex-linked dominant, WBC = white blood cell.

Table 15–3. TUBULAR, TUBULOINTERSTITIAL, VASCULAR, OBSTRUCTIVE, AND NEOPLASTIC DISEASES OF THE KIDNEYS

Most Common...	Answer and Explanation
cause of ARF	*ischemic ATN*
cause of ischemic ATN	*prerenal azotemia* [Prerenal azotemia is associated with a reduced GFR and the potential for ischemic tubular damage.]
causes of nephrotoxic ATN	**drugs** (e.g., **aminoglycosides,** cisplatin, cyclosporine), *radiocontrast agents*
patterns of ATN	**ischemic ATN** and *nephrotoxic ATN* [The majority of cases of ischemic ATN are oliguric. The former produces multifocal areas of coagulation necrosis of tubules with sloughing of cells into the lumen, tubulorrhexis (disruption of the tubular BM), and pigmented renal tubular casts.]
histologic pattern of nephrotoxic ATN	*coagulation necrosis of the proximal tubule cells with sparing of the BM*
mechanisms of oliguria in ATN	*tubular cells blocking the lumen, vasoconstriction of the afferent arterioles, increased interstitial pressure from fluid leaking out through damaged BMs*
tests used in the work-up of oliguria	*FENa, UOsm, random UNa,* and *UA* [*Good tubular function* (ability to concentrate urine): FENa <1, UOsm >500 mOsm/kg, UNa <40 mEq/L, UA without renal tubular casts. *Tubular dysfunction* (loss of concentration): FENa >1, UOsm <350 mOsm/kg, UNa >40 mEq/L, UA with renal tubular casts]
causes of oliguria with preserved tubular function	**prerenal azotemia** (normal UA), *acute GN* (RBC casts)
causes of oliguria with tubular dysfunction	**ATN** (renal tubular casts), *postrenal azotemia* (normal UA)
causes of CRF	**DM nephropathy** (KW disease), *hypertension, GN.*

Table 15–3. TUBULAR, TUBULOINTERSTITIAL, VASCULAR, OBSTRUCTIVE, AND NEOPLASTIC DISEASES OF THE KIDNEYS *Continued*

Most Common...	Answer and Explanation
lab findings in CRF	*hyperkalemia* (peaked T waves), *increased AG metabolic acidosis, hypocalcemia* (hypovitaminosis D), *hyperphosphatemia, prolonged BT* (dysfunctional platelets), *normocytic anemia* (decreased erythropoietin), *isosthenuria, broad and waxy casts*
bone findings in CRF	*osteomalacia* (due to hypocalcemia), *osteoporosis* (bone is a buffer), *osteitis fibrosa cystica* (secondary hyperparathyroidism from hypocalcemia)
cardiac findings in CRF	*fibrinous pericarditis, CHF, accelerated atherosclerosis, hypertension*
GI findings in CRF	*hemorrhagic gastritis, PUD*
causes of acute interstitial nephritis	**APN** (most commonly due to *Escherichia coli*), *drug-induced* (e.g., methicillin)
cause of APN	*ascending infection* [This most commonly occurs from VUR, due to an incompetent ureterovesical junction. Infection spreads into the tubules (microabscesses) and interstitium of the kidneys.]
S/S and lab findings in APN	*sudden onset of spiking fever, flank pain, dysuria, pyuria, WBC casts*
causes of CPN	**reflux** (VUR), *obstruction* (tumors, prostatic hyperplasia, stones) [Kidneys are shrunken and reveal irregular scarring overlying blunted calyces, atrophy of tubules (look like thyroid follicles) and glomeruli.]
S/S and lab findings in acute drug-induced interstitial nephritis	*fever, rash, oliguria, renal azotemia, eosinophilia, eosinophiluria* [It is a type IV cellular immune reaction.]
cause of chronic drug-induced interstitial nephritis	*analgesic nephropathy* due to a combination of *acetaminophen* (FR injury of tubules and interstitium) and *aspirin* (reduced intrarenal prostaglandin [vasodilator] synthesis leading to ischemia in the renal medulla)

Table continued on following page

Table 15–3. TUBULAR, TUBULOINTERSTITIAL, VASCULAR, OBSTRUCTIVE, AND NEOPLASTIC DISEASES OF THE KIDNEYS *Continued*

Most Common...	Answer and Explanation
S/S of analgesic nephropathy	*woman with a long history of pain* (e.g., headaches) who *presents with hypertension and chronic renal disease*
causes of renal papillary necrosis	**analgesic nephropathy** [Other causes include *DM, APN, sickle cell trait/disease.* It presents with renal colic.]
causes of urate nephropathy	**treatment of disseminated cancers** (increased production of purines), *lead poisoning* (increases urate absorption)
renal findings in multiple myeloma	*nephrocalcinosis* (hypercalcemia-induced), *hypersensitivity reaction to BJ protein*
renal disease in essential HN	*BNS* [BNS is due to hyaline arteriolosclerosis leading to tubular atrophy, glomerular sclerosis, and fibrosis in the renal cortex (kidney is small and has a cobblestoned surface).]
lab findings in BNS	**proteinuria,** *hematuria, renal azotemia*
cause of malignant HN	**pre-existing BNS** [Other causes: *PSS, HUS, TTP*]
G/M findings of malignant HN	*enlarged kidneys with flea-bitten appearance, fibrinoid necrosis of large and small vessels, necrotizing arteriolitis* (cause of flea-bitten appearance), *glomerulitis, "onion skinning" of the arterioles*
S/S of malignant HN	**diastolic BP >130 mm Hg** [Other causes include *papilledema, convulsions* (cerebral edema), *headache.*]
cause of renal infarctions	*emboli from the left heart* [Infarcts are pale and wedge-shaped.]
cause of diffuse cortical necrosis	*pregnancy complicated by DIC* [It is a diffuse pale infarction of the renal cortex.]
kidney finding in urinary tract obstruction	*hydronephrosis* [There is dilatation of the renal pelvis with flattening and compression atrophy of the cortex and medulla.]
causes of hydronephrosis	**renal calculi in the ureter** [Other causes include *obstruction at ureterovesical junction* (cancer, stone), *urethral obstruction* (BPH).]

Table 15–3. TUBULAR, TUBULOINTERSTITIAL, VASCULAR, OBSTRUCTIVE, AND NEOPLASTIC DISEASES OF THE KIDNEYS *Continued*

Most Common...	Answer and Explanation
metabolic abnormalities predisposing to renal calculi	**hypercalciuria** [Other risk factors: low urine volume, reduced urine citrate (normally chelates calcium)]
renal stones	**calcium oxalate** [Other stones include *calcium phosphate, magnesium ammonium phosphate* (struvite stone, "staghorn calculus"), *uric acid*. More common in men than women]
S/S of a renal calculus	*sudden onset of colicky pain in the flank with radiation into the groin* (hematuria commonly present)
initial tests used to identify stones	**UA** (confirms hematuria, possibly identifies crystals), *KUB* (most stones are radiopaque), *renal ultrasonography* if KUB test is negative
confirmatory test for a stone	*stone analysis by x-ray diffraction*
cause of a "staghorn calculus"	*ammonium-producing bacterial infection* (urease producers like *Proteus*)
treatment of a calcium stone	**increased water intake,** *hydrochlorothiazide* (increases calcium reabsorption)
hamartoma of the kidney	*angiomyolipoma* (associated with tuberous sclerosis)
malignant kidney tumor in adults	*renal adenocarcinoma* (Grawitz tumor, hypernephroma) [Usually they are >3 cm.]
causes of a renal adenocarcinoma	**smoking,** *von Hippel-Lindau disease, APKD*
S/S of a renal adenocarcinoma	**hematuria,** *flank mass, pain* [*Ectopic hormone relationships*: erythropoietin (polycythemia), PTH-like peptide: hypercalcemia. They *invade the renal vein* and *metastasize* to **lungs,** bone, and skin.]
malignant kidney tumor in children	*Wilms' tumor* (nephroblastoma) [Some cases have an AD inheritance.]

Table continued on following page

**Table 15–3. TUBULAR, TUBULOINTERSTITIAL,
VASCULAR, OBSTRUCTIVE, AND NEOPLASTIC DISEASES
OF THE KIDNEYS** *Continued*

Most Common...	Answer and Explanation
G/M findings of a Wilms' tumor	*gross:* large, hemorrhagic tumor *micro:* they are composed of embryonic cells, rhabdomyoblasts, and primitive glomeruli [They commonly metastasize to the lungs.]
S/S of a Wilms' tumor	**unilateral palpable mass,** *hypertension, aniridia* (absent iris; in AD chromosome 11 disease only), *hematuria*

Question: Which of the following are expected in CRF? **SELECT 5**
(A) BUN:creatinine ratio ~10:1
(B) FENa <1
(C) UOsm <350 mOsm/kg
(D) Hypocalcemia
(E) Hypophosphatemia
(F) Normocytic anemia
(G) Waxy casts

Answers: (A), (C), (D), (F), (G): The FENa (B) should be >1 (tubular dysfunction) and the serum phosphorus (E) normal to elevated.

AD = autosomal dominant, AG = anion gap, APKD = adult polycystic kidney disease, APN = acute pyelonephritis, ARF = acute renal failure, ATN = acute tubular necrosis, BJ = Bence-Jones, BM = basement membrane, BNS = benign nephrosclerosis, BP = blood pressure, BPH = benign prostatic hyperplasia, BT = bleeding time, CHF = congestive heart failure, CPN = chronic pyelonephritis, CRF = chronic renal failure, DIC = disseminated intravascular coagulation, DM = diabetes mellitus, FENa = fractional excretion of sodium, FR = free radical, GFR = glomerular filtration rate, GI = gastrointestinal, G/M = gross and microscopic, GN = glomerulonephritis, HN = hypertension, HUS = hemolytic uremic syndrome, KUB = kidney/ureter/bladder radiographs, KW = Kimmelstiel-Wilson; mOsm = milliosmole, PSS = progressive systemic sclerosis, PTH = parathyroid hormone, PUD = peptic ulcer disease, RBC = red blood cell, S/S = signs and symptoms, TTP = thrombotic thrombocytopenic purpura, UA = urinalysis, UNa = urine sodium, UOsm = urine osmolality, VUR = vesicoureteral reflux, WBC = white blood cell.

**Table 15–4. LOWER URINARY TRACT AND MALE
GENITALIA DISORDERS**

Most Common...	Answer and Explanation
LUT congenital anomaly	*hypospadias* [In this condition, the urethra opens on the undersurface of the penis.]

Table 15–4. LOWER URINARY TRACT AND MALE GENITALIA DISORDERS *Continued*

Most Common...	Answer and Explanation
cause of bladder diverticula	*obstruction of the urethra* (e.g., BPH)
cause of malacoplakia of the bladder	*chronic Escherichia coli infection* [Raised yellow plaques contain histiocytes with Michaelis-Gutmann bodies (calcium phosphate).]
cause of acute cystitis	*ascending infection secondary to E. coli*
viral cause of hemorrhagic cystitis	*adenovirus*
types of bladder cancer	**transitional cell carcinoma** (usually papillary) [Other types include *squamous cell carcinoma (Schistosoma haematobium)*, adenocarcinoma, *embryonal rhabdomyosarcoma* (most common sarcoma in children).]
causes of transitional cell carcinoma of the bladder	**smoking** [Other causes include *aniline dyes, cyclophosphamide* (also hemorrhagic cystitis), *phenacetin.* Hematuria is the most common presentation.]
cause of acute prostatitis	*E. coli*
cause of chronic prostatitis	*abacterial in most cases*
benign disorder of the prostate	BPH [It is due to a slight excess of dihydrotestosterone enhanced by estrogen. It is age-dependent and does not evolve into cancer.]
location for BPH	*transitional zone closest to the prostatic urethra*
S/S and lab findings in BPH	*signs of obstruction* (trouble initiating the stream, dribbling, incomplete emptying, nocturia), *hematuria*
cancer in males	*prostate adenocarcinoma* [It is age-dependent and more common in blacks than whites. Age is the most significant risk factor, followed by family history.]
location for prostate cancer	*peripheral zone of the prostate* (palpable by DRE)

Table continued on following page

Table 15–4. LOWER URINARY TRACT AND MALE
GENITALIA DISORDERS Continued

Most Common...	Answer and Explanation
screening program for prostate cancer	*DRE and PSA annually beginning at 50 years of age* [DRE does not falsely increase PSA (PAP is no longer used).]
spread of prostate cancer	*perineural invasion, lymphatic to regional lymph nodes, hematogenous* (bone)
confirmatory test for prostate cancer	*transrectal ultrasonography with needle biopsies of suspicious sites*
site and effect of prostate cancer in bone	*vertebral column where it produces an osteoblastic response with elevation of alkaline phosphatase*
grading system for prostate cancer	*Gleason system*
cause of left scrotal enlargement resembling a "bag of worms"	*a varicocele* [It is always left-sided (testicular vein drains into the left renal vein, not the inferior vena cava) and is a common cause of male infertility.]
cause of scrotal enlargement	*hydrocele* [It is due to persistence of the tunica vaginalis.]
cause of abrupt testicular pain	*torsion of the testicle* (loss of cremasteric reflex)
causes of acute epididymitis	*<35 years: Neisseria gonorrhoeae, Chlamydia trachomatis* *>35 years: E. coli, Pseudomonas aeruginosa*
location for a cryptorchid testis	*inguinal canal*
complication of a cryptorchid testis	*potential for infertility and seminoma* [The risk for seminoma applies to both the affected testicle and the normal testicle.]
causes of orchitis	**extension of acute epididymitis,** *syphilis, mumps, HIV*
tumor of the epididymis	*adenomatoid tumor* [It is benign and derives from mesothelial cells.]
cause of a painless mass in the testicle	*malignancy, most commonly a seminoma* [Seminomas respond best to radiation and have the best prognosis.]

Table 15–4. LOWER URINARY TRACT AND MALE
GENITALIA DISORDERS *Continued*

Most Common...	Answer and Explanation
testicular cancer in children	*yolk sac tumor* (endodermal sinus tumor) [They secrete AFP as a tumor marker.]
testicular cancer in older men	*metastatic malignant lymphoma*
tumor markers used in the work-up of testicular cancer	*AFP* (yolk sac tumor origin), β-*hCG* (syncytio-trophoblast origin)
testicular cancers producing gynecomastia	*choriocarcinoma secreting* β-*hCG* [It is the most aggressive of the testicular cancers.]
testicular cancer containing derivatives from more than one germ layer	**teratoma** (more common in infants and children), *teratocarcinoma* (mixture of embryonal and teratoma; more often in adults)
cancer/risk factors for the penis	*squamous cell carcinoma; risk factors:* **lack of circumcision,** *Bowen's disease* (shaft of the penis), *erythroplasia of Queyrat* (red lesions on the glans)
source of energy for sperm	*fructose in the seminal vesicles*
components of semen	*spermatozoa* (from seminiferous tubules), *coagulant* (from seminal vesicles), *enzymes to liquefy semen* (prostate gland)
primary causes of male hypogonadism	**decreased testosterone synthesis in Leydig cells** [Other causes include *seminiferous tubule failure to produce sperm* (e.g., Klinefelter's syndrome), *abnormal androgen receptors* (e.g., testicular feminization).]
lab findings in pure seminiferous tubule failure	*high FSH* (loss of inhibin from Sertoli cells), *normal LH* (Leydig cells are synthesizing testosterone), *normal serum testosterone, decreased sperm count*
lab findings in pure Leydig cell failure	*normal FSH* (inhibin present), *high LH* (testosterone decrease), *low sperm count*
lab findings in Klinefelter's syndrome	*high FSH* (loss of inhibin), *high LH* (low testosterone), *azoospermia* (no active seminiferous tubules)

Table continued on following page

Table 15–4. LOWER URINARY TRACT AND MALE GENITALIA DISORDERS *Continued*

Most Common...	Answer and Explanation
causes of male impotence	**stress** [Other causes include *low testosterone* (old age), *vascular disease* (e.g., atherosclerosis), *neurogenic disease* (e.g., autonomic neuropathy in DM; parasympathetic system erects and sympathetic system ejects).]
sign of stress-induced impotence	*patients still have nocturnal erections* [The other types lose this finding.]

Question: In an 80-year-old man with low back pain and point tenderness over the vertebral bodies, which of the following would be your initial step in the work-up?
- (A) PSA
- (B) Bone scan
- (C) Serum alkaline phosphatase
- (D) DRE
- (E) Bone marrow biopsy

Answer: (D): The patient most likely has prostate cancer metastatic to the vertebral column, hence a DRE (D) is the first step. The other tests except for choice (E) should follow.

AFP = alpha-fetoprotein, β-hCG = beta-human chorionic gonadotropin, BPH = benign prostatic hyperplasia, DM = diabetes mellitus, DRE = digital rectal exam, FSH = follicle-stimulating hormone, HIV = human immunodeficiency virus, LH = luteinizing hormone, LUT = lower urinary tract, PAP = prostatic acid phosphatase, PSA = prostate-specific antigen, S/S = signs and symptoms.

CHAPTER

16

FEMALE REPRODUCTIVE AND BREAST PATHOLOGY

CONTENTS

Table 16–1. SEXUALLY TRANSMITTED DISEASES

Most Common...	Answer and Explanation
STD	*Chlamydia trachomatis infection* [It frequently coexists with GC.]
STD associated with *C. trachomatis*	**urethritis** (not detected with a Gram stain) [Other STDs: *PID, cervicitis* (red inclusions in endocervical cells), *proctitis, prostatitis, epididymitis, ophthalmia neonatorum*]
STD causing ophthalmia neonatorum	*C. trachomatis infection* [It develops 1 week after delivery.]
topical agent used to prevent both GC and *C. trachomatis* conjunctivitis in newborns	*erythromycin drops protect against GC and Chlamydia* [Silver nitrate only protects against GC. Chemical conjunctivitis is most common in the first 24–48 hours.]
treatment for STDs due to *C. trachomatis*	*doxycycline*
STD producing urethritis/PID in the first week after exposure	*GC* [It is a gram-negative, coffee bean–shaped diplococcus. *C. trachomatis* is symptomatic 7–10 days after sexual exposure.]
STDs associated with GC	**urethritis, cervicitis** [Other STDs include *PID* (late menses or shortly after), *vulvovaginitis* (prepubescent females who lack estro-

Table continued on following page

Table 16–1. SEXUALLY TRANSMITTED DISEASES *Continued*

Most Common...	Answer and Explanation
continued	gen), *proctitis, ophthalmia neonatorum* (first week), *pharyngitis, disseminated GC, Bartholin's gland abscess, epididymitis, prostatis.*]
method of diagnosing GC	*urethral swabs* (male/female), *cervical swab* with direct inoculation of Thayer-Martin plate (chocolate agar)
cause of treatment failure in GC	*chromosomal mutations and β-lactamase production* (plasmid mediated)
treatment of GC	*ceftriaxone* (for GC) + *doxycycline* (for *Chlamydia*)
drug used for GC treatment failures	*spectinomycin*
causes of the Fitz-Hugh–Curtis syndrome	**C. trachomatis** and *GC* [The syndrome occurs as a complication of PID. It is a perihepatitis (adhesions between liver capsule and peritoneum) in the RUQ that develops from pus collecting under the diaphragm.]
S/S of disseminated GC	**tenosynovitis** (wrist, foot), *septic arthritis* (knee, wrist, foot), *dermatitis* (pustules on wrist, foot)
complications of GC and *C. trachomatis* infections	*sterility* (male/female), *ectopic pregnancy*
cause of genital herpes	*HSV type 2*
S/S of primary/ recurrent herpes genitalis	*primary disease:* fever, regional lymphadenopathy, painful ulcerating vesicles *recurrent herpes:* not systemic; vesicles located on the penis, labia, vulva, cervix (mucopurulent cervicitis)
finding on a Tzanck preparation [scraping at the base of a herpes vesicle] in HSV-2	*multinucleated squamous cells with eosinophilic nuclear inclusions surrounded by a clear space*
drug used to reduce recurrences of herpes genitalis	*acyclovir*

Table 16–1. SEXUALLY TRANSMITTED DISEASES *Continued*

Most Common...	Answer and Explanation
cause of veneral warts (condyloma acuminatum)	*HPV types 6 and 11* [They are fern-like lesions that develop in the moist anogenital areas. They are usually flat condylomas on the cervix.]
histologic finding in HPV	*koilocytosis* [Koilocytosis is where the nucleus of squamous cells is pyknotic and surrounded by a clear halo.]
HPV type associated with cervical, anal, and vaginal squamous cancers	**HPV 16,** *18,* and *31*
treatment for veneral warts	*topical podophyllin*
cause of LGV	*C. trachomatis subspecies*
S/S of LGV	*genital papules* (no ulceration), *painful lymphadenopathy with draining sinuses* (granulomatous microabscesses), *lymphedema of scrotum or vulva, rectal strictures in women*
cause of chancroid	*Haemophilus ducreyi* [It is a gram-negative rod that has a "school of fish" orientation on Gram stain.]
S/S of chancroid	*painful genital ulcer with suppurative inguinal lymph nodes*
cause of granuloma inguinale	*Calymmatobacterium granulomatis* (Donovan's bacillus) [It is a gram-negative coccobacillus found in macrophages.]
S/S of granuloma inguinale	*creeping ulcers that heal by scarring*
cause of syphilis	*Treponema pallidum*, a spirochete
S/S in primary syphilis	*solitary painless chancre on the shaft of the penis or on the labia*
cause of syphilitic lesions	*endarteritis obliterans* [It is a vasculitis with a heavy plasma cell infiltrate that produces ischemic necrosis of tissue.]

Table continued on following page

Table 16–1. SEXUALLY TRANSMITTED DISEASES *Continued*

Most Common...	Answer and Explanation
S/S of secondary syphilis	*diffuse maculopapular rash* (also includes palms/soles), *condyloma latum* (raised pink lesions in moist anogenital areas), *generalized lymphadenopathy*
S/S of latent syphilis	*asymptomatic* [Women can transmit disease to their fetuses.]
S/S of tertiary syphilis	**aortitis involving the arch of the aorta,** *neurosyphilis* (see Chapter 20), *gummas*
tests for all stages of syphilis	*dark-field microscopy* (gold standard), *direct IF, RPR, VDRL, FTA-ABS* (confirmatory test)
cause of a false-positive syphilis serologic result	*anticardiolipin antibodies reacting against the cardiolipin antigen in the RPR or VDRL test system* [SLE should always be excluded, since some patients have anticardiolipin antibodies.]
cause of a false-negative syphilis serologic result	*antibody excess* (prozone) [This is particularly true in secondary syphilis. Dilution of the serum will optimize the concentration of antibodies and antigens in the test system, leading to agglutination.]
effect of treatment of syphilis on the RPR, VDRL, FTA-ABS	*nontreponemal tests will either become nonreactive or low-titered, while the FTA-ABS is always positive* (a positive test may indicate active or inactive disease)
treatment of syphilis	*penicillin*
S/S of a Jarisch-Herxheimer reaction	*generalized rash, fever, and headache after treatment of syphilis with penicillin* [It is a hypersensitivity reaction noted particularly in the treatment of secondary syphilis. It is due to the proteins released from dead treponemes and is not an allergic reaction against penicillin.]
cause of bacterial vaginosis	*Gardnerella vaginalis* [It is a gram-negative rod.]
pathogenesis of bacterial vaginosis	*alteration of the vaginal pH* (raised to 5–5.5) *due to a reduction in lactobacilli* (acid producers of the vagina) [It is not an inflammatory vaginitis.]

Table 16–1. SEXUALLY TRANSMITTED DISEASES *Continued*

Most Common...	Answer and Explanation
S/S and lab findings in bacterial vaginosis	*malodorous discharge* (amine smell with KOH), *no inflammation, presence of clue cells* (squamous cells with adherent bacteria)
treatment of bacterial vaginosis	*metronidazole* [Treatment of the partner does not reduce the incidence of recurrence.]
S/S and lab findings in vaginal candidiasis	*pruritic vaginitis, red inflamed mucosa, cottage cheese discharge, yeasts, and pseudohyphae on a KOH prep* [It commonly occurs in diabetes, pregnancy, and after taking antibiotics.]
treatment of vaginal candidiasis	*fluconazole* (PO or intravaginal)
protozoal cause of vaginitis	*Trichomonas vaginalis*
S/S and lab findings in *Trichomonas* vaginitis	*pruritic vaginitis, inflamed mucosa, greenish-frothy discharge, dysuria* (urethritis), *motile organisms in a hanging drop preparation of discharge.*
treatment of *Trichomonas* vaginitis	*metronidazole* (treat both partners)

Question: Which of the following STDs are associated with ulcerations on the external genitalia? **SELECT 4**
  (A) Bacterial vaginosis
  (B) LGV
  (C) Primary syphilis
  (D) Granuloma inguinale
  (E) GC infection
  (F) *C. trachomatis* infection
  (G) Chancroid
  (H) Herpes genitalis

Answers: (C), (D), (G), (H): Bacterial vaginosis is noninflammatory. GC *(C. trachomatis)* infections have urethral exudates but no ulcerations. LGV has papules but no ulcers.

FTA-ABS = fluorescent *Treponema* antibody absorption test, GC = gonococcus *(Neisseria gonorrhoeae),* HPV = human papillomavirus, HSV = herpes simplex virus, IF = immunofluorescence, KOH = potassium hydroxide, LGV = lymphogranuloma venereum, PID = pelvic inflammatory disease, PO = per os, RPR = rapid plasma reagin, RUQ = right upper quadrant, SLE = systemic lupus erythematosus, S/S = signs and symptoms, STD = sexually transmitted disease, VDRL = Veneral Disease Research Laboratory.

Table 16–2. VULVAR, VAGINAL, AND CERVICAL DISEASES

Most Common...	Answer and Explanation
cause of a Bartholin's gland abscess	*Neisseria gonorrhoeae*
causes of leukoplakia in elderly women	**lichen sclerosis** (atrophic dystrophy), *squamous hyperplasia* (epithelium may be dysplastic)
cancers of the vulva	**SCC** (labia), malignant melanoma (labia, clitoris)
cause of vulvar squamous dysplasia	**HPV types 16,** *18, or 31; atypical squamous hyperplasia*
causes of SCC of the vulva	**HPV** (see above) [Other causes: *smoking, immunosuppression, atypical squamous hyperplasia*]
G/M findings of extramammary Paget's disease of the vulva	*erythroleukoplakia with large, pale-staining, mucin-positive cells* (adenocarcinoma) *limited to the epidermis*
S/S of the Rokitansky-Kuster-Hauser syndrome	*primary amenorrhea; absence of the vagina and upper uterus*
location of a Gartner duct cyst	*anterolateral aspect of the vulva or lateral wall of the vagina* [It is of wolffian duct origin.]
cause of vaginal adenosis	*DES exposure in utero* [It is the precursor lesion for clear cell adenocarcinoma of the vagina.]
S/S of DES exposure	*infertility* (DES inhibits differentiation of müllerian structures), *transverse vaginal ridge, cervical stenosis/incompetence, hypoplastic uterus*
cancer of the vagina	*SCC extending down from a primary cervical SCC*
sarcoma in a female child	*embryonal rhabdomyosarcoma* (sarcoma botryoides) *arising in the vagina* (bloody, grape-like mass)
screening test for cervical dysplasia/cancer	*cervical Pap* (i.e., Papanicolaou) *smear* [It has markedly reduced the incidence of cervical cancer.]

Table 16–2. VULVAR, VAGINAL, AND CERVICAL DISEASES *Continued*

Most Common...	Answer and Explanation
cells evaluated in a cervical Pap smear	*superficial squamous cells* (estrogen stimulated), *intermediate squamous cells* (progesterone stimulated), *parabasal cells* (unstimulated squamous cells), *ECCs*
indicator cell of an adequately performed cervical Pap smear	*ECCs* [ECCs indicate that the transformation zone (junction of endocervix with cervix) has been sampled, which is the primary site of dysplasia.]
method of evaluating hormonal status in a cervical Pap smear	*100-cell count of superficial, intermediate, and parabasal cells* (maturation index)
maturation index of a non-pregnant woman, pregnant woman, and woman without estrogen stimulation	*non-pregnant woman:* superficial 70%, intermediate 30%, parabasal 0% *pregnant woman:* 100% intermediate *woman without estrogen:* predominantly parabasal cells (atrophic smear)
systems for reporting cervical Pap smears	**Papanicolaou** (class I [normal] to class V [invasive]), *cervical intraepithelial neoplasia* (CIN I [mild dysplasia], II [moderate], III [severe carcinoma in situ]), *Bethesda system* (descriptive report)
benign cervical lesion	*cervical polyp* [It is non-neoplastic and the most common cause of postcoital bleeding.]
pathogens causing cervicitis [cervical inflammation with discharge]	*post-partum:* staphylococci, streptococci *pregnancy:* group B streptococcus *(Streptococcus agalactiae)* *non-pregnant:* HSV-2 (cervical ulcerations, excessive discharge), *Escherichia coli*
cause of microglandular hyperplasia of the endocervix	*birth control pills*
causes of cervical dysplasia/cancer	*early age of intercourse, multiple partners, smoking, oral contraceptive use, immunosuppression, infection with HPV types 16, 18, 31*

Table continued on following page

Table 16–2. VULVAR, VAGINAL, AND CERVICAL DISEASES *Continued*

Most Common...	Answer and Explanation
age brackets for CIN I, CIN II/III, invasive SCC	*CIN I: 20–30 years old; CIN II/III: 30–40 years old; invasive SCC: 40–60 years old* [It takes ~10 years to progress from CIN I to CIN III and ~10 years from CIN III to invasive SCC.]
test performed after an abnormal cervical Pap smear report	*colposcopy* [This test involves direct visualization of the cervix after it has been saturated with acetic acid.]
types of cervical SCC	**large cell nonkeratinizing,** *large cell keratinizing, small cell*
symptom of a cervical SCC	metrorrhagia (interval bleeding)
COD in cervical SCC	*local extension into the retroperitoneum with obstruction of the ureters and death from renal failure*
method of spread of cervical SCC	*down into the vagina, out into the lateral walls, and distant spread*

Question: Which of the following cancers are more likely to be adenocarcinomas rather than SCCs? **SELECT 3**
  (A) Extramammary Paget's disease
  (B) Vulvar cancer
  (C) Vaginal cancer
  (D) DES-related cancer
  (E) Cervical cancer
  (F) Breast cancer

Answers: (A), (D), (F): All the other choices listed are more likely to be SCCs.

CIN = cervical intraepithelial neoplasia, COD = cause of death, DES = diethylstilbestrol, ECC = endocervical cell, G/M = gross and microscopic, HPV = human papillomavirus, HSV = herpes simplex virus, SCC = squamous cell carcinoma, S/S = signs and symptoms.

Table 16–3. UTERINE AND FALLOPIAN TUBE DISORDERS

Most Common...	Answer and Explanation
sequence of events leading to menarche	*breast development* (thelarche), *growth spurt, pubic hair, axillary hair, menarche*

Table 16–3. UTERINE AND FALLOPIAN TUBE DISORDERS *Continued*

Most Common...	Answer and Explanation
cause of true and pseudoprecocious puberty [secondary sex characteristics before 8 years old]	**midline hypothalamic hamartoma,** *congenital adrenal hyperplasia,* respectively
hormones involved in the proliferative and secretory phases of the menstrual cycle	*estrogen* (proliferative phase with gland hyperplasia) and *progesterone* (secretory phase with gland tortuosity and secretions), respectively
clinical/histologic evidence of ovulation	*rise in basal body temperature of 0.6°F; subnuclear vacuoles beneath the glandular cells*
cause of mittelschmerz	*ovulation* [Bleeding from the ruptured follicle causes localized peritoneal irritation.]
hormonal effects of estrogen during the menstrual cycle	*negative feedback on FSH* (prepares the follicle) and a *positive feedback on LH* (estrogen surge at midcycle causes a rise in LH, which initiates ovulation on day 14)
hormonal effects of progesterone during the menstrual cycle	*it has a negative feedback on both FSH and LH* [maintains the corpus luteum and androgen (DHEA, androstenedione, testosterone)/progesterone synthesis in the theca interna around the developing follicle]
location for fertilization	*ampulla of the fallopian tube* [It takes ~5–6 days to implant in the endometrial mucosa (~day 21).]
hormone maintaining the corpus luteum in pregnancy	β-*hCG* [It keeps the corpus luteum synthesizing 17-hydroxyprogesterone for 8–10 weeks. The placenta then takes over progesterone synthesis and the corpus luteum involutes.]
source of estradiol	*aromatization* (aromatase located in granulosa cells in the developing follicle) *of testosterone synthesized in the theca interna*
source of estriol	**metabolite of estradiol,** *primary estrogen of pregnancy*

Table continued on following page

Table 16–3. UTERINE AND FALLOPIAN TUBE
DISORDERS *Continued*

Most Common...	Answer and Explanation
source of androgens	*testosterone:* 50% from peripheral conversion of androstenedione, 25% from ovary, 25% from adrenal cortex; *androstenedione:* 50% from ovary, 50% from adrenal cortex; *DHEA-sulfate:* 95% adrenal cortex
binding protein for estrogen/testosterone	*SHBG* [It has a greater affinity for testosterone than for estrogen.]
cause/effect of an increase in SHBG	*increased estrogen, lower free testosterone levels,* respectively
cause/effect of a decrease in SHBG	*androgens, obesity, hypothyroidism; increased free testosterone levels* (potential for hirsutism), respectively
effects of combination birth control pills on the menstrual cycle	*estrogen inhibits FSH and low baseline levels prevent estrogen surge and the LH surge; progestin arrests the proliferative phase and inhibits LH*
S/S and lab findings in menopause	**secondary amenorrhea,** *hot flushes, decreased vaginal secretions, night sweats; increase in FSH, decrease in estradiol*
cause of DUB [bleeding related to a hormone imbalance]	*anovulatory cycles* [There is estrogen but not enough progesterone. Estrogen increases glandular tissue, which eventually sloughs off due to poor support. Ovulatory causes of DUB: irregular shedding, inadequate luteal phase.]
cause of primary amenorrhea [no menses by 16 years of age]	*constitutional delay* (genetic)
genetic cause of primary amenorrhea	*Turner's syndrome* [Estradiol is decreased and the gonadotropins increased (hypergonadotropic hypogonadism).]
end-organ cause of primary amenorrhea	**imperforate hymen,** *Rokitansky-Kuster-Hauser syndrome* (see above)
cause of primary amenorrhea associated with anosmia and color blindness	*Kallmann's syndrome* [The syndrome is characterized by a defect in the release of GnRH and absence of the olfactory bulb. Estradiol and gonadotropins are decreased (hypogonadotropic hypogonadism).]

Table 16–3. UTERINE AND FALLOPIAN TUBE
DISORDERS *Continued*

Most Common...	Answer and Explanation
cause of secondary amenorrhea [absence of menses for 3 months]	*pregnancy* (always order a β-hCG test)
end-organ cause of secondary amenorrhea	*Asherman's syndrome* [This is due to repeated D&Cs with removal of the stratum basalis.]
ovarian cause of secondary amenorrhea	*menopause*
tests used to evaluate hypogonadism	**β-hCG** (rule out pregnancy), *progesterone challenge* [The absence of bleeding after progesterone indicates a hypothalamic/pituitary, ovarian, or end-organ problem.]
cause of primary/ secondary dysmenorrhea	*increased uterine synthesis of prostaglandin F, endometriosis*, respectively
causes of acute endometritis	**post-partum,** *post-abortion*
causes of chronic endometritis [presence of plasma cells]	*chronic PID, post-partum, IUD use*
pathogen producing chronic endometritis in IUD users	*Actinomyces israelii* [It is a gram-positive filamentous bacterium with sulfur granules.]
cause of septic pelvic thrombophlebitis	*thrombosis of the ovarian vein post-partum or postsurgically* [Infusion of heparin causes the fever to disappear in 24–48 hours.]
symptom produced by endometrial polyps	*menorrhagia* (excessive bleeding during normal menses) [It is a benign polyp that is not precancerous.]
causes of endometrial hyperplasia	**unopposed estrogen** (e.g., estrogen therapy in osteoporosis), *obesity, polycystic ovarian syndrome, granulosa cell tumor of the ovary* [Patients present with vaginal bleeding.]

Table continued on following page

Table 16–3. UTERINE AND FALLOPIAN TUBE
DISORDERS *Continued*

Most Common...	Answer and Explanation
types of endometrial hyperplasia	*simple* (large, dilated glands), *complex* (branching glands, crowding, often associated with atypical hyperplasia) [Cystic atrophy occurs in those lacking estrogen stimulation.]
S/S and G/M findings in adenomyosis	*dysmenorrhea, dyspareunia* (painful intercourse), *menorrhagia; myometrial hypertrophy; presence of glands and stroma in the myometrial tissue* (this is not endometriosis), respectively
causes of endometriosis	**reverse menses with tissue refluxing into the abdominal cavity** [Other theories: *coelomic epithelial metaplasia, vascular/lymphatic dissemination*]
sites of endometriosis	**ovaries** ("chocolate cysts") [Other sites include *uterine ligaments* (dyspareunia), *pouch of Douglas* (painful defecation), *small bowel* (obstruction), *fallopian tubes* (ectopic pregnancy).]
symptom of endometriosis	*chronic pelvic pain*
G/M findings of endometriosis	*presence of functioning glands and stroma outside the confines of the uterus that look like powder burns; glands, stroma, and hemosiderin are present*
method of diagnosing endometriosis	*laparoscopy*
overall benign tumor in women	*uterine leiomyomas* ("fibroids") [They may be subserosal, intramural, or submucosal in location.]
S/S and G/M findings in uterine leiomyomas	*menorrhagia* (submucosal location), *dysmenorrhea, obstructive delivery; nonencapsulated swirling mass with fibrosis, degeneration, hyalinization; benign smooth muscle without atypical mitoses*
frequency of gynecologic cancers in descending order	**endometrial adenocarcinoma,** *ovarian cancer, cervical cancer*

Table 16–3. UTERINE AND FALLOPIAN TUBE DISORDERS *Continued*

Most Common...	Answer and Explanation
COD due to gynecologic cancers in descending order	**ovarian cancer,** *cervical cancer, endometrial cancer*
causes of endometrial carcinoma	**unopposed estrogen** (e.g., early menarche, late menopause, nulliparity, estrogen therapy), *obesity, breast cancer, low fiber/high saturated fat diet, DM, hypertension*
S/S and G/M findings of endometrial carcinoma	*postmenopausal vaginal bleeding; polypoid mass; well to intermediately differentiated adenocarcinoma with or without benign* (adenoacanthoma)/*malignant squamous epithelium* (adenosquamous)
distant metastatic site of endometrial cancer	*lungs*
uterine sarcoma	*leiomyosarcoma* [Most arise de novo and not from a leiomyoma.]
criteria for malignancy of a smooth muscle tumor	**number of mitoses per high-power field** (5 or more per 10 HPF), *necrosis*
cause of EP	**previous PID,** *endometriosis*
S/S of an EP	**hypogastric pain** [Other S/S include *vaginal bleeding, missed period, hypovolemic shock* (intraperitoneal bleeding).]
COD in early pregnancy	*ruptured EP*
method of diagnosing EP	**β-hCG** (does not localize site of implantation), *transvaginal ultrasonogram, culdocentesis* (needle in pouch of Douglas; finding of unclotted blood), *laparoscopy*
infection of the fallopian tubes	*PID*

Table continued on following page

MOST COMMONS IN PATHOLOGY AND LABORATORY MEDICINE

Table 16–3. UTERINE AND FALLOPIAN TUBE
DISORDERS *Continued*

Question: Which of the following predispose to cancer? **SELECT 4**
(A) Endometrial polyps
(B) Cervical polyps
(C) Endometrial hyperplasia
(D) Adenomyosis
(E) Uterine leiomyomas
(F) Pelvic irradiation
(G) Vaginal adenosis
(H) Microglandular hyperplasia of the endocervix
(I) Simple hyperplasia of the vulva

Answers: (C), (F), (G), (I): Endometrial hyperplasia predisposes to
adenocarcinoma; pelvic irradiation to mixed müllerian tumors of the
endometrium (adenocarcinoma + sarcoma); vaginal adenosis to clear
cell adenocarcinoma (DES-related); and simple hyperplasia of the
vulva to SCC.

β-hCG = beta-human chorionic gonadotropin, COD = cause of death,
D&C = dilatation and curettage, DES = diethystilbestrol, DHEA = dehydroepiandrosterone, DM = diabetes mellitus, DUB = dysfunctional uterine bleeding, EP = ectopic pregnancy, FSH = follicle-stimulating hormone, G/M = gross and microscopic, GnRH = gonadotropin-releasing
hormone, IUD = intrauterine device, LH = luteinizing hormone, PID =
pelvic inflammatory disease, SCC = squamous cell carcinoma, SHBG =
sex hormone–binding globulin, S/S = signs and symptoms.

Table 16–4. OVARIAN AND PLACENTAL DISORDERS

Most Common...	Answer and Explanation
infection of the ovaries	*tubo-ovarian abscess associated with PID*
cause of ovarian enlargement in a non-pregnant and a pregnant woman	*follicular cyst, corpus luteum cyst,* respectively [Both of these are non-neoplastic cysts.]
cause of POS	*excessive production of LH leading to increased synthesis of ovarian androgens* (hirsutism), *which in turn are aromatized to estrogens* (endometrial hyperplasia), *which have a negative feedback on FSH and positive feedback on LH, thereby continuing the cycle*

Table 16–4. OVARIAN AND PLACENTAL DISORDERS *Continued*

Most Common...	Answer and Explanation
ovarian findings in POS	*enlarged ovaries with subcortical cysts* [Suppression of FSH by estrogen leads to degeneration of the follicles.]
S/S of POS	*obesity, hirsutism, infertility, menstrual irregularities* (usually oligomenorrhea [infrequent menses])
lab findings in POS	*LH:FSH ratio >3:1; increased androstenedione, testosterone, estrone* (weak estrogen)
risk factors for ovarian cancer	**increased ovulation** (nulliparity, late menopause) [Other risk factors: *genetic disorders* (e.g., gonadal dysgenesis), *low fiber/high fat diet*. Oral contraceptives protect against ovarian cancer (decreased ovulation).]
oncogenes involved with ovarian cancer	*ras oncogene* and *p53 suppressor gene*
types of metastasis in ovarian cancer	**seeding,** *lymphatic spread*
types of ovarian tumors in descending order of frequency	**surface derived,** *germ cell, sex cord/stromal*
benign/malignant tumor under each category of ovarian tumor	**surface derived**: serous cystadenoma/cystadenocarcinoma *germ cell:* cystic teratoma/dysgerminoma *sex cord-stromal:* fibroma/granulosa cell tumor
ovarian tumors with increased bilaterality	*serous cystadenoma and serous cystadenocarcinoma*
ovarian tumor with psammoma bodies	*serous cystadenocarcinoma*
ovarian tumor in young girls	*endodermal sinus tumor* (yolk sac tumor; secretes AFP)
ovarian tumors with calcifications	**cystic teratoma** (bone and/or teeth), *gonadoblastoma* (combined germ cell/sex cord-stromal tumor), *fibroma*
ovarian tumor associated with Turner's syndrome	*dysgerminoma* [It is the female counterpart of a seminoma in a male.]

Table continued on following page

Table 16–4. OVARIAN AND PLACENTAL DISORDERS *Continued*

Most Common...	Answer and Explanation
ovarian tumor associated with pseudomyxoma peritonei	*mucinous cystadenocarcinoma* (seeding of mucinous implants)
ovarian tumor type associated with hyperthyroidism	*germ cell tumor* with *struma ovarii* [Struma ovarii is a teratoma with thyroid tissue.]
germ cell tumor associated with endometriosis/ endometrial carcinoma	*endometrioid carcinoma* (particularly the clear cell variant)
ovarian tumor producing endometrial hyperplasia	*granulosa cell tumor* [It is the most common estrogen-secreting ovarian tumor (sex cord-stromal tumor).]
ovarian tumor associated with Meigs' syndrome	*fibroma* [It is a benign sex cord-stromal tumor. Meigs' syndrome is ovarian fibroma, ascites, and right-sided pleural effusion.]
ovarian tumors associated with Walthard's rests, Schiller-Duval bodies, and Call-Exner bodies	*Brenner's tumor* (benign; surface derived), *endodermal sinus tumor* (malignant; germ cell), *granulosa cell tumor* (low-grade malignant; sex cord-stromal), respectively
ovarian tumors with androgen production	*Sertoli-Leydig cell tumor* (alias androblastoma, arrhenoblastoma), *Leydig cell tumor* (alias hilar cell tumor; contains crystalloids of Reinke)
cause of a Krukenberg tumor	*metastasis from a primary gastric adenocarcinoma* (signet ring type; bilateral ovarian metastases)
metastasis to the ovaries	*breast cancer*
ovarian tumor marker	*CA 125*
causes of hirsutism [excess hair]	**idiopathic** (increased production of ovarian-derived testosterone) [*Others: adrenogenital syndrome, POS, progestins, minoxidil, obesity, hypothyroidism*]

Table 16–4. OVARIAN AND PLACENTAL DISORDERS *Continued*

Most Common...	Answer and Explanation
causes of virilization [male secondary sex characteristics]	*ovarian:* Sertoli-Leydig cell, Leydig cell tumors *adrenal:* Cushing's syndrome, adrenogenital syndrome
lab tests used to localize the cause of hyperandrogenicity	*total testosterone with fractionation* (free testosterone): if increased, an ovarian source is likely *DHEA-S:* if increased, an adrenal source is likely
drugs used to treat hirsutism	**spironolactone** (blocks hair follicle androgen receptors) [Other drugs: *birth control pills* (block LH), *dexamethasone* (blocks ACTH)]
cell secreting β-hCG and HPL	*syncytiotrophoblast* [The syncytiotrophoblast and cytotrophoblast line the chorionic villi.]
cause of painless vaginal bleeding in pregnancy	*placenta previa* [The placenta is implanted over the cervical os.]
cause of painful vaginal bleeding in pregnancy	*abruptio placentae* [There is premature separation of the placenta with a resultant retroplacental clot. Hypertension is commonly present in the patient.]
complication with placenta accreta	*massive postpartum vaginal bleeding* [The placenta directly implants into the myometrium without a decidua basalis. A hysterectomy must be performed to stop the bleeding.]
causes of an enlarged placenta	**DM,** *Rh HDN, syphilis*
twin placentas associated with monozygotic twins	*monochorionic placentas* (monoamniotic [both in the same sac], diamniotic [individual sacs]) [Dichorionic placentas may be dizygotic or monozygotic.]
twin placenta with Siamese twins	*monochorionic monoamniotic placenta*
cause of chorioamnionitis	*PROM with ascending infection by group B streptococcus* (*Streptococcus agalactiae*)
S/S of pre-eclampsia	*hypertension, proteinuria, pitting edema, convulsions* (connotes eclampsia)

Table continued on following page

Table 16–4. OVARIAN AND PLACENTAL DISORDERS *Continued*

Most Common...	Answer and Explanation
cause of pre-eclampsia	*abnormal placentation with uterine ischemia* (overriding effect of AT II over prostaglandins)
lab findings in eclampsia	*proteinuria; increase in serum BUN, creatinine, uric acid; decrease in creatinine clearance; HELLP syndrome* (**h**emolytic anemia, **el**evated transaminases, **l**ow **p**latelets)
treatment of convulsions in eclampsia	**magnesium sulfate,** *terbutaline* (tocolytic agent), *low-dose aspirin*
vessel arrangement in the umbilical cord	*two umbilical arteries and one umbilical vein* [A single artery is associated with congenital abnormalities.]
site of origin of AF	*fetal kidneys* [AF is predominantly fetal urine. It has an alkaline pH and "ferns" when dried on a glass slide.]
causes of polyhydramnios	*abnormalities in swallowing:* TE fistula, duodenal atresia; *DM, open neural tube defects*
cause of oligohydramnios	*fetal renal abnormalities* (e.g., cystic disease of the kidneys)
cause of bilirubin pigment in AF	*HDN*
surfactant, its source, its function	*lecithin* (phosphatidylcholine), *type II pneumocytes, lowers alveolar surface tension,* respectively
stimuli for surfactant synthesis	*glucocorticoids, thyroxine*
causes of surfactant deficiency	**prematurity** [Other causes include *DM* (hyperglycemia in the mother causes the fetus to release insulin, which inhibits surfactant synthesis), *cesarean section* (no stress on the baby with release of cortisol).]

Table 16–4. OVARIAN AND PLACENTAL DISORDERS *Continued*

Most Common...	Answer and Explanation
cause of a high/low maternal AFP	*open neural tube defects, Down syndrome,* respectively [AFP levels are dependent on gestational age.]
fetal/maternal sites for synthesis of estriol in sequence	*maternal placenta* (pregnenolone) → *fetal adrenal cortex* (converted to DHEA-S) → *fetal liver* (16-hydroxylase converts compound to 16-OH-DHEA-S) → *maternal placenta* (sulfatase cleaves off sulfate and compound is aromatized to estriol) → *maternal liver* (conjugates free estriol; excreted in the bile/urine)
types of gestational neoplasms	**hydatidiform moles** (benign; **complete** [46,XX,XX of paternal origin; no embryo], partial [trisomy; may contain an embryo]) [Other types: *invasive mole* (benign), *choriocarcinoma* (malignant)]
G/M findings in complete mole	*grape-like appearance from swollen, avascular chorionic villi lined by hyperplastic trophoblastic tissue*
presentation of a complete mole	**pre-eclampsia in the first trimester,** *lack of fetal movement, uterus too large for gestational age*
tumor marker of molar pregnancies	β-*hCG* [After evacuation of a mole, the β-hCG levels are followed until they become normal.]
causes of a choriocarcinoma	**complete mole** [Other causes include *spontaneous abortion, normal pregnancy.* They consist only of trophoblastic tissue (no chorionic villi are present).]
sites of metastasis of a choriocarcinoma	**lungs,** *vagina*
treatment of choriocarcinomas	*methotrexate, actinomycin D* [The gestationally derived choriocarcinomas have an excellent prognosis, even in the presence of metastases.]

Table continued on following page

Table 16–4. OVARIAN AND PLACENTAL DISORDERS *Continued*

Question: Which of the following ovarian tumors are germ cell tumors? **SELECT 3**
(A) Cystic teratoma
(B) Serous cystadenoma
(C) Brenner's tumor
(D) Endometrioid carcinoma
(E) Granulosa cell tumor
(F) Fibroma
(G) Yolk sac tumor
(H) Sertoli-Leydig cell tumor
(I) Dysgerminoma
(J) Mucinous cystadenoma

Answers: (A), (G), (I): Choices (B), (C), (D), and (J) are surface-derived tumors; choices (E), (F), and (H) are sex cord/stromal tumors.

ACTH = adrenocorticotropic hormone, AF = amniotic fluid, AFP = alpha-fetoprotein, AT II = angiotensin II, β-hCG = beta-human chorionic gonadotropin, BUN = blood urea nitrogen, DHEA-S = dehydroepiandrosterone sulfate, DM = diabetes mellitus, FSH = follicle-stimulating hormone, G/M = gross and microscopic, HDN = hemolytic disease of the newborn, HPL = human placental lactogen, LH = luteinizing hormone, PID = pelvic inflammatory disease, POS = polycystic ovarian syndrome, PROM = premature rupture of membranes, S/S = signs and symptoms, TE = tracheoesophageal.

Table 16–5. BREAST DISORDERS

Most Common...	Answer and Explanation
breast mass in a woman <50 and >50 years old	*fibrocystic change* (FCC), *infiltrating ductal carcinoma*, respectively
tumor in a woman <35 years old	*fibroadenoma* [It is a benign tumor derived from stromal cells.]
cause of a bloody nipple discharge in women <50 and >50 years old	*intraductal papilloma, infiltrating ductal carcinoma*, respectively
pathologic cause of galactorrhea	*prolactinoma* [They arise in the anterior pituitary gland.]
disease involving the nipple	*Paget's disease of breast*
disease involving the lactiferous duct	*intraductal papilloma*

Table 16–5. BREAST DISORDERS *Continued*

Most Common...	Answer and Explanation
diseases involving the large ducts	*infiltrating ductal carcinoma, FCC*
diseases involving the terminal lobules	*lobular carcinoma, sclerosing adenosis*
components of FCC	**cysts** (large, small), **fibrosis,** *sclerosing adenosis* (proliferation of small ductules/acini), *ductal hyperplasia* (papillomatosis [benign papillary proliferation], apocrine metaplasia [bright red epithelium], atypical hyperplasia [precancerous])
cause of acute mastitis	*Staphylococcus aureus in a lactating woman*
cause of fat necrosis	*trauma to the breast* [It undergoes fibrosis and dystrophic calcification, hence simulating breast cancer.]
G/M and S/S of a fibroadenoma	*popcorn-shaped mass with stromal proliferation compressing ducts into slit-like spaces* (intracanalicular pattern); *freely moveable mass*
overall cancer in women	*infiltrating ductal carcinoma* [It is the second most common cause of death due to cancer. Incidence is increasing (due to mammography).]
initial step in working up a breast mass	*fine needle aspiration*
risk factors for breast cancer	**age** >50 (most important) [Other risk factors include *family history* (first-degree relatives: mother, sister), *excessive estrogen exposure, history of endometrial carcinoma or previous breast cancer.*]
genetic association with breast cancer	*BRCA1 gene on chromosome 17, BRCA2 gene on chromosome 13* [These genes can be identified to evaluate women for cancer risk.]
oncogene relationships with breast cancer	*ras oncogene* (point mutation), *p53 suppressor gene* (point mutation), *erbB2 oncogene* (amplification)

Table continued on following page

Table 16–5. BREAST DISORDERS *Continued*

Most Common...	Answer and Explanation
S/S of breast cancer	**painless mass in the upper outer quadrant,** *skin retraction, nipple retraction, axillary lymphadenopathy, peau d'orange* (orange skin appearance; plugs of tumor in dermal lymphatics)
use of mammography	*to detect nonpalpable breast masses*
G/M appearance of infiltrating ductal carcinoma	*stellate-shaped, indurated, gray-white tumor that is gritty on cut section*
cancer with an eczematous appearance of the nipple	*Paget's disease* [It is an underlying breast cancer that is infiltrating the nipple and skin.]
cancer with a lymphocytic infiltrate and pushing margins	*medullary carcinoma* [It is a bulky tumor with large cells, a lymphocytic infiltrate, and pushing rather than infiltrating margins.]
cancer with erythematous skin and peau d'orange	*inflammatory carcinoma* [It has the poorest prognosis.]
cancer that has an increased incidence of bilaterality	*lobular carcinoma involving the terminal lobules*
cancer with the slowest progression into an invasive cancer	*lobular carcinoma*
malignant stromal cancer	*cystosarcoma phylloides* (cystic with leaf-like extensions) [The stroma is malignant and the epithelial component is benign. It is a bulky, usually low-grade malignancy that spares the axillary lymph nodes.]
factors affecting prognosis in breast cancer	**status of the axillary lymph nodes** [Other prognostic factors include *ERA-PRA status* (postmenopausal patients are more likely positive; positive assays indicate a better remission rate; patients are candidates for tamoxifen [anti-estrogen] therapy), *cancer grade, erbB2 oncogene status* (poor prognosis if present). Node involvement depends on tumor size (>2 cm imposes increased risk).]

Table 16–5. BREAST DISORDERS *Continued*

Most Common...	Answer and Explanation
treatment of breast cancer	**modified radical mastectomy** (nipple/areolar complex, all breast tissue, pectoralis minor, axillary lymph nodes in continuity), *lumpectomy with low axillary node dissection followed by radiation.* [They have similar 5-year survival rates.]
metastatic sites of breast cancer	**bone** (particularly the vertebral column) [Other sites of metastasis: *lungs, brain, ovaries*]
overall 5-year survival rate for breast cancer	*60%*
time periods for physiologic gynecomastia [development of male breast tissue]	*birth, puberty, old age* [Gynecomastia can be unilateral or bilateral. In most cases, the tissue should not be surgically removed.]
cause of gynecomastia	*increased estrogen stimulation*
pathologic cause of gynecomastia	*alcoholic cirrhosis* [Cirrhotic livers are unable to metabolize estrogens and 17-ketosteroids (aromatized into estrogen).]

Question: Which of the following are risk factors for breast cancer? **SELECT 5**

    (A) Fibroadenoma
    (B) Atypical ductal hyperplasia
    (C) Breast feeding
    (D) Age
    (E) Aunt with breast cancer
    (F) Sister with breast cancer
    (G) Early menarche/late menopause
    (H) Endometrial cancer
    (I) Cervical cancer

Answers: (B), (D), (F), (G), (H): Choices (A), (C), (E), and (I) are not risk factors for breast cancer. Second-degree relatives (aunts) with cancer do not represent a risk factor.

ERA = estrogen receptor assay, G/M = gross and microscopic, PRA = progesterone receptor assay, S/S = signs and symptoms.

CHAPTER

17

ENDOCRINE PATHOLOGY

CONTENTS

Table 17–1. GENERAL CONCEPTS, PITUITARY DISORDERS

Most Common...	Answer and Explanation
functional type of endocrine disorder	*hypofunctioning gland* (e.g., **autoimmune destruction,** decreased stimulation)
causes of a hyperfunctioning endocrine gland	**benign adenoma,** *primary hyperplasia, cancer*
endocrine gland with a primary cancer	*thyroid gland*
lab tests for hypofunctioning endocrine glands	*stimulation tests* (e.g., ACTH stimulation test in hypocortisolism)
lab tests for hyperfunctioning endocrine glands	*suppression tests* (e.g., dexamethasone suppression test for hypercortisolism) [Most hyperfunctioning glands are nonsuppressible (autonomous). Exceptions: prolactinoma, pituitary Cushing's syndrome]
cause of hypopituitarism in children	*craniopharyngioma* [It is a benign tumor (cystic, calcifications) derived from Rathke's pouch remnants.]
causes of hypopituitarism in adults	**nonfunctioning pituitary adenomas,** *Sheehan's postpartum necrosis* (cessation of lactation; pituitary infarction)

Table continued on following page

Table 17–1. GENERAL CONCEPTS,
PITUITARY DISORDERS *Continued*

Most Common...	Answer and Explanation
sequence of trophic hormone loss in hypopituitarism	*FSH and LH* (amenorrhea, impotence) → *GH* (dwarfism in child) → *TSH* (hypothyroidism) → *ACTH* (hypocortisolism) → *prolactin* (cessation of lactation in breast-feeding women)
imaging test for pituitary disorders	*MRI*
cause of anosmia, color blindness, and hypogonadism	*Kallmann's syndrome* [It is due to a deficiency of GnRH.]
defect in African pygmies	*low somatomedin* (SMM; GH normally stimulates its synthesis and release in the liver), *normal GH*
defect in Laron dwarfism	*end-organ unresponsiveness to GH* (normal or increased) *with reduced synthesis of SMM*
test for ACTH reserve in the anterior pituitary	*metyrapone* [Metyrapone blocks 11-hydroxylase in the adrenal cortex hence decreasing cortisol, 11-hydroxylase (deoxycortisol → cortisol), increasing ACTH (loss of negative feedback), and increasing deoxycortisol, which is proximal to the enzyme block.]
stimulation tests for GH deficiency	**sleep** (GH is normally released early in the morning), *arginine*
stimulation test for FSH and LH	*GnRH stimulation* [In hypopituitarism, FSH and LH are not increased.]
test for differentiating secondary from primary hypocortisolism (Addison's disease)	*prolonged ACTH stimulation test* [In secondary hypocortisolism (hypopituitarism), the urine finding for 17-hydroxycorticoids eventually increases. In Addison's disease, the 17-hydroxycorticoids do not increase (gland is destroyed).]
types of diabetes insipidus (DI)	**central** (deficiency of ADH), *nephrogenic* (end-organ unresponsiveness to ADH)
symptoms/lab findings of DI	*polyuria, increased thirst, hypernatremia* (high POsm), *dilute urine* (UOsm often <100 mOsm/kg)
causes of polyuria other than DI	**diuretics** (e.g., thiazides) [Other causes include *osmotic diuresis* (e.g., glucosuria), *hypercalcemia, psychogenic polydipsia* (excessive water drinker).]

Table 17–1. GENERAL CONCEPTS, PITUITARY DISORDERS *Continued*

Most Common...	Answer and Explanation
lab findings in DI pre- and post-ADH injection after water deprivation	*(see table below)*

	POsm/UOsm post water deprivation	UOsm post ADH
CDI	increased/ decreased	UOsm increased >50% over UOsm post water deprivation
NDI	increased/ decreased	UOsm increased <45% over UOsm post water deprivation

[Note: In CDI, the urine becomes concentrated after giving ADH, while in NDI, the degree of concentration is less, depending on the severity of the disease.]

Most Common...	Answer and Explanation
lab findings in psychogenic polydipsia post-water deprivation and ADH injection	*(see table below)*

POsm/UOsm post water deprivation	UOsm post ADH
normal/ increased	UOsm not significantly increased

[Note: Restricting water produces normal urine concentration and a POsm that is at the upper limit of normal.]

Most Common...	Answer and Explanation
S/S of acromegaly [excess GH and SMM]	*children:* gigantism (increased linear growth since the epiphyses are not fused) *adults:* increased size of hands and feet, skull and jaw; visceromegaly, hypertension, DM, heart failure (most common cause of death)
pituitary tumor	*prolactinoma*
S/S of a prolactinoma	*female:* secondary amenorrhea (prolactin inhibits GnRH), galactorrhea *male:* impotence
causes of galactorrhea other than prolactinoma	*primary hypothyroidism* (low T$_4$ increases TRH, which stimulates prolactin), *drugs* (estrogen, tricyclics), *pregnancy, pituitary stalk transection* (loss of inhibitory effect of dopamine on prolactin)
treatment of prolactinomas	*bromocriptine,* which is a dopamine analogue

Table continued on following page

Table 17–1. GENERAL CONCEPTS, PITUITARY DISORDERS *Continued*

Question: Which of the following are expected lab abnormalities in adults (male and female) with severe hypopituitarism? **SELECT 3**
(A) Hyperglycemia
(B) Low estradiol
(C) Normal sperm count
(D) Low serum T_4
(E) Hyperkalemia
(F) Increased urine sodium loss
(G) Increased urine 17-hydroxycorticoids after prolonged ACTH stimulation
(H) Increased plasma ACTH

Answers: (B), (D), (G): Estradiol is decreased owing to a decrease in gonadotropins, and T_4 is decreased owing to a decrease in TSH. Prolonged ACTH stimulation stimulates the atrophic adrenal cortex to begin synthesizing cortisol again. Hypoglycemia rather than hyperglycemia (A) occurs owing to a decrease in GH and cortisol, both of which enhance gluconeogenesis. Since ACTH does not stimulate aldosterone, electrolyte abnormalities (E), (F) are not as severe as in Addison's disease, which would result in sodium loss in the urine, hyperkalemia, and increased plasma ACTH (H) owing to the decrease in cortisol. There is a low sperm count (C).

ACTH = adrenocorticotropic hormone, ADH = antidiuretic hormone, CDI = central diabetes insipidus, FSH = follicle-stimulating hormone, GH = growth hormone, GnRH = gonadotropin-releasing hormone, LH = luteinizing hormone, MRI = magnetic resonance imaging, NDI = nephrogenic diabetes insipidus, POsm = plasma osmolality, S/S = signs and symptoms, T_4 = thyroxine, TRH = thyrotropin-releasing hormone, TSH = thyroid-stimulating hormone, UOsm = urine osmolality.

Table 17–2. THYROID DISEASES

Most Common...	Answer and Explanation
tests included in a thyroid profile	*serum T_4, resin T_3 uptake* (RTU), T_4 *binding ratio* (T_4BR = RTU/30%), *free-T_4 index* (FT$_4$-I), *TSH* (best overall test)
cause of an elevated/decreased serum T_4	*increased free T_4 hormone level* (e.g., hyperthyroidism) *or an increase in TBG or decreased free T_4 level* (e.g., hypothyroidism) *or decrease in TBG* [Adding TBG to plasma automatically leads to T_4 binding to one third of its binding sites without altering free T_4 hormone levels. Any increase or decrease in TBG will increase or decrease the total T_4, which measures T_4 bound to TBG and free T_4.]

Table 17–2. THYROID DISEASES *Continued*

Most Common...	Answer and Explanation
cause of an increase/decrease in TBG	*estrogen, androgen,* respectively
effect of an increase/decrease in TBG on the serum TSH	*no change in the TSH, since the free T_4 is normal*
use of the RTU	*it reflects the number of binding sites available on TBG when $^*T_3$ is added to a tube of patient plasma. Any leftover $^*T_3$ is bound to a resin, measured (only the $^*T_3$ bound to the resin, not the TBG), and reported as a percent (normally 30%)* [In hyperthyroidism (more than one third of TBG binding sites are saturated) and hypothyroidism (less than one third of TBG binding sites are occupied), the RTU is increased (more $^*T_3$ left over) and decreased (less $^*T_3$ left over), respectively. If TBG is increased or decreased, the RTU is decreased (less $^*T_3$ left over) or increased (more $^*T_3$ left over), respectively.]
use of the T_4BR	*the patient's RTU result is converted into the T_4BR by dividing the measured RTU by 30% (e.g., patient RTU = 15%, T_4BR = 0.5 [15/30]). The T_4BR is multiplied by the total serum T_4 to obtain the FT_4-I, which is the amount of unbound, free T_4 in plasma*
uses of the serum TSH	*if decreased, the patient may have hyperthyroidism or hypopituitarism; if increased, the patient has primary hypothyroidism*
uses of I_{131}	*if increased, the gland is increasing the synthesis of thyroid hormone (e.g., Graves' disease); if decreased, the gland is either inflamed (e.g., acute thyroiditis) or underactive (e.g., hypothyroidism)* [It is also used in distinguishing "cold" from "hot" thyroid nodules (see below).]
cause of a midline cystic mass in the neck	*thyroglossal duct cyst* [It is leftover duct material from caudal descent of the thyroid in the fetus.]
cause of acute thyroiditis	*bacterial infection* (e.g., group A *Streptococcus, Staphylococcus aureus*)

Table continued on following page

Table 17–2. THYROID DISEASES *Continued*

Most Common...	Answer and Explanation
cause of subacute thyroiditis	*viral infection* (e.g., coxsackievirus) [A granulomatous reaction is present in the tissue.]
thyroiditis	*Hashimoto's thyroiditis* [It is an autoimmune disease with destruction of the thyroid.]
S/S of acute/ subacute thyroiditis	*painful thyroid, signs of hyperthyroidism from release of hormone from damaged thyroid tissue*
G/M findings in Riedel's thyroiditis	*fibrotic gland with infiltration of surrounding structures by fibrous tissue*
cause of hypothyroidism	*Hashimoto's thyroiditis* [Anti-microsomal and thyroglobulin antibodies, cytotoxic T cells, and blocking autoantibodies against the TSH receptor are operative in decreasing T_4 synthesis.]
G/M findings in Hashimoto's thyroiditis	*enlarged, pale gray to yellow gland that has an intense lymphocytic/plasma cell infiltrate with germinal follicles and destruction of gland parenchyma and colloid*
S/S of hypothyroidism	*symmetrically enlarged, painless gland;* **weakness** *(proximal muscle myopathy; elevated CK), coarse yellow skin (beta-carotenemia), dry/brittle hair, periorbital puffiness (GAG deposition), delayed recovery of Achilles reflex, cold intolerance, diastolic hypertension, pretibial myxedema, depression, menorrhagia*
lab findings in primary hypothyroidism	**high serum TSH,** *low serum T_4, low RTU, low FT_4-I, low I_{131}, high serum CH* (reduced LDL receptor synthesis), *high serum CK* (myopathy)
treatment of hypothyroidism	*levothyroxine* [The goal is to lower the serum TSH into the normal range.]
cause of hyperthyroidism	*Graves' disease* [It is an autoimmune disease with autoantibodies against the TSH receptor (TSI [stimulates hormone synthesis]; type II hypersensitivity).]
causes of hyperthyroidism other than Graves' disease	*toxic nodular goiter* (Plummer's disease), *acute/subacute thyroiditis, iatrogenic*

Table 17–2. THYROID DISEASES *Continued*

Most Common...	Answer and Explanation
G/M findings in Graves' disease	*diffusely enlarged, congested gland with scant colloid and papillary infolding into the acini*
S/S unique to Graves' disease	*lid stare, exophthalmos, pretibial myxedema*
S/S in all causes of hyperthyroidism	*sinus tachycardia, atrial fibrillation, angina, systolic hypertension, heat intolerance, weight loss, diarrhea, proximal muscle weakness, lid stare*
lab findings in hyperthyroidism	**low serum TSH,** *high serum T_4, high RTU, high FT_4-I, high I_{131}* (Graves', toxic nodular goiter), *low I_{131}* (thyroiditis, patient taking excess hormone), *low CH* (increased LDL receptor synthesis), *hyperglycemia* (increased glycogenolysis and gluconeogenesis), *lymphocytosis, hypercalcemia* (increased bone turnover)
treatment of Graves' disease	β-*blockers* (decrease catecholamine effects), *antithyroid medications* (e.g., propylthiouracil [only drug that can be used in pregnancy]), **ablation with I_{131}** (most common), *surgery*
causes of a goiter [enlarged thyroid gland due to excess colloid]	**iodide deficiency** [Other causes: *goitrogenic diets* (e.g., turnips), *enzyme deficiencies*]
cause of a multinodular goiter	*relative deficiency of thyroid hormone with alternating hyperplasia and involution* (low T_4) → *stimulate TSH* → *hyperplasia and increase in T_4 synthesis* → *drop in TSH and gland involution* (cysts, atrophy) → *gland failure with drop in T_4 and increase in TSH with repetition of the cycle*
complications with multinodular goiters	**hemorrhage into a cyst** [Other complications: *hypothyroidism, toxic nodular goiter* (Plummer's disease; this is not Graves' disease)]
causes of a "cold" solitary thyroid nodule in a woman	**non-neoplastic cyst** (60%), *follicular adenoma* (25%), *cancer* (15%) ["Cold" nodules connote no uptake of I_{131} into the nodule (nonfunctioning tissue).]

Table continued on following page

Table 17–2. THYROID DISEASES *Continued*

Most Common...	Answer and Explanation
cause of a "hot" nodule	*toxic nodular goiter* [Only the hot nodule takes up the I_{131}, since the remainder of the gland is not synthesizing hormone.]
risk factors for a nodule representing cancer	*previous history of radiation to the head/ neck area, child, adult male, palpable lymph nodes*
benign thyroid tumor	*encapsulated, follicular adenoma* [They are "cold" nodules and may progress to a follicular carcinoma.]
thyroid cancer	*papillary adenocarcinoma* [It has the best prognosis of the thyroid cancers.]
G/M findings of papillary adenocarcinoma	*indurated, solitary or multifocal, gray-white tumor with papillary fronds, empty-appearing nuclei* (Orphan Annie nuclei), *psammoma bodies, and lymphatic invasion with spread to cervical lymph nodes*
G/M findings of follicular thyroid cancer	*encapsulated mass or invasive cancer with well-differentiated thyroid follicles invading the capsule* (encapsulated type) *and blood vessel lumens. Lymphatic invasion and lymph node metastasis is uncommon.*
cell of origin of medullary carcinoma of the thyroid	*parafollicular C cells* [Parafollicular cells synthesize calcitonin, the tumor marker for the cancer. Most cases are sporadic and a small percentage are in the AD MEN IIa and IIb syndromes.]
microscopic finding in medullary carcinoma distinguishing it from other thyroid cancers	*amyloid deposits derived from calcitonin*
cause of primary malignant lymphoma of the thyroid	*pre-existing Hashimoto's thyroiditis*

Table 17–2. THYROID DISEASES *Continued*

Question: In a pregnant woman with a normal physical exam, you would **LEAST** expect which of the following lab results?
(A) High serum T$_4$
(B) Low RTU
(C) Low T$_4$BR
(D) Low TSH
(E) Normal FT$_4$-I

Answer: (D): A pregnant woman has an increase in estrogen, which increases TBG, thereby increasing serum T$_4$ and decreasing RTU and T$_4$BR. The FT$_4$-I is normal, since the high serum T$_4$ multiplied by the low T$_4$BR normalizes the FT$_4$-I, representing the free T$_4$ (unbound) concentration. Since free T$_4$ is not altered by changes in TBG, the TSH is normal.

AD = autosomal dominant, CH = cholesterol, CK = creatine kinase, GAG = glycosaminoglycan, G/M = gross and microscopic, I$_{131}$ = radioactive iodine uptake, LDL = low-density lipoprotein, MEN = multiple endocrine neoplasia, S/S = signs and symptoms, T$_3$ = triiodothyronine, T$_4$ = thyroxine, *T$_3$ = radioactive T$_3$, TBG = thyroid-binding globulin, TSH = thyroid-stimulating hormone, TSI = thyroid-stimulating immunoglobulin.

Table 17–3. PARATHYROID AND CALCIUM DISORDERS

Most Common...	Answer and Explanation
functions of PTH	*increase renal reabsorption of calcium* (distal tubule), *decrease reabsorption of phosphate and bicarbonate* (proximal tubule), *increase synthesis of 1α-hydroxylase* (second hydroxylation of vitamin D), and *increase resorption of bone to maintain the ionized calcium level*
functions of vitamin D	*increase small bowel absorption of calcium and phosphorus; mineralize cartilage and bone*
cause of hypercalcemia in the ambulatory population	*primary hyperparathyroidism* (HPTH)
causes of primary HPTH	**parathyroid adenoma**, *primary hyperplasia, cancer*

Table continued on following page

Table 17–3. PARATHYROID AND CALCIUM
DISORDERS *Continued*

Most Common...	Answer and Explanation
G/M findings in a parathyroid adenoma	*encapsulated proliferation of neoplastic chief cells surrounded by inactive glandular tissue* (increased intervening fat) and *inactive remaining parathyroid glands*
S/S of primary HPTH	**asymptomatic** (most common), *renal stones* (most common symptomatic presentation), *PUD* (calcium stimulates gastrin release), *pancreatitis* (calcium activates pancreatic enzymes), *constipation, polyuria* (nephrocalcinosis), *metastatic calcification* (skin, cornea, kidneys), *bone lesions* (osteitis fibrosa cystica), *mental disorders*
lab findings in primary HPTH	*hypercalcemia, hypophosphatemia, high PTH, normal anion gap metabolic acidosis* (loss of HCO_3^- in the urine is counterbalanced by a gain in Cl^- ions), *hypercalciuria, phosphaturia, short QT interval on an ECG*
radiographic findings in primary HPTH	*subperiosteal resorption of bone in the fingers, cystic lesions in the jaw and other sites with hemorrhage and fibrosis* (osteitis fibrosa cystica, "brown tumors")
cause of hypercalcemia in a hospitalized patient	*malignancy-induced hypercalcemia* [Hypercalcemia may occur by either metastasis to bone with release of calcium or secretion of a PTH-like peptide (increases calcium and decreases phosphorus reabsorption in the kidneys).]
cancers secreting PTH-like peptide	*renal adenocarcinoma, squamous carcinoma of the lung, breast cancer*
lab findings in malignancy-induced hypercalcemia	*hypercalcemia, low PTH* (hypercalcemia suppresses endogenous PTH)
causes of hypercalcemia other than primary HPTH or malignancy	*sarcoidosis, multiple myeloma, thiazides, vitamin D toxicity*
treatment of hypercalcemia	**induce a diuresis with isotonic saline followed by a loop diuretic** [*Others:* plicamycin, calcitonin, bisphosphonates]

Table 17–3. PARATHYROID AND CALCIUM
DISORDERS *Continued*

Most Common...	Answer and Explanation
cause of hypocalcemia	*hypoalbuminemia* [Since 40% of the total calcium is bound to albumin, the total calcium is decreased. The ionized calcium is normal.]
pathologic cause of hypocalcemia in a hospitalized patient	*hypomagnesemia* [Magnesium normally enhances PTH activity, increases PTH release from the gland, and acts as a cofactor for adenylate cyclase, so its deficiency hinders PTH function.]
causes of hypomagnesemia	**diuretics,** *diarrhea, alcoholism, drugs* (e.g., aminoglycosides, cisplatin)
causes of primary hypoparathyroidism	**previous thyroid surgery,** *autoimmune destruction*
sign of hypoparathyroidism	*tetany* (low ionized calcium; circumoral paresthesias, Trousseau's sign [carpopedal spasm] with a blood pressure cuff, Chvostek's sign [facial muscle twitching with tapping of the facial nerve])
lab findings in primary hypoparathyroidism	*hypocalcemia, low ionized calcium, hyperphosphatemia, low PTH*
cause of pseudohypoparathyroidism	*AD disease with a defective receptor for PTH* (type I) or *postreceptor problem* (type II)
S/S of pseudohypoparathyroidism	*tetany, mental retardation, short fourth and fifth metacarpal bones* ("knuckle-knuckle-dimple-dimple" sign), *calcification of basal ganglia*
lab findings in pseudohypoparathyroidism	*hypocalcemia, hyperphosphatemia, normal to high PTH, increased urine cAMP after PTH infusion in type II and no increase in type I*
cause of tetany when the total calcium is normal	*alkalosis* [Alkalosis increases the number of negative charges on albumin, hence increasing the amount bound to albumin. This lowers the ionized calcium level, without affecting the total calcium, which measures both bound and free calcium.]

Table continued on following page

MOST COMMONS IN PATHOLOGY AND LABORATORY MEDICINE

Table 17–3. PARATHYROID AND CALCIUM DISORDERS Continued

Most Common...	Answer and Explanation
causes of hypocalcemia other than hypoparathyroidism or hypoalbuminemia	*vitamin D deficiency* (renal failure, malabsorption, liver disease), *acute pancreatitis* (enzymatic fat necrosis)
cause of secondary HPTH	*chronic renal failure* with production of hypovitaminosis D leading to hypocalcemia, a stimulus for PTH synthesis (all four glands are hyperplastic)

Question: Which of the following distinguish primary HPTH from malignancy-induced hypercalcemia? **SELECT 3**
(A) Serum PTH
(B) Short QT interval
(C) Metabolic acidosis
(D) Lytic lesions in bone
(E) Association with MEN syndromes I and IIa

Answers: (A), (C), (E): Primary HPTH, unlike malignancy-induced hypercalcemia, produces a normal AG metabolic acidosis (C), owing to loss of bicarbonate in the urine, and is associated with a high PTH (A) and MEN I and IIa syndromes (E). Both causes of hypercalcemia have short QT intervals (B) and lytic lesions (D) in bone, not the malignancy-induced hypercalcemia that metastasizes to bone, not the PTH-like peptide cause).

AD = autosomal dominant, AG = anion gap, cAMP = cyclic adenosine monophosphate, ECG = electrocardiogram, G/M = gross and microscopic, MEN = multiple endocrine neoplasia, PTH = parathormone, PUD = peptic ulcer disease, S/S = signs and symptoms.

Table 17–4. ADRENAL DISEASES, MULTIPLE ENDOCRINE NEOPLASIA SYNDROMES, ECTOPIC HORMONE SYNDROMES

Most Common...	Answer and Explanation
enzymes in the zona glomerulosa	*21-, 11-, 18-hydroxylase enzymes*, the latter converting corticosterone to aldosterone
enzymes in the zona fasciculata and reticularis	21-, 17-, 11-hydroxylase enzymes [17-Hydroxylase enzymes enable these zones to synthesize the 17-KS (androstenedione, DHEA) and 17-hydroxyprogesterone, which is ultimately converted into cortisol.]

Table 17–4. ADRENAL DISEASES, MULTIPLE ENDOCRINE NEOPLASIA SYNDROMES, ECTOPIC HORMONE SYNDROMES *Continued*

Most Common...	Answer and Explanation
cause of primary aldosteronism (Conn's syndrome)	*adenoma arising in the zona glomerulosa* (see Chapter 5)
cause of Cushing's syndrome	*exogenous administration of glucocorticoids*
pathologic causes of Cushing's syndrome	**pituitary** (sometimes called Cushing's disease), *adrenal, and ectopic Cushing's* (usually a small cell carcinoma of the lung) *syndrome*
S/S of Cushing's syndrome	**weight gain** [Other S/S include *purple striae, diastolic hypertension, truncal obesity, thin extremities, hirsutism, "moon face," "buffalo hump," DM.*]
screening tests for Cushing's syndrome	**24-hour urine for free (unbound) cortisol** (increased), *low-dose dexamethasone suppression test* (no suppression of cortisol), *plasma ACTH* (lowest in adrenal Cushing's, highest in ectopic Cushing's), *loss of the diurnal cortisol rhythm* (high in both AM and PM; normally, high in AM and low in PM)
confirmatory tests for Cushing's syndrome	**high-dose dexamethasone suppression test** (suppression of cortisol in pituitary Cushing's [partially autonomous] but not the others); *CT scan of the pituitary and adrenals localizes the disease*
cause of Nelson's syndrome	*bilateral adrenalectomy in a patient who has a pituitary adenoma* [The drop in cortisol causes further enlargement of the pituitary adenoma with associated headache and hyperpigmentation from excessive release of ACTH.]
tumor of the adrenal medulla in children	*neuroblastoma* [It is a malignant tumor of neural crest origin (S100 antigen positive). Deletion on chromosome 1 leads to amplification of the *n-myc* oncogene.]
microscopic findings in a neuroblastoma	*malignant neuroblasts* (small, dark cells) *forming Homer-Wright rosettes*

Table continued on following page

Table 17–4. ADRENAL DISEASES, MULTIPLE ENDOCRINE NEOPLASIA SYNDROMES, ECTOPIC HORMONE SYNDROMES *Continued*

Most Common...	Answer and Explanation
signs of a neuroblastoma	**hypertension,** *unilateral abdominal mass*
lab findings in a neuroblastoma	*increased urine for VMA, metanephrines, HVA*
sites of metastasis	**bone** [Other sites: *lymph nodes, liver, skin.* Age is the most important prognostic factor (best prognosis if age is <1 year old).]
adrenal medulla tumor in adults	*pheochromocytoma* [~90% are benign, located in the adrenal medulla, and unilateral.]
clinical associations of a pheochromocytoma	*MEN IIa and IIb, von Hippel-Lindau disease, neurofibromatosis*
G/M findings in a pheochromocytoma	*gray tumor that turns brown with exposure to oxidants* (chromaffin tumor), *cysts with hemorrhage, pleomorphic cells often confused with malignancy*
S/S of a pheochromocytoma	**hypertension,** *palpitations, headache, drenching sweats*
lab findings in a pheochromocytoma	**increased urine for metanephrines (best test) and VMA,** *lack of suppression with clonidine, hyperglycemia, neutrophilic leukocytosis* (decreases adhesion molecule synthesis)
cause of acute adrenal insufficiency	*abrupt withdrawal of glucocorticoids*
causes of chronic primary adrenal insufficiency	**autoimmune destruction** (Addison's disease), *TB* (Third World countries)
S/S of Addison's disease	**weakness, hypotension** (salt loss from aldosterone deficiency), *hyperpigmentation* (increased ACTH stimulation of melanocytes)

Table 17–4. ADRENAL DISEASES, MULTIPLE ENDOCRINE NEOPLASIA SYNDROMES, ECTOPIC HORMONE SYNDROMES *Continued*

Most Common...	Answer and Explanation
lab findings in Addison's disease	*hyponatremia, hyperkalemia, normal anion gap metabolic acidosis, fasting hypoglycemia, high plasma ACTH, no cortisol response to prolonged ACTH stimulation, eosinophilia* (loss of cortisol)
cause of the Waterhouse-Friderichsen syndrome	*disseminated Neisseria meningitidis* [This leads to DIC, bilateral adrenal hemorrhage, shock, and death.]
disorders in the MEN I syndrome	*pituitary adenoma, parathyroid adenoma* (hypercalcemia), *pancreatic tumor* (usually Zollinger-Ellison or insulinoma), *PUD*
disorders in the MEN IIa syndrome	*parathyroid adenoma* (hypercalcemia), *pheochromocytoma* (usually bilateral), *medullary carcinoma of the thyroid*
disorders in the MEN IIb syndrome	*pheochromocytoma, medullary carcinoma of the thyroid, mucosal neuromas*
tumor secreting ADH, ACTH	*small cell carcinoma of the lung*
tumor secreting PTH-like peptide, erythropoietin	*renal adenocarcinoma*
tumor secreting an insulin-like factor, erythropoietin	*hepatocellular carcinoma*
lung tumor secreting PTH-like peptide	*primary squamous cell carcinoma*
tumor secreting β-hCG	*choriocarcinoma*: gestationally derived in women, testicular cancer in men
tumor location for secreting serotonin and producing the carcinoid syndrome	*carcinoid tumor of the terminal ileum of the small intestine with metastasis to the liver*

Table continued on following page

Table 17–4. ADRENAL DISEASES, MULTIPLE ENDOCRINE NEOPLASIA SYNDROMES, ECTOPIC HORMONE SYNDROMES *Continued*

Question: Which of the following lab or clinical findings are more compatible with Cushing's syndrome than with primary aldosteronism? **SELECT 2**
  (A) Hyperglycemia
  (B) Hypokalemia
  (C) Metabolic alkalosis
  (D) Diastolic hypertension
  (E) Purple striae

Answers: (A), (E): Primary aldosteronism has an increase only in aldosterone, not cortisol, so hyperglycemia (A) and purple striae [E; to rupture in stretch marks) are not present. Cushing's patients do produce weak mineralocorticoids (not aldosterone), so they do have similar lab findings to those of primary aldosteronism regarding electrolyte and acid base disorders [(B), (C)], and they also have hypertension (D).

ACTH = adrenocorticotropic hormone, ADH = antidiuretic hormone, β-hCG = beta-human chorionic gonadotropin, CT = computed tomography, DHEA = dehydroepiandrosterone, DIC = disseminated intravascular coagulation, DM = diabetes mellitus, HVA = homovanillic acid, G/M = gross and microscopic, KS = ketosteroids, MEN = multiple endocrine neoplasia, PTH = parathormone, PUD = peptic ulcer disease, S/S = signs and symptoms, TB = tuberculosis, VMA = vanillylmandelic acid.

Table 17–5. DIABETES MELLITUS, ISLET CELL TUMORS, HYPOGLYCEMIA

Most Common...	Answer and Explanation
type of DM	*type II DM* [It is subclassified into **obese,** non-obese, or maturity-onset types.]
differences between type I and II DM	*age at diagnosis* (I: <20 yrs old, II: >30 yrs old), *body habitus* (I: thin, II: obese), *pathogenesis* (I: insulin lack [anti-islet cell and insulin antibodies], II: relative insulin deficiency, insulin resistance [receptor deficiency, post-receptor defect]), *HLA relationships* (I: Dr3, Dr4, DQ; II: none), *family history* (I: none, II: multifactorial inheritance), *ketoacidosis* (I: may occur, II: does not occur), *treatment* (I: insulin dependent, II: diet, oral drugs, insulin in some cases)
causes of secondary DM	*pancreatic disease, endocrine* (Cushing's pheochromocytoma, acromegaly), *genetic, drugs* (e.g., pentamidine)

Table 17–5. DIABETES MELLITUS, ISLET CELL TUMORS, HYPOGLYCEMIA *Continued*

Most Common...	Answer and Explanation
pathologic processes in DM	*NEG, osmotic damage*
disorders associated with NEG	*hyaline arteriolosclerosis, enhanced athero-sclerosis* (increases oxidized LDL)
pathogenesis of osmotic damage	*glucose is converted into sorbitol by aldose reductase; sorbitol is osmotically active and draws water into the cell*
disorders associated with osmotic damage	*cataracts, peripheral neuropathy* (Schwann cells destroyed), *retinal microaneurysms* (peri-cytes destroyed)
diseases in which DM is the most common cause	*peripheral neuropathy, nontraumatic ampu-tation of the leg, blindness, chronic renal dis-ease*
benefits of tight glucose control	*reduction in risk for* (descending order) **reti-nopathy,** *peripheral neuropathy, nephropa-thy*
causes of hyperglycemia in DKA	**increased gluconeogenesis** (glucagon), *in-creased glycogenolysis* (glucagon, catechola-mines)
cause of lipolysis in DKA	*activation of hormone-sensitive lipase in adi-pose* tissue (glucagon, catecholamines) *with release of FAs and glycerol*
cause of ketoacidosis in DKA	*increased β-oxidation of FAs with increased formation of acetyl CoA, which is converted by the liver into AcAc, acetone, β-OHB*
fate of glycerol in DKA	*converted in the liver into glycerol 3-PO$_4$, which is converted into DHAP and used as a substrate for gluconeogenesis*
cause of an increase in VLDL and chylomicrons in DKA	*decreased capillary lipoprotein lipase activ-ity owing to the absence of insulin*
cause of volume loss in DKA	*osmotic diuresis from glucosuria and loss of water, sodium, and potassium*
cause of HNKC	*type II DM* [There is enough insulin to pre-vent ketogenesis but not enough to prevent hyperglycemia.]

Table continued on following page

Table 17–5. DIABETES MELLITUS, ISLET CELL TUMORS, HYPOGLYCEMIA *Continued*

Most Common...	Answer and Explanation
causes of diabetic nephropathy	*glomerular hyperfiltration* (increased GFR), *increased glomerular capillary permeability* (NEG), *hyaline arteriolosclerosis of afferent/ efferent arterioles* (NEG)
types of retinopathy in DM	*nonproliferative* (microaneurysms), *proliferative* (capillary proliferation with retinal detachment, exudates, hemorrhage)
type of peripheral neuropathy in DM	*distal sensorimotor neuropathy*
causes of pressure ulcers on the feet in DM	**peripheral neuropathy** (cannot feel pressure), *complicated by ischemia and infection*
disorders associated with autonomic neuropathy in DM	*bradycardia → tachycardia, hypotension, impotence, gastric hypomotility, diarrhea*
fungus associated with frontal lobe abscesses in DKA	*Mucor* [It proliferates in the sinuses and extends into the brain through the cribriform plate (rhinocerebral mucormycosis).]
bacteria associated with malignant external otitis in DM	*Pseudomonas aeruginosa*
lab test used to evaluate long-term glycemic control in DM	*HbA1C* [It evaluates the last 4–8 weeks of glycemic control.]
cutoff point for a fasting glucose level in diagnosing DM	*≥126 mg/dL* (used to be 140 mg/dL), *confirmed on a subsequent day by a value ≥126 mg/dL*
cutoff point for diagnosing DM on a random glucose test	*symptoms of polyuria, polydipsia, weight loss with a random glucose level ≥200 mg/dL*
2-hour cutoff point for diagnosing DM after a 2-hour OGTT (75 g)	*≥200 mg/dL* on two separate occasions
screening test used for GDM in pregnancy	*50 g glucose challenge between 24th and 28th week; a value ≥140 mg/dL after 1 hour is a positive test and is confirmed with a 3-hour OGTT using 100 g of glucose*

Table 17–5. DIABETES MELLITUS, ISLET CELL
TUMORS, HYPOGLYCEMIA *Continued*

Most Common...	Answer and Explanation
COD in DM	*AMI*
maternal/fetal disorders associated with GDM	*maternal:* ~35% chance of developing DM in 5–10 years *fetal:* RDS, congenital heart disease, macrosomia, open neural tube defects
complications associated with IGT	*peripheral vascular disease, peripheral neuropathy, 30% develop DM in 10 years*
type of insulin regimen used in treating type I DM	*split routine with NPH and regular insulin in the* AM *and* PM
cause of hypoglycemia	*insulin-induced in a type I diabetic*
types of hypoglycemia	*fed state* (adrenergic symptoms), *fasting* (neuroglycopenia; tired, neurologic findings)
causes of fed state hypoglycemia	**insulin-dependent DM,** *dumping syndrome* (post-Billroth II operation), *leucine sensitivity* (children; leucine stimulates insulin release)
causes of fasting hypoglycemia	*alcohol* (pyruvate converted into lactate by the increase in NADH in alcohol metabolism), *liver disease* (decreased gluconeogenesis and glycogen stores), *carnitine deficiency* (reduced β-oxidation of FAs, hence all tissues compete for glucose for fuel), *von Gierke's disease* (absent glucose 6-phosphatase), *insulinoma*
test used to document hypoglycemia	*72-hour fast and satisfying Whipple's triad* (symptoms, hypoglycemia, symptoms relieved by glucose)
islet cell tumor	*insulinoma* [A generally benign tumor, it presents with fasting hypoglycemia and increased serum insulin and C-peptide levels.]
S/S of a glucagonoma	*malignant tumor of α-islet cells associated with DM and a rash* (necrolytic migratory erythema)
S/S of somatostatinoma	*malignant tumor of δ-islet cells associated with DM, steatorrhea, gallstones, and achlorhydria*

Table continued on following page

Table 17–5. DIABETES MELLITUS, ISLET CELL TUMORS, HYPOGLYCEMIA *Continued*

Most Common...	Answer and Explanation
S/S of a VIPoma (pancreatic cholera, Verner-Morrison syndrome)	*malignant tumor of islets with excessive production of vasoactive intestinal peptide leading to secretory diarrhea and achlorhydria*

Question: Which of the following biochemical processes are occurring in a patient with DKA? **SELECT 4**
- (A) Anaerobic glycolysis
- (B) Gluconeogenesis
- (C) Fatty acid synthesis
- (D) Glycogenolysis
- (E) Lipogenesis
- (F) Inactivation of hormone-sensitive lipase
- (G) Inactivation of PFK
- (H) Synthesis of AcAc

Answers: (B), (D), (G), (H): In the absence of insulin and presence of glucagon and other counterregulatory hormones, gluconeogenesis (B), β-oxidation of FAs, glycogenolysis (D), activation of hormone sensitive lipase (lipolysis), and ketogenesis occur. Insulin enhances PFK (G), lipogenesis (E), FA synthesis (C), glycogen synthesis, and aerobic glycolysis (A).

AcAc = acetoacetic acid, AMI = acute myocardial infarction, β-OHB = beta-hydroxybutyric acid, COD = cause of death, DHAP = dihydroxyacetone phosphate, DKA = diabetic ketoacidosis, DM = diabetes mellitus, FA = fatty acid, GDM = gestational diabetes mellitus, GFR = glomerular filtration rate, HbA1C = hemoglobin A1C, HLA = human leukocyte antigen, HNKC = hyperosmotic non-ketotic coma, IGT = impaired glucose tolerance, LDL = low-density lipoprotein, NADH = nicotinamide adenosine dinucleotide (reduced form), NEG = non-enzymatic glycosylation, NPH = neutral protamine Hagedorn (insulin), OGTT = oral glucose tolerance test, PFK = phosphofructokinase, RDS = respiratory distress syndrome, S/S = signs and symptoms, VIP = vasoactive intestinal polypeptide, VLDL = very low density lipoprotein.

CHAPTER

MUSCULOSKELETAL AND SOFT TISSUE PATHOLOGY

CONTENTS

Table 18–1. SYNOVIAL FLUID ANALYSIS, JOINT, LIGAMENT, TENDON DISORDERS

Most Common...	Answer and Explanation
function of SF	*lubricant, nourishment for articular cartilage*
routine tests of SF	*cell count* (<200 WBCs/µL) *and differential, culture, crystal analysis, mucin clot test*
monoclinic [needle-shaped] SF crystals	**MSU,** *CPP*
triclinic [rhomboid-shaped] crystal	*CPP*
appearance of MSU when aligned parallel to the slow axis of the compensator	*yellow monoclinic crystal* (background is red) [These characteristics define a negatively bi-refringent crystal.]
appearance of CPP when aligned parallel to the slow axis of the compensator	*blue monoclinic or triclinic crystal* [These characteristics define a positively birefringent crystal.]
test evaluating SF viscosity	*mucin clot test* [Acid added to a tube of SF clots hyaluronic acid; poor clot formation indicates joint inflammation.]

Table continued on following page

Table 18–1. SYNOVIAL FLUID ANALYSIS, JOINT, LIGAMENT, TENDON DISORDERS *Continued*

Most Common...	Answer and Explanation
classification of joint disorders	**group I** (noninflammatory), *group II* (inflammatory), *group III* (septic), *group IV* (hemorrhagic, trauma)
noninflammatory joint diseases	**OA,** *neuropathic joint*
joint disease and disabling joint disease	*OA* [OA is a female-dominant disease, characterized by progressive and disabling degeneration of the articular cartilage.]
joints involved in OA	**weight-bearing joints** (hip, knee) and *hands* (**DIP** and PIP joints; genetic predisposition), *vertebral column*
secondary causes of OA	**trauma** [Other causes: *Legg-Perthes, obesity, hemochromatosis*]
G/M findings in OA	**wearing down of articular cartilage,** *cartilage fibrillation* (perpendicular clefts), *subchondral bone cysts, osteophytes at the joint margins* (reactive bone formation), *secondary synovial inflammation*
S/S of OA	**arthralgia** [Other findings include *Heberden's node of DIP joint* (osteophyte), *Bouchard's node of PIP joint, compression neuropathies from vertebral involvement.*]
radiographic findings in OA	*narrow joint space, osteophytes, subchondral bone cysts*
causes of a neuropathic (Charcot) joint	**DM** [Other causes include *syringomyelia, tabes dorsalis.* Combination of insensitivity to pain and ischemia.]
cause of primary gout	*multifactorial inheritance*
causes of secondary gout	*DM, alcoholism, diuretics, PRV*
primary causes of an increase in uric acid synthesis	*decrease in HGPRT, increase in PRPP* [Uric acid is a byproduct of purine metabolism.]
cause of hyperuricemia in gout	*decreased excretion of uric acid in the kidneys*

Table 18–1. SYNOVIAL FLUID ANALYSIS, JOINT, LIGAMENT, TENDON DISORDERS *Continued*

Most Common...	Answer and Explanation
cause of hyperuricemia in the Lesch-Nyhan syndrome (SXR)	*complete absence of HGPRT*
joint involved in the initial attack of acute gouty arthritis	*first metatarsophalangeal joint* (big toe) [This is called *podagra*.]
cause of joint inflammation in acute gouty arthritis	*interaction of MSU with neutrophils and release of leukocyte-derived chemotactic factor*
lab test used to diagnose gout	*SF analysis with demonstration of negatively birefringent crystals* [Hyperuricemia does not define gout.]
abnormality in chronic gout	*tophus formation* [A tophus is deposits of MSU in tissue (multinucleated granulomatous reaction) around the joint and other sites.]
complications of gout	*disabling arthritis, renal disease* (urate nephropathy)
associations with gout	*chronic lead exposure* (lead enhances uric acid reabsorption), *alcohol ingestion* (lactic and ketoacids compete with uric acid for renal excretion)
drugs used in treating acute gouty arthritis	**indomethacin** (anti-inflammatory agent), *colchicine* (blocks leukocyte-derived chemotactic factor)
drug reducing uric acid synthesis	*allopurinol* [It blocks xanthine oxidase.]
uricosuric agents	**probenecid,** *sulfinpyrazone* [Low-dose aspirin reduces uric acid excretion and high doses are uricosuric.]
S/S of CPPD (pseudogout)	*chondrocalcinosis involving the knee* (inflammatory arthritis with CPP crystals and linear deposits of CPP in articular cartilage)
seronegative (RF negative) spondyloarthropathy	*AS* [It is an inflammatory arthritis most commonly afflicting young men who are HLA B27 positive.]

Table continued on following page

Table 18–1. SYNOVIAL FLUID ANALYSIS, JOINT, LIGAMENT, TENDON DISORDERS *Continued*

Most Common...	Answer and Explanation
joints and other sites targeted in AS	**sacroiliac joint,** *vertebral column* ("bamboo spine"), *aorta* (aortitis with aortic insufficiency), *uveal tract* (uveitis with blurry vision)
S/S of AS	**morning stiffness in the sacroiliac joint** that improves with exercise [Other S/S include *diminished anterior flexion* (eventual restrictive lung disease), *aortic insufficiency, visual problems.*]
S/S of Reiter's syndrome	*conjunctivitis, urethritis* (*Chlamydia trachomatis*) or enterocolitis [*Shigella, Campylobacter, Yersinia*], *HLA B27–positive arthritis*
S/S of psoriatic arthritis	*morning stiffness similar to RA, sausage-shaped DIP joints with nail pitting and erosive joint disease, sometimes associated with HLA B27*
IBD associated with HLA B27–positive arthritis	*UC*
nongonococcal cause of septic arthritis	*Staphylococcus aureus*
cause of septic arthritis in urban populations in the United States	*Neisseria gonorrhoeae* [It most commonly occurs in women during menses or pregnancy.]
S/S of disseminated gonorrhoeae	**tenosynovitis** (wrists, ankles), *septic arthritis* (knee, wrists, ankles), *dermatitis* (pustules: wrists, ankles)
complement deficiencies in disseminated gonococcemia	*C5–C8* [These components are necessary for phagocytosis of the organisms.]
cause of Lyme disease	*tick-transmitted* (*Ixodes*) *Borrelia burgdorferi* (spirochete) [The white-tailed deer is the animal reservoir for the organism.]

Table 18–1. SYNOVIAL FLUID ANALYSIS, JOINT, LIGAMENT, TENDON DISORDERS *Continued*

Most Common...	Answer and Explanation
skin lesion in early Lyme disease	*erythema chronicum migrans* [It is a red, expanding lesion with concentric circles emanating from the site of the tick bite. Doxycycline is the treatment of choice.]
late manifestations of Lyme disease	**joint disease** (knee) [Other late findings: *Bell's palsy* (seventh nerve; most common cranial nerve), *myocarditis, heart block.* Ceftriaxone is the treatment of choice.]
secondary infection transmitted by *Ixodes*	*babesiosis, an intraerythrocytic protozoal disease caused by Babesia microti*
dislocation in newborns	*congenital hip dislocation* [It is more common in girls than boys. There is a limitation of abduction on the affected side.]
cause of pain and swelling of the proximal tibial apophysis	*Osgood-Schlatter disease* [It is a childhood disease characterized by an inflammatory reaction at the insertion of the patellar tendon on the apophysis. It is self-limited, but produces knobby-appearing knees.]
cause of the carpal tunnel syndrome	*entrapment of the median nerve in the transverse carpal ligament* [It occurs in those who use their hands a lot (e.g., barbers), RA, amyloidosis, hypothyroidism, pregnancy.]
S/S of carpal tunnel syndrome	*pain, numbness, or tingling of the plantar surface of the thumb, index finger, middle finger and radial side of the fourth finger* [Thenar atrophy may occur.]
cause of intervertebral disc disease	*degeneration of the fibrocartilage and nucleus pulposus* [A ruptured disc may herniate posteriorly and compress the nerve root and/or spinal cord. Pain radiating from low back, to the buttocks, down the leg, and below the knee (sciatica) commonly occurs.]
S/S of herniation of an L3-L4 disc	*absent knee jerk and weak quadriceps*

Table continued on following page

Table 18–1. SYNOVIAL FLUID ANALYSIS, JOINT, LIGAMENT, TENDON DISORDERS *Continued*

Most Common...	Answer and Explanation
S/S of herniation of an L4-L5 disc	*normal knee and Achilles reflex, weakness of dorsiflexion of the great toe, sensory changes in the anterolateral leg and webbed space next to the great toe*
S/S of herniation of an L5-S1 disc	*absent Achilles reflex, sensory changes on the lateral and posterior calf and plantar aspect of the foot*

Question: Which of the following are more likely present in OA rather than RA? **SELECT 4**
- (A) Narrow joint space
- (B) Osteophytes
- (C) Pannus
- (D) Autoantibody against IgG
- (E) Subchondral bone cysts
- (F) Morning stiffness >1 hour
- (G) DIP involvement
- (H) PIP involvement
- (I) MCP involvement
- (J) Noninflammatory joint disease

Answers: (B), (E), (G), (J): Both diseases have narrowing of the joint space and involvement of the PIP joint. RA, an inflammatory joint disease, has RF (IgM antibody against IgG), pannus, and morning stiffness > 1 hour.

AS = ankylosing spondylitis, CPP = calcium pyrophosphate, CPPD = calcium pyrophosphate dihydrate crystal deposition arthropathy, DIP = distal interphalangeal, DM = diabetes mellitus, G/M = gross and microscopic, HGPRT = hypoxanthine-guanine phosphoribosyltransferase, HLA = human leukocyte antigen, IBD = inflammatory bowel disease, Ig = immunoglobulin, MCP = metacarpal-phalangeal, MSU = monosodium urate, OA = osteoarthritis, PIP = proximal interphalangeal, PRPP = 5-phospho-α-D-ribosyl-1-pyrophosphate, PRV = polycythemia rubra vera, RA = rheumatoid arthritis, RF = rheumatoid factor, SF = synovial fluid, S/S = signs and symptoms, SXR = sex-linked recessive, UC = ulcerative colitis, WBC = white blood cell.

Table 18–2. BONE/CARTILAGE DISORDERS

Most Common...	Answer and Explanation
hereditary bone disease	*osteogenesis imperfecta* [It is an AD or AR disease with a defect in synthesis of type I collagen.]
S/S of osteogenesis imperfecta	**pathologic fractures** ("brittle bone" disease), *blue sclera, deafness, defective dentine in the teeth*
signs of achondroplasia	*AD disease with normal-sized head and vertebral column but shortened arms and legs due to impaired enchondral ossification and premature closure of the epiphyseal plates of the long bones*
S/S of osteopetrosis	*AD or AR disease associated with pathologic fractures* ("marble bone disease"), *anemia (marrow replaced by bone), visual and hearing loss* (cranial nerve compression) *due to a defect in osteoclasts and "too much bone"*
metabolic bone disease	*osteoporosis* [It refers to an overall reduction in mineralized bone.]
causes of osteoporosis	**estrogen deficiency** [Other causes include *endocrine disorders* (e.g., Cushing's, hyperthyroidism, primary HPTH), *immobilization, drugs* (e.g., heparin, corticosteroids), *renal failure* (metabolic acidosis, secondary HPTH), *lack of gravity.*]
cause of osteoporosis in estrogen deficiency	*estrogen normally dampens the release of osteoclast-activating factor (OAF) from osteoblasts after PTH interacts with its receptor on osteoblasts; a lack of estrogen results in greater breakdown of bone by osteoclasts than formation of bone by osteoblasts*
fractures associated with postmenopausal osteoporosis	**compression fractures of the vertebra,** *Colles' fracture*

Table continued on following page

Table 18–2. BONE/CARTILAGE DISORDERS *Continued*

Most Common...	Answer and Explanation
lab test used to diagnose osteoporosis	*dual photon absorptiometry* [It is a noninvasive test that measures bone density.]
lab tests used to measure bone turnover in osteoporosis	*osteocalcin, pyridinium collagen cross-links* [The former is released from increased osteoclastic resorption of bone and the latter is a constituent of bone collagen that is released with bone resorption.]
recommendations for the prevention of postmenopausal osteoporosis	**estrogen with or without progesterone** (protects against endometrial cancer) [Other recommendations: *exercise* (weight bearing), *calcium* 1000 mg/d, and *vitamin D* 400 U/d. Estrogen also protects the patient from CAD.]
drugs used in the treatment of osteoporosis	*bisphosphonates* (inhibit bone resorption), *calcitonin*
cause of osteoporosis in men	*low testosterone levels* [Osteoporosis occurs later since men have a greater skeletal mass than women. Hip fractures are the most common complication.]
cause of osteomyelitis in children/young adults	*Staphylococcus aureus*
site in bone targeted by osteomyelitis	*metaphysis* [The metaphysis has the richest blood supply.]
G/M features of osteomyelitis	*liquefactive necrosis with production of devitalized bone* (sequestrum) and *reactive bone formation* (involucrum) *if the condition becomes chronic*
complications of osteomyelitis	*draining sinus tracts, nidus for septicemia, squamous cancer in the sinus tract, amyloidosis*
type of osteomyelitis in sickle cell anemia	*Staphylococcus aureus* [*Salmonella*, though common in the setting of sickle cell disease, is still not the most common overall osteomyelitis.]

Table 18–2. BONE/CARTILAGE DISORDERS *Continued*

Most Common...	Answer and Explanation
cause of Pott's disease	*TB* [It refers to a TB infection involving the vertebral column leading to destruction of bone and extension of inflammation along the sheath of the psoas muscle.]
bone lesions present in congenital syphilis	*osteochondritis,* with new bone formation around long bones leading to *saber shins* with forward bowing of the tibia
femoral fracture	*femoral neck fracture* [It most commonly occurs in the elderly patient with osteoporosis.]
wrist bone fracture leading to aseptic necrosis	*scaphoid* (navicular) *fracture*
fracture associated with falling on the outstretched hand	*Colles' fracture of the distal radius* [Radiologically, it produces a "dinner fork" deformity of the proximal radial fragment, which is displaced upward and backward.]
cause of pathologic fractures [fracture in diseased bone]	*metastatic disease to bone*
site/causes of avascular (aseptic) necrosis of bone	*femoral head,* most commonly secondary to a *femoral head fracture* [Other causes: steroids, sickle cell disease, osteoporosis, Legg-Perthes disease]
osteochondrosis [aseptic necrosis of ossification centers] in children	*Legg-Perthes disease involving the femoral head* [It is more common in boys between 3 and 10 years of age and presents with a painless limp.]
test used to identify aseptic necrosis	*MRI* [It shows increased density in the area of involvement.]
cause of Paget's disease of bone	*? viral infection targeting osteoclasts leading to an initial phase of increased osteoclastic activity followed by increased osteoblastic activity*
S/S of Paget's disease of bone	**pathologic fractures** (pelvis, femur), *bone pain, high output failure* (AV communications in bone), *osteogenic sarcoma, head enlargement* (increased hat size, deafness)

Table continued on following page

Table 18–2. BONE/CARTILAGE DISORDERS *Continued*

Most Common...	Answer and Explanation
G/M findings in Paget's disease of bone	*thick, soft bone with a loss of lamellar structure* (mosaic bone), *which renders it susceptible to fracture*
initial lab findings in Paget's disease of bone	*increased alkaline phosphatase* (osteoblastic bone formation), *usually in an asymptomatic, elderly male*
treatment of Paget's disease of bone	**bisphosphonates,** calcitonin
S/S of Albright's syndrome	*polyostotic fibrous dysplasia* (benign bone disease), *café-au-lait pigmentation, precocious puberty, usually in females*
cancer associated with hypertrophic osteoarthropathy	*primary lung cancer* [Hypertrophic osteoarthropathy refers to periosteal inflammation with new bone formation and arthritis, which may or may not be associated with clubbing of the fingers.]
benign bone tumor in children producing nocturnal pain relieved by aspirin	*osteoid osteoma* [It involves the cortical aspect of the proximal femur. It has a radiolucent nidus surrounded by dense sclerotic bone on a radiograph.]
primary bone tumors in order of increasing age	*Ewing's sarcoma* (first and second decade), *osteogenic sarcoma* (10–25 years old), *chondrosarcoma* (>30 years old), *multiple myeloma* (>50 years old)
primary malignant bone tumors in descending order of frequency	**multiple myeloma,** *osteogenic sarcoma, chondrosarcoma, Ewing's sarcoma, giant cell tumor of bone*
malignancy of bone	*metastatic breast cancer*
benign bone tumor	*osteochondroma* [It is a benign cartilaginous tumor arising as an outgrowth from the metaphysis of bone. It is capped by benign proliferating cartilage.]
bone tumors arising in the epiphysis of bone	**giant cell tumor of bone** (adult female–dominant tumor arising in the distal end of femur/proximal tibia), *chondroblastoma* (benign cartilaginous tumor; "popcorn appearance" on radiograph)

Table 18–2. BONE/CARTILAGE DISORDERS *Continued*

Most Common...	Answer and Explanation
malignant tumors in children with a "round cell" infiltrate resembling ALL	**metastatic neuroblastoma,** *Ewing's sarcoma, metastatic malignant lymphoma* (lymphoblastic lymphoma, Burkitt's lymphoma)
classic radiographic findings in osteogenic sarcoma	*"sunburst appearance"* in soft tissue surrounding the tumor (calcified malignant osteoid), *Codman's triangle* (lifting of the periosteum due to tumor infiltrating out of the metaphysis into soft tissue)
classic radiographic finding in Ewing's sarcoma	*concentric "onion skin layering" due to new bone formation around the primary tumor* (usually in the tibia or flat bones of the pelvis)
location of an osteogenic sarcoma	*distal femur or proximal tibia* [Both of these sites are around the knee.]
risk factors for osteogenic sarcoma	*Paget's disease, radiation, retinoblastoma* (chromosome 13 relationship)
bone tumor associated with Gardner's polyposis syndrome	*osteoma* [It is a benign tumor most commonly located in the **sinuses,** jaws, facial bones.]
primary bone tumor located in the vertebra	*osteoblastoma* ("giant osteoid osteoma")
malignant cartilaginous tumor and its location	*chondrosarcoma* [It is most often located in the **pelvis** and *upper end of the femur.*]
risk factors for chondrosarcoma	*multiple osteochondromas* (osteochondromatosis; AD disease), *Ollier's disease* (multiple enchondromas [arise in the medullary cavity])
bone tumor with multinucleated giant cells	*giant cell tumor* [It is a benign tumor arising in the epiphysis of bone in young to middle-aged women. Mononuclear fibroblast-like cells are the neoplastic component, while the multinucleated giant cells are benign.]

Table continued on following page

Table 18–2. BONE/CARTILAGE DISORDERS *Continued*

Most Common...	Answer and Explanation
malignant bone tumor in young children presenting as an infectious disease	*Ewing's sarcoma* [It occurs young males and presents with fever, anemia, elevated ESR, and heat and swelling overlying the affected bone.]

Question: Which of the following bone disorders are more common in patients under 20 years of age? **SELECT 5**
- (A) Osteochondroma
- (B) Multiple myeloma
- (C) Chondrosarcoma
- (D) Legg-Perthes disease
- (E) Giant cell tumor
- (F) Osteoid osteoma
- (G) Ewing's sarcoma
- (H) Paget's disease
- (I) Osteogenic sarcoma

Answers: (A), (D), (F), (G), (I): Multiple myeloma, chondrosarcoma, and Paget's disease are more common in patients >30 years of age.

AD = autosomal dominant, ALL = acute lymphoblastic leukemia, AR = autosomal recessive, AV = arteriovenous, CAD = coronary artery disease, ESR = erythrocyte sedimentation rate, G/M = gross and microscopic, HPTH = hyperparathyroidism, MRI = magnetic resonance imaging, PTH = parathormone, S/S = signs and symptoms, TB = tuberculosis.

Table 18–3. MUSCLE AND SOFT TISSUE DISORDERS

Most Common...	Answer and Explanation
features of type I muscle fibers	*slow twitch fibers* (red muscle), *rich in mitochondria, good for sustained contractions without fatigue but they do not hypertrophy, low in glycogen, increased enzymes in aerobic glycolysis with conditioning*
features of type II muscle fibers	*fast twitch fibers* (white muscle), *poor in mitochondria, rich in glycogen, hypertrophy with exercise*
symptom of muscle disease	*weakness*
causes of muscle weakness	*UMN or LMN disease* (e.g., ALS), *defects in the neuromuscular synapse* (e.g., MG), *primary muscle disease* (e.g., DMD)

Table 18–3. MUSCLE AND SOFT TISSUE DISORDERS
Continued

Most Common...	Answer and Explanation
causes of neurogenic atrophy	*destruction of the motor neuron* (e.g., polio, ALS), *degeneration of the axon* (e.g., distal sensorimotor peripheral neuropathy in DM)
muscular dystrophy (MD) in children	*DMD* [It is an SXR disease, with a defect in dystrophin. Becker's type is a weaker variant. There is degeneration of type I and II fibers.]
S/S of DMD	*muscle weakness/wasting in the pelvic girdle beginning at 2–5 years of age, waddling gait, heart failure, pseudohypertrophy of calf muscles* (fatty infiltration of muscle tissue)
lab findings in DMD	*increased serum CK and aldolase* [The dystrophin defect can be detected prenatally.]
adult MD	*myotonic dystrophy* [It is an AD disease with a triplet repeat defect.]
S/S of myotonic dystrophy	*facial weakness, inability to relax muscles* (myotonia), *frontal balding, cataracts, testicular atrophy, cardiac disease*
cause of the "floppy infant syndrome"	*congenital myopathies* (e.g., central core disease [absent central core in type I fibers], nemaline rod myopathy [rod-like structures in type I fibers])
infectious causes of myositis	*viral* (e.g., coxsackievirus, influenza), *bacterial* (*Clostridium perfringens*), *parasitic* (*Toxoplasma gondii, Taenia solium, Trichinella spiralis*)
drugs causing myositis	*alcohol, clofibrate, L-tryptophan, penicillamine*
acid-base causes of myositis	*severe hypokalemia, severe hypophosphatemia*
cause of MG	*autoantibodies against the acetylcholine receptor* (type II hypersensitivity)
source of antibodies in MG	*B cells in germinal follicles that develop in the thymus*
S/S of MG	**ptosis** [Other S/S include *muscle weakness that worsens with exercise, diplopia, respiratory failure.*]

Table continued on following page

Table 18–3. MUSCLE AND SOFT TISSUE DISORDERS
Continued

Most Common...	Answer and Explanation
findings in the thymus in MG	**B cell hyperplasia** (85%), *thymoma* (15%)
initial lab tests performed in MG	*Tensilon test* (edrophonium) [The drugs block acetylcholinesterase, thereby increasing ACh in the synapse and improving muscle strength. Others: measuring serum autoantibodies; electromyography]
treatment of MG	**acetylcholinesterase inhibitors** (e.g., pyridostigmine), *corticosteroids, thymectomy*
cancer associated with the Eaton-Lambert syndrome	*primary small cell cancer of the lung* [The syndrome resembles MG in that there is muscle weakness, but the Tensilon test is negative and muscle strength increases with exercise.]
cause of botulism	*Clostridium botulinum* [It is due to ingestion of preformed toxins (food poisoning) in adults or colonization of the bowel with subsequent toxin formation in infants (via honey in milk).]
site of action of botulinum toxin	*blocks the release of ACh, producing a descending paralysis* [The pupils are dilated.]
drug blocking the release of ACh	*aminoglycosides*
fibromatosis [non-neoplastic proliferation of connective tissue]	*Dupuytren's contracture* [It involves the palmar fascia and causes contraction of the fourth and fifth fingers. It is common in alcoholics.]
fibromatosis associated with Gardner's polyposis syndrome	*desmoid tumor* [It usually occurs in the anterior abdominal wall.]
fibromatosis associated with methysergide	*retroperitoneal fibrosis* [This often leads to hydronephrosis.]
benign soft tissue tumor	*lipoma* [It arises from adipose cells.]
benign soft tissue tumor in the GI tract	*leiomyoma* [It is most commonly located in the stomach.]

Table 18–3. MUSCLE AND SOFT TISSUE DISORDERS
Continued

Most Common...	Answer and Explanation
benign soft tissue tumor of the heart in children	*rhabdomyoma* [It is associated with tuberous sclerosis, an AD disease.]
benign soft tissue tumor of the heart in adults	*myxoma* [It most commonly occurs in the left atrium.]
risk factors for producing sarcomas	*ionizing radiation* (e.g., malignant fibrous histiocytoma, osteogenic sarcoma), *viruses* (e.g., herpesvirus 8 in Kaposi's sarcoma), *genetic predisposition* (e.g., neurofibrosarcoma in neurofibromatosis)
sarcoma [malignant tumor arising from mesenchymal tissue] in children	*embryonal rhabdomyosarcoma* (sarcoma botryoides) [It arises in the vagina in girls and prostate in boys.]
sarcoma in adults	**malignant fibrous histiocytoma,** *liposarcoma* (second most common)

Question: Which of the following disorders is associated with normal muscle strength?
(A) Polymyositis
(B) Parkinson's disease
(C) DMD
(D) Eaton-Lambert syndrome
(E) MG
(F) Hypokalemia
(G) Myotonic dystrophy
(H) Primary hypothyroidism
(I) Hypophosphatemia

Answer: (B): Parkinson's disease is associated with muscle rigidity leading to bradykinesia, which is misinterpreted by the patient as representing muscle weakness. All the other choices listed are associated with muscle weakness.

ACh = acetylcholine, AD = autosomal dominant, ALS = amyotrophic lateral sclerosis, CK = creatine kinase, DM = diabetes mellitus, DMD = Duchenne's muscular dystrophy, GI = gastrointestinal, LMN = lower motor neuron, MG = myasthenia gravis, S/S = signs and symptoms, SXR = sex-linked recessive, UMN = upper motor neuron.

CHAPTER

DERMATOPATHOLOGY

CONTENTS

Table 19–1. TERMS, ECZEMA, AND MACULOPAPULAR DISORDERS

Most Common...	Answer and Explanation
skin diseases seen in clinical practice	**superficial dermatophyte infections,** *acne vulgaris, seborrheic dermatitis*
initial test used to identify superficial dermatophyte infections	*scraping of the lesion followed by KOH digestion of the keratin material, followed by examination under the microscope for yeasts and hyphae* [A *Wood's lamp* (UVA light) is used to detect fluorescent metabolites of fungi.]
test used to identify viral inclusions in vesicular lesions	*Tzanck preparation* [The test is performed by taking scrapings from the base of an unroofed vesicle, which are stained and examined for inclusions (e.g., HSV I and II and varicella have intranuclear inclusions in multinucleated cells).]
epidermal layer involved in hyperkeratosis	*stratum corneum* (anucleate cells with keratin) [An increase in thickness of this layer produces a scaly appearance of the skin called hyperkeratosis.]
cause of acanthosis [increased skin thickness]	*hyperkeratosis*

Table continued on following page

Table 19–1. TERMS, ECZEMA, AND
MACULOPAPULAR DISORDERS *Continued*

Most Common...	Answer and Explanation
epidermal layer involved in rete ridge hyperplasia	*stratum basalis* [It is the actively dividing layer of the epidermis. Rete ridge hyperplasia refers to a sawtooth appearance of the basal layer.]
cause of spongiosis in the epidermis	*fluid accumulation between keratinocytes* [It may lead to vesicle formation (fluid-filled blister <5 mm).]
appearance of a macule	*pigmented or red flat lesion on the skin surface*
appearance of a papule	*peaked or dome-shaped lesion on the skin surface*
appearance of a bulla	*fluid-filled blister >5 mm*
appearance of a pustule	*blister filled with an exudate*
term applied to inflammation of the skin	*dermatitis,* of which eczema is the most common cause [Eczema is subdivided into acute, subacute, and chronic types. It is usually accompanied by pruritus.]
appearance of acute eczema	*weeping, erythematous rash with vesicle formation*
appearance of chronic eczema	*thickened, dry, hyperkeratotic skin* (lichenification) *due to constant scratching*
cause of atopic dermatitis	*genetic predisposition for type I, IgE-mediated hypersensitivity reactions* [Disease in these patients is called atopic.]
cause of pruritus in atopic dermatitis	*a lower itch threshold than normal* ("itch that rashes" rather than the "rash that itches")
locations for atopic dermatitis	*cheeks, trunk, extensor surfaces in infants, moving to the flexor creases as the child grows older*
type of contact dermatitis [dermatitis due to exposure to antigen or irritating substances]	*irritant contact dermatitis* [It is a nonimmunologic reaction due to a local toxic effect on skin (e.g., detergent).]

Table 19–1. TERMS, ECZEMA, AND
MACULOPAPULAR DISORDERS *Continued*

Most Common...	Answer and Explanation
type of hypersensitivity reaction causing allergic contact dermatitis	*type IV cellular immune reaction* (e.g., poison ivy, reaction to nickel, reaction to certain chemicals)
test used to document allergic contact dermatitis	*patch test* [In this test, the suspected offending agent is placed on normal skin and kept in place with a patch to see if a skin reaction occurs.]
drugs that produce a contact photodermatitis	**tetracycline,** *sulfonamides, thiazides* [It is a type IV cellular immune reaction secondary to UVB light.]
cause of dandruff and cradle cap	*seborrheic dermatitis due to a superficial dermatophyte infection (Malassezia furfur)*
cause of tinea capitis [dermatophyte infection of scalp]	*Trichophyton tonsurans* [It infects the inner hair shaft (hair breaks off, producing alopecia). The Wood's lamp test is negative. *Microsporum canis* infects the outer shaft and is Wood's lamp positive.]
cause of tinea corporis [dermatophyte infection of skin]	*Trichophyton rubrum*
appearance of tinea corporis	*circular, pruritic lesions with a pale center and a red, crusted leading edge* (part that should by scraped for KOH study)
group of drugs used to treat tinea corporis	*topical imidazole derivatives*
drug used to treat nail and hair dermatophyte infections	*oral griseofulvin*
cause of tinea versicolor	*M. furfur involving the stratum corneum* [The skin has uneven areas of hyper- and hypopigmentation. It has a "spaghetti (hyphae) and meatball (yeasts)" appearance in a KOH preparation.]

Table continued on following page

Table 19–1. TERMS, ECZEMA, AND
MACULOPAPULAR DISORDERS *Continued*

Most Common...	Answer and Explanation
skin diseases produced by *Candida albicans*	**diaper rash,** *onychomycosis* (nail infections) [*Candida albicans* produces budding yeasts and pseudohyphae in a KOH preparation.]
cause of condyloma acuminatum	*HPV types 6 and 11* [These are also called venereal warts and occur in the moist ano-genital area. They are treated with topical podophyllin.]
cause of molluscum contagiosum	*poxvirus* [The lesions are raised, bowl-shaped, and have a central area of depression (umbilicated) filled with keratin containing the viral particles.]
S/S of rubeola	*fever, conjunctivitis, Koplik spots in the mouth* (red with a white center), *followed by a blanching maculopapular rash beginning at the hairline and extending over the body* [The virus is not teratogenic.]
S/S of rubella	*fever, headache, arthralgias, painful postau-ricular lymphadenopathy followed by a mac-ulopapular rash beginning on the head and spreading downward* [The virus is terato-genic.]
cause of erythema infectiosum (fifth disease)	*parvovirus B19* [The maculopapular rash be-gins on the face ("slapped face" appearance) and extends over the trunk.]
cause of roseola	*herpesvirus 6* [It begins with high fever, often causing febrile convulsions, which drops after 3–4 days and is followed by a maculo-papular rash that begins on the trunk and spreads to the limbs.]
cause of TSS	*toxin producing Staphylococcus aureus* [It is most frequently associated with tampon-wearing menstruating women.]
S/S of TSS	*high fever, mental confusion, diarrhea, hypo-tension, pharyngitis, erythematous maculo-papular rash that occurs on the hands and feet and resolves with desquamation*
treatment of TSS	*nafcillin*
cause of scarlet fever	*group A Streptococcus (S. pyogenes)* [It is a gram-positive coccus that produces an eryth-rogenic toxin.]

Table 19–1. TERMS, ECZEMA, AND MACULOPAPULAR DISORDERS *Continued*

Most Common...	Answer and Explanation
S/S of scarlet fever	*erythematous, maculopapular, blanching rash that begins on the trunk and limbs and resolves with desquamation; on the face, it produces circumoral pallor and a "strawberry tongue."*
complications associated with scarlet fever	**poststreptococcal GN,** *rheumatic fever*
types of skin reactions produced by drugs	**maculopapular rashes,** *urticaria* (raised, pruritic lesions)

Question: A baseball player develops a dermatitis on his face, neck, nape of his neck, dorsum of his hands, and forearms. Which of the following is the **MOST LIKELY** cause?
(A) Viral infection
(B) Bacterial infection
(C) Drug
(D) Autoimmune disease
(E) Fungal infection

Answer: (C): The rash is in sun-exposed areas, so it probably represents a contact photodermatitis due to a drug (e.g., tetracycline).

GN = glomerulonephritis, HPV = human papillomavirus, HSV = herpesvirus, Ig = immunoglobulin, KOH = potassium hydroxide, S/S = signs and symptoms, TSS = toxic shock syndrome, UV = ultraviolet.

Table 19–2. PAPULOSQUAMOUS, VESICULOBULLOUS, AND PUSTULAR SKIN DISORDERS

Most Common...	Answer and Explanation
cause and complication of actinic keratosis	*UVB light leading to squamous dysplasia and the potential for squamous cancer of the skin* [The lesions have a gray-white hyperkeratotic appearance.]
appearance of lichen planus	*pruritic lesion with papules on the wrists, lower back, and scalp, and, in the mouth, a leukoplakic, net-like lesion called Wickham's striae*

Table continued on following page

Table 19–2. PAPULOSQUAMOUS, VESICULOBULLOUS, AND PUSTULAR SKIN DISORDERS *Continued*

Most Common...	Answer and Explanation
causes of psoriasis	*unregulated proliferation of keratinocytes and microcirculatory abnormalities in the superficial dermis often associated with a genetic predisposition and an environmental trigger* (e.g., streptococcal pharyngitis)
appearance of psoriatic plaques	*raised, well-demarcated, flat, salmon-colored plaques covered by silver-white scales, which, when picked off, exhibit pinpoint bleeding* (Auspitz's sign)
nail findings in psoriasis	*pitting of the nails*
microscopic findings in psoriasis	*hyperkeratosis, parakeratosis* (persistence of nuclei in the stratum corneum), *absence of the granular cell layer, rete ridge hyperplasia, extension of the papillary dermis with vessel proliferation beneath the thinnest portions of the epidermis* (reason for Auspitz's sign)
locations for psoriasis	**scalp,** *forearms, knees*
treatment of psoriasis	*topical steroid creams*
S/S of pityriasis rosea	*initial, oval, pink patch on the trunk called a "herald patch," followed in a few days by a papular rash in a "Christmas tree" distribution on the trunk*
appearance of varicella (chickenpox)	*macules, vesicles, pustules that are in different stages of development that begin on the trunk and extend to the extremities and face*
complications associated with varicella	**persistence into adult life** (herpes zoster), *cerebellar inflammation* (self-limited), *Reye's syndrome* (child takes aspirin), *pneumonia*
S/S of *herpes zoster*	*recurrent, painful eruption of vesicles that follow a dermatome of a sensory nerve* (virus is dormant in the sensory dorsal root ganglia) [It may or may not be associated with an underlying malignancy.]
cause of impetigo	*Staphylococcus aureus* [The lesions are honey-colored and crusted in appearance. It may also be due to *Streptococcus pyogenes*.]

Table 19–2. PAPULOSQUAMOUS, VESICULOBULLOUS, AND PUSTULAR SKIN DISORDERS *Continued*

Most Common...	Answer and Explanation
cause of the scalded skin syndrome	*toxin producing S. aureus*
cause of pemphigus vulgaris	*IgG antibodies directed against the intercellular attachments between keratinocytes above the basal cell layer* (type II hypersensitivity) [This produces flaccid bullae that develop above the basal cells (they look like tombstones) that contain fluid and acantholytic keratinocytes (lost their attachments to each other).]
locations for pemphigus vulgaris	**oral mucosa,** *skin* [The lesions separate easily from the basal layer when gently touched (Nikolsky's sign). Steroids are essential for treatment.]
cause of bullous pemphigoid	*IgG antibodies directed against the basement membrane* (type II hypersensitivity) *causing bullae to develop that are subepidermal, do not contain acantholytic cells, and do not exhibit Nikolsky's sign*
cause of dermatitis herpetiformis (DH)	*IC deposition of IgA immune complexes at the tips of the dermal papilla, leading to subepidermal bullae filled with neutrophils*
association of DH	*celiac disease* [It is an autoimmune disease with antibodies against gluten (gliadin fraction).]
cause of erythema multiforme	*immunologic reaction targeting the skin and mucous membranes* (Stevens-Johnson syndrome) *characterized by bull's-eye appearing lesions* [Inciting causes include infections (e.g., *Mycoplasma pneumoniae*), drugs (e.g., penicillin), other autoimmune diseases (e.g., SLE).]
cause of acne vulgaris	*abnormal keratinization of the follicular epithelium* (obstructs the follicle), *increased androgen-induced sebum formation, bacterial lipase* (produced by the gram-positive anaerobe *Propionibacterium acnes*) *production of irritating fatty acids that cause inflammation*

Table continued on following page

Table 19–2. PAPULOSQUAMOUS, VESICULOBULLOUS, AND PUSTULAR SKIN DISORDERS *Continued*

Most Common...	Answer and Explanation
causes of acne vulgaris	**hormones** (e.g., testosterone, progesterone, corticosteroids), *lithium, occupational factors* (e.g., grease) [Dietary factors are noncontributory, including chocolate and nuts.]
cause of acne rosacea	*inflammatory reaction of the pilosebaceous units of the face leading to pustules, rhinophyma* (hyperplasia of sebaceous glands in the nose), and *flushing of the cheeks*

Question: Which of the following skin disorders exhibit hyperkeratosis? **SELECT 3**
(A) Pemphigus vulgaris
(B) Lichen planus
(C) Psoriasis
(D) Acne vulgaris
(E) Actinic keratosis
(F) Impetigo
(G) Varicella
(H) Dermatitis herpetiformis

Answers: (B), (C), (E): Choices A, F, G, and H are vesiculobullous lesions, while acne is a pustular disease.

IC = immunocomplex, Ig = immunoglobulin, SLE = systemic lupus erythematosus, S/S = signs and symptoms, UV = ultraviolet.

Table 19–3. URTICARIA, CELLULITIS, ATROPHY, NODULAR, CYSTIC, AND MELANOCYTIC DISORDERS OF THE SKIN AND PORPHYRIA

Most Common...	Answer and Explanation
cause of urticaria	*type I, IgE-mediated hypersensitivity reaction due to the release of histamine from mast cells in the skin* [They are raised, pruritic lesions. Inciting agents include food, drugs, insect bites, UVB light.]
cause of angioedema	*diffuse swelling of the skin due to edema in the deep subcutaneous tissue* (e.g., C1 esterase inhibitor deficiency; see Chapter 4, ACE inhibitors)

**Table 19–3. URTICARIA, CELLULITIS, ATROPHY,
NODULAR, CYSTIC, AND MELANOCYTIC DISORDERS OF
THE SKIN AND PORPHYRIA** *Continued*

Most Common...	Answer and Explanation
cause of cellulitis	*Streptococcus pyogenes* (group A strepto-cocci) [They produce hyaluronidase, leading to superficial spread of the infection.]
cause of erysipelas	*Streptococcus pyogenes* [Erysipelas is a raised, erythematous, hot cellulitis ("brawny edema") that may involve any part of the body.]
microscopic findings in SLE involving the skin	*epidermal atrophy, vacuolar degeneration of the basal cell layer and hair shafts* (IC directed against the BM; basis of the band test, a direct IF test that detects the ICs at the dermal-epidermal junction), *lymphoid infiltrate in the above areas*
cause of chromoblastomycosis	*traumatic implantation of the pigmented fungus into the subcutaneous tissue* (usually a splinter) *leading to a granulomatous reaction*
cause of sporotrichosis	*traumatic implantation of the fungus* (usually a thorn prick in a rose gardener) *leading to draining lymphocutaneous nodules* [Oral potassium iodide is used for treatment.]
cause of leprosy	*direct contact or droplet infection of Mycobacterium leprae*
findings in tuberculoid leprosy	*intact cellular immunity* (positive lepromin skin test), *no viable organisms in the granulomatous lesions, autoamputation of the digits*
findings in lepromatous leprosy	*lack of cellular immunity* (negative lepromin skin test; no granulomas), *numerous organisms* (uninvolved area beneath the epidermis overlying the macrophages containing the organisms is called the Grenz zone), *classic leonine facies*
treatment for leprosy	*dapsone*
benign skin lesion simulating a well-differentiated squamous cell carcinoma	*keratoacanthoma* [It develops rapidly within a few months and has a crateriform appearance and keratinocytes that appear to be invading the dermis. The lesion normally regresses with scarring.]

Table continued on following page

Table 19–3. URTICARIA, CELLULITIS, ATROPHY, NODULAR, CYSTIC, AND MELANOCYTIC DISORDERS OF THE SKIN AND PORPHYRIA *Continued*

Most Common...	Answer and Explanation
appearance of erythema nodosum	*painful, raised nodule on the anterior aspect of the shins* [It is a localized inflammation of subcutaneous fat. Inciting agents include systemic fungal infections (e.g., coccidioido-mycosis), TB, streptococcal infections, and drugs.]
skin cancers associated with UVB light	**BCC** (also the most common overall skin cancer; invades but does not metastasize), *SCC, malignant melanoma*
appearance of a BCC	*raised, crateriform lesion with red walls* (blood vessels), and *an ulcerated center most commonly located on the face* (e.g., inner aspect of the nose, around the orbit, upper lip)
microscopic appearance of a BCC	*multifocal tumor with cords of basophilic staining cells originating from the basal cell layer infiltrating the dermis where they form nests of neoplastic cells*
causes of SCC of the skin other than UVB light	**immunosuppression** (most common cancer), *chronic draining sinuses, keloids in third-degree burns, arsenic poisoning, radiation therapy*
cause of a cystic mass on the scalp that drains keratin material	*pilar cyst derived from the epidermis of a hair follicle* [Located elsewhere, they are called *epidermal inclusion cysts.*]
cause of vitiligo	*autoimmune destruction of melanocytes leaving areas of depigmentation*
appearance of seborrheic keratosis	*raised, pigmented lesion with a "stuck on" appearance*
cause of a sudden increase in the number of seborrheic keratoses in an adult	*this is called the Leser-Trélat sign and may indicate the presence of an underlying gastric adenocarcinoma*
appearance of acanthosis nigricans	*pigmented, verrucoid-appearing lesion commonly located in the axilla*
systemic associations of acanthosis nigricans	*gastric adenocarcinoma, insulin receptor deficiency leading to DM*

Table 19–3. URTICARIA, CELLULITIS, ATROPHY, NODULAR, CYSTIC, AND MELANOCYTIC DISORDERS OF THE SKIN AND PORPHYRIA Continued

Most Common...	Answer and Explanation
cause of pigmented macular lesions in sun-exposed areas	*freckles* (ephelides) [They are not premalignant.]
benign tumor of melanocytes	*nevocellular nevus* [These tumors are of neural crest origin and are S100-antigen positive.]
order of histologic development of nevocellular nevi	*junctional nevus* (young child; nevus cells located in the basal cell layer; flat lesion) → *compound nevus* (older child; raised pigmented, verrucoid lesion; nevus cells at the junction and within the dermis) → *intradermal nevus* (puberty, adult; pigmented lesion; nevus cells only in the dermis)
nevus with the potential for developing into a malignant melanoma	*dysplastic nevus*
malignant tumor of melanocytes	*malignant melanoma,* which includes **SSC** (lower extremities, back), *nodular melanoma, LMM* (face of elderly patients), *and ALM* (under nails, soles of the feet, palms)
risk factors for malignant melanoma	**severe sunburn at an early age,** *dysplastic nevi, first-degree relative with a melanoma, xeroderma pigmentosum* (AR disease; no DNA repair enzymes), *fair skin*
natural history of an SSC and LMM	*they enter a radial growth phase, where tumor spreads either along the epidermis or within the superficial dermis* [They do not metastasize in this phase. They then enter a *vertical growth phase* and invade into reticular dermis, thereby increasing the risk for metastasis.]
natural history of a nodular and acral lentiginous melanoma	*they lack a radial growth phase and go directly into a vertical phase*

Table continued on following page

Table 19-3. URTICARIA, CELLULITIS, ATROPHY, NODULAR, CYSTIC, AND MELANOCYTIC DISORDERS OF THE SKIN AND PORPHYRIA *Continued*

Most Common...	Answer and Explanation
malignant melanoma in blacks	*acral lentiginous melanoma*
staging systems for malignant melanoma	**Breslow** (direct measurement of level of invasion; invasion <0.76 mm is not associated with metastasis; invasion >1.7 mm has the potential for metastasis; best staging system), *Clark system* (divided into levels I through V)
site of metastasis for malignant melanoma	*regional lymph nodes*
initial treatment of a lesion suspected of being a malignant melanoma	*total excision*
danger signs that a pigmented lesion may be a malignant melanoma	*increase in size, irregular borders, areas of depigmentation or ulceration*
porphyrias in the United States	**PCT** (acquired disease), *AIP* (AD disease; unusual for an enzyme deficiency disorder)
enzyme deficiency in PCT	*uroporphyrinogen decarboxylase* [It catalyzes the conversion of uroporphyrinogen III into coproporphyrinogen III.]
S/S of PCT	*bullous skin lesions on exposure to light* (porphyrins are light sensitive), *hyperpigmentation, hypertrichosis* (vellus type hair), *fragile skin, wine-red color of urine on voiding*
lab findings in PCT	**increased urine uroporphyrin I** (-ogen compounds are colorless and must be oxidized to have color), *normal porphobilinogen levels*
enzyme deficiency in AIP	*uroporphyrinogen synthase* [It catalyzes the reaction that converts porphobilinogen (PBG) into uroporphyrinogen III. Heme has a negative feedback on ALA synthase; therefore, if decreased (drug metabolism), it will precipitate an acute attack by enhancing its activity and causing a build-up of porphyrins prior to the enzyme block.]

Table 19–3. URTICARIA, CELLULITIS, ATROPHY, NODULAR, CYSTIC, AND MELANOCYTIC DISORDERS OF THE SKIN AND PORPHYRIA *Continued*

Most Common...	Answer and Explanation
S/S of AIP	*sudden onset of colicky abdominal pain often misinterpreted as a surgical abdomen, hence the reason for a "bellyful of scars,"* neurologic problems (neuropathies, dementia) *often precipitated by drugs that enhance the liver cytochrome system* (e.g., alcohol, barbiturates), *thereby decreasing heme*
lab findings in AIP	*increased urine PBG* (colorless at first, but later turns color with exposure to light [porphobilin is formed]; "window sill test"), *low enzyme activity can be detected even in asymptomatic periods*
treatment of AIP	*avoid drugs that enhance the cytochrome system and heme infusions, which will inhibit ALA synthase*

Question: In a 56-year-old black man with metastatic malignant melanoma to the lungs and brain, the most likely primary site would be which of the following?
(A) GI tract
(B) Back
(C) Lungs
(D) Brain
(E) Hands/feet

Answer: (E): Black patients with malignant melanoma most likely have acral lentiginous melanoma, in which the lesions are located under the nails or on the palms or soles of the feet.

ACE = angiotensin converting enzyme, AD = autosomal dominant, AIP = acute intermittent porphyria, ALA = aminolevulinic acid, ALM = acral lentiginous melanoma, AR = autosomal recessive, BCC = basal cell carcinoma, BM = basement membrane, DM = diabetes mellitus, GI = gastrointestinal, IC = immunocomplex, IF = immunofluorescent, Ig = immunoglobulin, LMM = lentigo maligna melanoma, PCT = porphyria cutanea tarda, SCC = squamous cell carcinoma, SLE = systemic lupus erythematosus, S/S = signs and symptoms, SSC = superficial spreading malignant melanoma, TB = tuberculosis, UV = ultraviolet.

CHAPTER
20

CENTRAL AND PERIPHERAL NERVOUS SYSTEM PATHOLOGY AND SPECIAL SENSES

CONTENTS

Table 20–1. CEREBRAL SPINAL FLUID ANALYSIS, OVERVIEW OF SIGNS/SYMPTOMS, HYDROCEPHALUS, CEREBRAL EDEMA, CONGENITAL DISORDERS

Most Common...	Answer and Explanation
cause of a bloody CSF tap	*iatrogenic* [Absence of a pink supranate after centrifugation of the tubes and a drop in the RBC count in successive tubes indicates a nonpathologic cause of blood in the CSF.]
cause of a yellow CSF	*xanthochromia which is the bilirubin breakdown product of blood from a pathologic bleed in the CNS* [It may also indicate a high CSF protein.]
causes of an increased CSF protein	**CNS inflammation** (increased vessel permeability) or *synthesis of IgG by plasma cells in the CNS* (e.g., demyelinating disease like MS)
causes of a low CSF glucose	*called hypoglycorrhachia, a low CSF glucose* (<40 mg/dL) *is due to **bacterial meningitis,** fungal meningitis, or metastatic disease to the meninges*

Table continued on following page

**Table 20–1. CEREBRAL SPINAL FLUID ANALYSIS,
OVERVIEW OF SIGNS/SYMPTOMS, HYDROCEPHALUS,
CEREBRAL EDEMA, CONGENITAL DISORDERS** *Continued*

Most Common...	Answer and Explanation
WBC response in the CSF to a viral versus a bacterial meningitis	*viral:* initially a neutrophilic response, which switches to a lymphocyte response in 24–48 hours *bacterial:* neutrophilic response; TB has a mononuclear response
lab test on CSF to detect bacterial/ fungal pathogens	*Gram stain of a cytocentrifuged specimen* [Latex agglutination and CIE are also used if Gram stains are negative. An India ink prep is a good initial screen for *Cryptococcus.*]
differences between serum and CSF	*protein:* CSF <serum; *glucose:* CSF 60% of serum level; *chloride:* CSF >serum; *cell count:* CSF only 0–5 cells/μL (no neutrophils)
S/S of CNS disease	*focal neurologic abnormalities, headache, mental status alterations, dizziness*
pathologic processes targeting neurons	*central chromatolysis* (secondary to axonal injury; central loss of Nissl bodies), *red neurons* (apoptosis of neurons in hypoxia/ischemia), *neurofibrillary tangle* (paired neurofilaments), *senile plaque* (presynaptic axon terminals surrounding core of β-amyloid), *inclusions* (e.g., Negri bodies [rabies], Lewy bodies [Parkinson's disease])
functions of astrocytes	*repair* (called gliosis; does not involve collagen), *maintain the blood-brain barrier*
pathologic processes involving astrocytes	*neoplastic transformation* (astrocytoma), *gliosis* (CNS repair), *gemistocytes* (reactive astrocytes), *polyglucosan bodies* (product of old age)
functions of oligodendrocytes	*synthesize myelin in the CNS* (Schwann cells are responsible in PNS)
pathologic processes involving oligodendrocytes	*neoplastic transformation* (oligodendroglioma), *infected by viruses* (e.g., rubeola, papovavirus), *demyelination* (viral infections)
functions of microglial cells	*phagocytic function* (derive from monocytes)

Table 20–1. CEREBRAL SPINAL FLUID ANALYSIS, OVERVIEW OF SIGNS/SYMPTOMS, HYDROCEPHALUS, CEREBRAL EDEMA, CONGENITAL DISORDERS *Continued*

Most Common...	Answer and Explanation
pathologic processes involving microglial cells	*reservoir cell for HIV, gitter cells* (activated cell seen after an infarction), *rod cells* (cell associated with syphilis)
function of ependymal cells	*line the ventricles*
pathologic processes involving ependymal cells	*neoplastic transformation* (ependymomas)
causes of hydrocephalus [enlarged ventricles]	**obstruction of CSF from ventricles into sub-arachnoid space** (noncommunicating hydrocephalus; stenosis of the aqueduct of Sylvius), *increased production of CSF* (e.g., choroid plexus papilloma), *reduced resorption of CSF by the arachnoid granulations* (communicating hydrocephalus; scarring post-meningitis)
cause of hydrocephalus in newborns	*stenosis of the aqueduct of Sylvius*
types of cerebral edema	*cytotoxic* (e.g., intracellular swelling in hyponatremia), *vasogenic* (e.g., increased vessel permeability in inflammatory processes)
S/S of increased intracranial pressure	**morning headache,** *papilledema, projectile vomiting, bradycardia, hypertension, brain herniations, noncardiogenic pulmonary edema*
signs of a cingulate gyrus herniation beneath the falx cerebri	*compression of the ACA leading to contralateral motor and sensory loss in the leg*
gross findings in uncal herniation through the tentorium cerebelli	*compression of the midbrain* (Duret's hemorrhages), *oculomotor nerve compression* (ipsilateral ophthalmoplegia [eye deviated down and out], ptosis, mydriasis), *abducens nerve compression* (lateral gaze paralysis), *compression of the PCA* (occipital lobe infarction)

Table continued on following page

Table 20–1. CEREBRAL SPINAL FLUID ANALYSIS, OVERVIEW OF SIGNS/SYMPTOMS, HYDROCEPHALUS, CEREBRAL EDEMA, CONGENITAL DISORDERS *Continued*

Most Common...	Answer and Explanation
gross findings of cerebellar tonsil herniation into the foramen magnum	*grooving of the cerebellar tonsils and compression of the medulla oblongata*
open neural tube defect	*spina bifida occulta* [There is a dimple or tuck of hair overlying L5-S1 due to failure of closure of the vertebral arch.]
gross findings in anencephaly	*defect in closure of the upper part of the neural tube with complete absence of the brain, a frog-like facial appearance, absent fetal adrenal cortex*
gross findings in a meningocele	*open neural tube defect with a midline cystic mass containing dura and arachnoid*
gross findings in a meningomyelocele	*open neural tube defect with a midline cystic mass containing dura, arachnoid, and spinal cord*
lab finding in open neural tube defects	*increased AFP in maternal serum or AF*
gross finding in syringomyelia	*fluid-filled cavity (syrinx) in the central portion of the cervical spinal cord* (see cord enlargement on an MR image)
S/S of syringomyelia	*Horner's syndrome* (meiosis, lid lag, anhidrosis), *destruction of the crossed lateral spinothalamic tracts* (loss of pain and temperature sensation in a cape-like distribution), *atrophy of the intrinsic muscles of the hand* (anterior horn destruction)
gross findings in the Arnold-Chiari syndrome	*elongation of medulla oblongata and cerebellar tonsils through the foramen magnum, platybasia* (flat base of skull), *meningomyelocele, hydrocephalus* (~50%), *syringomyelia*
gross findings in Dandy-Walker syndrome	*hypoplasia of the cerebellar vermis, cystic dilatation of the fourth ventricle, hydrocephalus*
phakomatoses [ectodermal and CNS abnormalities] in the CNS	**neurofibromatosis,** *Sturge-Weber syndrome, tuberous sclerosis*

Table 20–1. CEREBRAL SPINAL FLUID ANALYSIS, OVERVIEW OF SIGNS/SYMPTOMS, HYDROCEPHALUS, CEREBRAL EDEMA, CONGENITAL DISORDERS *Continued*

Most Common...	Answer and Explanation
S/S of neurofibromatosis	*AD disease with café-au-lait spots, axillary freckling, pigmented neurofibromas, brain tumors* (e.g., meningiomas, acoustic neuromas, optic gliomas), *pheochromocytoma* (hypertension)
S/S of Sturge-Weber syndrome	*port-wine stain in the trigeminal nerve distribution, ipsilateral AV malformations, pheochromocytoma*
S/S of tuberous sclerosis	*AD disease with mental retardation, hamartomas* (astrocytic proliferations in the subependymoma that look like candle drippings on the ventricle walls, angiomyolipomas of the kidneys), *adenoma sebaceum of skin, rhabdomyoma of heart*

Question: A normal intracranial pressure would be expected in a patient with which of the following?
(A) Lead encephalopathy
(B) Frontal lobe tumor
(C) CNS infarction
(D) Malignant hypertension
(E) Cerebral atrophy

Answer: (E): In cerebral atrophy, there is a loss of brain mass leading to enlarged ventricles without an increase in CSF fluid or pressure. All the other choices are associated with an increased intracranial pressure.

ACA = anterior cerebral artery, AD = autosomal dominant, AF = amniotic fluid, AFP = alpha-fetoprotein, AV = arteriovenous, CIE = counterimmunoelectrophoresis, CNS = central nervous system, CSF = cerebral spinal fluid, HIV = human immunodeficiency virus, Ig = immunoglobulin, MR = magnetic resonance, MS = multiple sclerosis, PCA = posterior cerebral artery, PNS = peripheral nervous system, RBC = red blood cell, S/S = signs and symptoms, TB = tuberculosis, WBC = white blood cell.

Table 20–2. CENTRAL NERVOUS SYSTEM INFECTIONS

Most Common...	Answer and Explanation
methods of transmission of CNS infection	**hematogenous,** *traumatic, ascending* (e.g., rabies), local extension (e.g., mastoiditis, sinusitis)

Table continued on following page

Table 20–2. CENTRAL NERVOUS SYSTEM INFECTIONS
Continued

Most Common...	Answer and Explanation
types of CNS infection	**leptomeningitis** (inflammation of the meninges), *encephalitis* (inflammation of the brain), *cerebral abscess*
S/S of leptomeningitis	*fever, headache, nuchal rigidity, altered sensorium*
CSF differences between viral and bacterial meningitis	*viral:* normal glucose, lymphocyte dominant smear *bacterial:* low glucose, neutrophil-dominant smear, positive Gram stain
cause of viral meningitis	*coxsackievirus*
viral cause of hemorrhagic necrosis of the temporal lobes	*HSV-1*
causes of bacterial meningitis in newborns	***group B Streptococcus*** *(S. agalactiae), Escherichia coli, Listeria monocytogenes*
cause of bacterial meningitis in children between 1 month and 18 years of age	*Neisseria meningitidis* [In children between 3 months and 6 years of age, it used to be *Haemophilus influenzae*, but immunization has dramatically reduced its incidence.]
cause of bacterial meningitis in adults	*Streptococcus pneumoniae*
complications of meningitis	**temporary paralysis,** *permanent deafness, mental retardation, hydrocephalus, epilepsy*
complications associated with TB meningitis	*a complication of primary TB in children, it involves the base of the brain and produces vasculitis* (stroke potential) *and scarring* (hydrocephalus potential)

Table 20–2. CENTRAL NERVOUS SYSTEM INFECTIONS
Continued

Most Common...	Answer and Explanation
CSF findings in TB meningitis	*high protein* (forms a pellicle), *low glucose, <500 cells/μL* (lymphocytes/monocytes), *low chloride*
types of neurosyphilis	**meningovascular** (vasculitis/meningitis; may present with strokes), *paretic form* (generalized atrophy; numerous organisms), *tabes dorsalis* (attacks posterior root ganglia and cord; wide-based gait, absent DTRs, Argyll-Robertson pupil, loss of proprioception)
systemic fungal cause of meningitis	*Cryptococcus neoformans,* particularly in immunocompromised hosts
S/S of encephalitis	**mental status alterations,** *drowsiness, headache*
cause of rabies in the United States	**skunk bite** [*Other bites:* raccoon (Northeast), bats, fox, coyotes, dogs (rare)]
S/S of rabies	*paresthesias around the wound site, excitability* (pain, convulsions, frothing of the mouth, hydrophobia) *followed by flaccid paralysis and death*
microscopic finding in rabies	*intracytoplasmic Negri bodies in neurons* (particularly Purkinje cells)
CNS viral infection in AIDS	*CMV*
encephalitis in newborns	*CMV* with periventricular calcifications
S/S of polio	*flaccid paralysis* (paraplegia, quadriplegia) *due to viral destruction of the anterior horn cells in the spinal cord*
vector of encephalitis due to arboviruses	*mosquito* [St. Louis encephalitis is the most common arbovirus infection.]
cause of a space-occupying lesion in the CNS in AIDs	*Toxoplasma gondii,* a sporozoan [It produces multiple, ring-enhanced lesions in the brain.]

Table continued on following page

Table 20–2. CENTRAL NERVOUS SYSTEM INFECTIONS
Continued

Most Common...	Answer and Explanation
cause of a frontal lobe abscess in DKA	*Mucor* [It invades the brain through the cribriform plate.]
type of malaria involving the CNS	*Plasmodium falciparum*
protozoan producing meningoencephalitis after swimming in fresh water	*Naegleria fowleri*
tapeworm infection involving the CNS	*cysticercosis due to Taenia solium* [Eggs ingested by humans from an infected human host become larvae, which invade the CNS, eyes, skin, and other sites.]
cause of a solitary cerebral abscess	*extension of infection from an adjacent focus of infection* (e.g., sinusitis, mastoiditis)
cause of multiple cerebral abscesses	*hematogenous spread* (e.g., cyanotic CHD, bronchiectasis)
gross appearance of a cerebral abscess	*cystic cavity with a shaggy lining*
sign of a cerebral abscess	*hemiplegia*
CSF findings in a cerebral abscess	*normal glucose, increased protein, increased leukocytes*

Question: Which of the following CSF findings is common to both bacterial and viral meningitis?
(A) High protein
(B) Lymphocytes
(C) Low glucose
(D) Positive Gram stain
(E) Positive latex agglutination

Answer: (A): Both types have a high CSF protein owing to increased vessel permeability. Choices C, D, and E are present in bacterial meningitis, and choice B in viral meningitis.

AIDS = acquired immunodeficiency syndrome, CHD = congenital heart disease, CMV = cytomegalovirus, CNS = central nervous system, CSF = cerebral spinal fluid, DKA = diabetic ketoacidosis, DTR = deep tendon reflex, HSV = herpes simplex virus, S/S = signs and symptoms, TB = tuberculosis.

Table 20–3. CENTRAL NERVOUS SYSTEM TRAUMA, STROKES, DEMYELINATING DISORDERS, DEGENERATIVE DISORDERS

Most Common...	Answer and Explanation
sign following a concussion	*transient loss of consciousness*
cause of a cerebral contusion [superficial damage to the brain]	*acceleration-deceleration injuries*
cause of a coup and contrecoup injury	*acceleration-deceleration injury causing a contusion at the site of impact* (coup injury) *and at a distant site from the point of injury* (contrecoup injury)
sites for contrecoup injuries	*tips of the frontal and temporal lobes*
fractures producing rhinorrhea [CSF coming out of the nose]	*orbital blow-out and basilar skull fractures*
types of traumatic CNS bleeds	*epidural and subdural hematoma*
cause of an epidural hematoma	*fracture of the temporoparietal bone with severance of the middle meningeal artery leading to separation of the dura from the periosteum by blood under arterial pressures*
S/S of an epidural hematoma	*immediate loss of consciousness followed by a lucid interval and then death by herniation in 5–6 hours*
cause of a subdural hematoma	*blunt trauma to the skull causing a tearing of the bridging veins between the dura and arachnoid membranes leading to a venous clot over one or both convexities of the brain*
S/S of a subdural hematoma	*fluctuating levels of consciousness*
imaging technique used to initially identify epidural and subdural hematomas	*CT scan*

Table continued on following page

**Table 20–3. CENTRAL NERVOUS SYSTEM TRAUMA,
STROKES, DEMYELINATING DISORDERS,
DEGENERATIVE DISORDERS** *Continued*

Most Common...	Answer and Explanation
CNS cells susceptible to tissue hypoxia	**neurons** (**hippocampus,** Purkinje in cerebellum, cerebral cortex), *oligodendrocytes, astrocytes*
CNS complications related to ischemia	*watershed infarcts between two overlapping arterial supplies, laminar necrosis of the cerebral cortex* (neuronal apoptosis in layers 3, 5, 6; leads to cerebral atrophy), *stroke*
types of strokes in descending order of frequency	**atherosclerotic,** *embolic, intracerebral, subarachnoid*
cause of an atherosclerotic stroke	*thrombosis overlying an atherosclerotic plaque in the proximal portion of the internal carotid artery near the bifurcation*
type of necrosis in an atherosclerotic stroke	*pale infarction due to liquefactive necrosis*
G/M findings of an atherosclerotic stroke	*gross:* cerebral edema, softening of the brain, eventual cystic space after 10 days *micro:* liquefactive necrosis, neutrophil invasion with replacement by activated microglial cells (gitter cells), reactive astrocytes (gemistocytes) at the margins of the infarct
S/S of an atherosclerotic stroke	*usually preceded by TIAs* (CH emboli from the carotid plaque) *in the same distribution as the stroke* *MCA stroke:* expressive aphasia (dominant hemisphere), contralateral hemiparesis and sensory changes in upper extremities *vertebrobasilar stroke:* vertigo, ataxia, ipsilateral sensory changes on the face, contralateral motor and sensory changes in the trunk and limbs
imaging technique used in confirming a stroke	*CT scan in the first 48 hours*
cause of an embolic stroke	*thromboemboli originating from the left heart leading to a hemorrhagic infarction, usually in the distribution of the MCA*

Table 20–3. CENTRAL NERVOUS SYSTEM TRAUMA, STROKES, DEMYELINATING DISORDERS, DEGENERATIVE DISORDERS *Continued*

Most Common...	Answer and Explanation
gross findings of an embolic stroke	*hemorrhage extending to the surface of the brain owing to the weak vessels in the gray matter that rupture when reperfusion occurs after the embolus is dissolved*
cause of an intracerebral bleed	*hypertension,* which produces *Charcot-Bouchard microaneurysms of the lenticulo-striate vessels* (branches of the MCA) that *rupture, producing a hematoma* (not an infarct)
sites of an intracerebral bleed	**putamen,** *thalamus, pons, cerebellum*
S/S of malignant hypertension in the CNS	*headache, grade IV hypertensive retinopathy* (papilledema, hard and soft exudates, hemorrhage)
cause of a subarachnoid hemorrhage	*ruptured congenital berry aneurysm located at the junction of the anterior communicating artery with the ACA*
S/S of a subarachnoid hemorrhage	**sudden onset of a very severe occipital headache,** *loss of consciousness, neurologic deficits*
risk factors for a subarachnoid hemorrhage	*hypertension, adult polycystic kidney disease, adult coarctation of the aorta,* all of which increase the risk for developing berry aneurysms
cause of lacunar infarcts in the CNS	**hypertension,** *DM* [Lacunar infarcts are usually secondary to hyaline arteriolosclerosis and fibrinoid necrosis of the vessels in the area of the basal ganglia, internal capsule, pons, and thalamus.]
S/S of lacunar infarcts	*pure motor or pure sensory strokes*
causes of demyelination	*destruction of oligodendrocytes* (Schwann cells in the PNS) or *autoimmune destruction of the myelin sheath*

Table continued on following page

**Table 20–3. CENTRAL NERVOUS SYSTEM TRAUMA,
STROKES, DEMYELINATING DISORDERS,
DEGENERATIVE DISORDERS** *Continued*

Most Common...	Answer and Explanation
demyelinating disease in the CNS	*MS* [It is an autoimmune disease that attacks the myelin sheath. Patients have an HLA Dr2 haplotype.]
viral etiology implicated in causing MS	*herpesvirus 6*
G/M findings in MS	*gross:* salmon-colored demyelinating plaques in the white matter with a predilection for the angles of the ventricles, optic nerves, cerebellar peduncles, and brain stem *micro:* loss of myelin, reactive gliosis, perivenular T cell lymphocyte/plasma cell infiltrate
S/S of MS	**paresthesias** [Other S/S include *scanning speech* (drunk sounding), *intention tremor, nystagmus, optic neuritis* (sudden loss of vision, retrobulbar pain), *ataxia, preservation of intellect, internuclear ophthalmoplegia* (demyelination of the medial longitudinal fasciculus), *muscle weakness.*]
CSF findings in MS	*increased protein, oligoclonal bands in the γ-globulin region* (monoclonal bands characteristic of demyelination), *increased lymphocytes* (T cells), *normal glucose, increased myelin basic protein* (encephalitogenic protein)
treatment for MS	*ACTH injections, interferon-β, methylprednisolone*
cause of adrenoleukodystrophy	*SXR disease with a deficiency of an enzyme that leads to inability to transport long chain fatty acids into peroxisomes for degradation* [This results in an abnormal myelin deposit in the posterior brain and adrenal insufficiency.]
cause of metachromatic leukodystrophy	*AR disease with a deficiency of arylsulfatase A, leading to an accumulation of sulfatides that produce an abnormal myelin*

Table 20–3. CENTRAL NERVOUS SYSTEM TRAUMA, STROKES, DEMYELINATING DISORDERS, DEGENERATIVE DISORDERS *Continued*

Most Common...	Answer and Explanation
cause of Krabbe's disease	*AR disease with a deficiency of galactocere-broside β-galactocerebrosidase and accumulation of galactocerebroside* [The galactocerebroside produces an abnormal myelin and is phagocytosed by histiocytes producing multinucleated cells called globoid cells.]
causes of dementia [loss of higher intellectual function]	*Alzheimer's disease* [Other causes: multi-infarct dementia, B_{12} deficiency, acute intermittent porphyria, primary hypothyroidism]
causes of Alzheimer's disease	*genetic* (chromosome 21 production of β-amyloid [toxic to neurons; in senile plaques]; chromosome 19 apolipoprotein gene E, allele ε4, which produces a protein with high affinity for β-amyloid; chromosome 14, which produces Tau-microtubule–associated proteins in neurofibrillary tangles), *low acetylcholine levels, aluminum toxicity*
G/M findings in Alzheimer's disease	*gross:* cerebral atrophy (neuronal degeneration) involving the **temporal,** frontal, and parietal lobes *micro:* **senile plaques** (most important marker), neurofibrillary granules, granulovacuolar degeneration
S/S of Alzheimer's disease	**loss of recent memory,** *depression, psychosis, agitation*
COD in adults with Down syndrome	*Alzheimer's disease*
cause of Parkinson's disease	*degeneration and depigmentation of the neurons in the substantia nigra and locus ceruleus leading to a deficiency of dopamine* [Dopamine is the principal neurotransmitter of the afferents in the nigrostriatal tract involved in voluntary muscle movement.]
G/M findings in Parkinson's disease	*gross:* depigmentation of the substantia nigra and locus ceruleus in the midbrain *micro:* as above plus the presence of Lewy bodies in the neurons

Table continued on following page

Table 20–3. CENTRAL NERVOUS SYSTEM TRAUMA, STROKES, DEMYELINATING DISORDERS, DEGENERATIVE DISORDERS *Continued*

Most Common...	Answer and Explanation
S/S of Parkinson's disease	**rigidity of muscles leading to cogwheel rigidity in arm movements, bradykinesia** (slow voluntary movement misinterpreted as muscle weakness), *resting tremor, stooped posture, festinating gait* (shuffling gait), *expressionless face*
acquired causes of Parkinson's disease	**drugs** (e.g., phenothiazines, MPTP) [Other causes: *CO poisoning* (destruction of the globus pallidus), *Wilson's disease*]
cause of HD	*AD disease with triplet repeats of CAG on chromosome 4, low GABA, and low ACh* [Grossly, the tail of the caudate nucleus is absent.]
S/S of HD	*late onset of chorea, extrapyramidal signs, and dementia*
S/S of Friedreich's ataxia	*an AR disease, it is associated with neurologic findings secondary to degeneration of the spinocerebellar tracts, posterior columns, and lateral corticospinal tracts* [Other findings: retinitis pigmentosum, cardiac disease, DM]
cause of ALS	*defect in the zinc/copper binding superoxide dismutase leading to FR damage to upper and lower motor neurons*
S/S of ALS	*LMN signs involving the intrinsic muscles of the hands and forearms and spastic changes* (UMN signs) *in the lower extremities*
childhood equivalent of ALS	*Werdnig-Hoffmann disease*
S/S of Wilson's disease	*an AR disease involving a defect in secretion of copper in bile, it is associated with chronic liver disease and deposition of free copper in the eye* (Kayser-Fleischer ring) *and lenticular nuclei resulting in extrapyramidal signs and dementia*

Table 20–3. CENTRAL NERVOUS SYSTEM TRAUMA, STROKES, DEMYELINATING DISORDERS, DEGENERATIVE DISORDERS *Continued*

Most Common...	Answer and Explanation
CNS findings in alcoholics	**Wernicke-Korsakoff syndrome** (thiamine deficiency), *cerebral and cerebellar atrophy*
G/M findings in Wernicke-Korsakoff syndrome	*gross:* hemorrhage into the mamillary bodies and periventricular tissue *micro:* neuronal loss, gliosis, ring hemorrhages in vessels
S/S of Wernicke-Korsakoff syndrome	*Wernicke:* confusion, ataxia, nystagmus, cranial nerve palsies *Korsakoff:* retrograde and antegrade amnesia, confabulation
CNS lesion in CO poisoning	necrosis of the globus pallidus

Question: Which of the following represent lesions that are primarily due to atherosclerosis? **SELECT 2**
- (A) Laminar necrosis
- (B) Hemorrhagic infarction
- (C) Intracerebral hematoma
- (D) Subarachnoid hemorrhage
- (E) Lacunar infarcts
- (F) Watershed infarcts
- (G) Internuclear ophthalmoplegia
- (H) Duret's hemorrhages
- (I) Senile plaques

Answers: (A), (F): Hemorrhagic infarctions are more common in embolic than atherosclerotic strokes. Choices C and E are due to hypertension. Choice G is specific for MS. Choice H is a lesion associated with uncal herniation. Choice I is associated with Alzheimer's disease.

ACA = anterior cerebral artery, ACh = acetylcholine, ACTH = adrenocorticotropic hormone, AD = autosomal dominant, ALS = amyotrophic lateral sclerosis, AR = autosomal recessive, CH = cholesterol, CNS = central nervous system, COD = cause of death, CSF = cerebral spinal fluid, CT = computed tomography, DM = diabetes mellitus, FR = free radical, GABA = γ-aminobutyric acid, G/M = gross and microscopic, HD = Huntington's disease, HLA = human leukocyte antigen, LMN = lower motor neuron, MCA = middle cerebral artery, MPTP = 1-methyl-4-phenyl-1,2,3,6-tetrahydropyridine (meperidine analogue), MS = multiple sclerosis, PNS = peripheral nervous system, S/S = signs and symptoms, SXR = sex-linked recessive, TIA = transient ischemic attack, UMN = upper motor neuron.

Table 20–4. CENTRAL NERVOUS SYSTEM TUMORS, CENTRAL AND PERIPHERAL NERVOUS SYSTEM DISORDERS IN ACQUIRED IMMUNODEFICIENCY SYNDROME, PERIPHERAL NERVOUS SYSTEM DISORDERS, EYE AND EAR DISORDERS

Most Common...	Answer and Explanation
primary brain tumors in children in descending order of frequency	**cerebellar astrocytoma,** *medulloblastoma, brain stem glioma, ependymoma of the fourth ventricle* [~70% are infratentorial.]
primary brain tumors in adults in descending order of frequency	**GBM,** *meningioma, acoustic neuroma* [~70% are supratentorial.]
risk factors for primary brain tumors	**AIDS,** *Turcot's syndrome* (AR polyposis syndrome), *neurofibromatosis*
site for a GBM	*frontal lobes in an adult*
G/M of a GBM	*gross:* it is a high-grade astrocytoma producing hemorrhagic necrosis in the frontal lobe and a tendency for crossing over the corpus callosum into the other hemisphere *micro:* hemorrhagic necrosis, proliferation of vascular channels
site of an oligodendroglioma	*frontal lobes in an adult* [It commonly calcifies.]
site of an ependymoma in children versus adults	*children:* fourth ventricle *adult:* filum terminale (myxopapillary appearance) [It is also the most common intraspinal tumor.]
location of a medulloblastoma	*a primitive, highly malignant neuroectodermal tumor, it locates in the midline of the cerebellar vermis*
primary CNS tumors that seed the neuraxis	*GBM and medulloblastoma*
syndrome associated with cerebellar hemangioblastomas	*von Hippel-Lindau disease* [It also has a high incidence of renal adenocarcinoma.]
benign CNS tumor in adults	*meningioma* [It arises from arachnoid granulations and is more common in women than men.]

**Table 20–4. CENTRAL NERVOUS SYSTEM TUMORS,
CENTRAL AND PERIPHERAL NERVOUS SYSTEM
DISORDERS IN ACQUIRED IMMUNODEFICIENCY
SYNDROME, PERIPHERAL NERVOUS SYSTEM
DISORDERS, EYE AND EAR DISORDERS** *Continued*

Most Common...	Answer and Explanation
risk factors for developing a meningioma	**neurofibromatosis,** *previous CNS radiation*
location for meningiomas	*parasagittal*
G/M of a meningioma	*gross:* popcorn-shaped lesion that often indents but does not invade the brain; it may infiltrate into the overlying skull (not a sign of malignancy) *micro:* swirling meningothelial cells surrounding psammoma bodies
S/S of a meningioma	*most common cause of new onset focal epileptic seizures in adults*
tumor derived from the notochord	*chordoma* [It is a malignant, midline, lobulated tumor most commonly occurring in the sacrococcygeal area. It contains cells that have droplets of mucus (called physaliferous cells).]
cause for the recent increase in primary CNS lymphomas	*AIDS* (both the HIV and EBV viruses are linked to these tumors) [Primary lymphomas in the CNS are multifocal, while metastatic lymphomas to the CNS (most common overall lymphoma) target the meninges.]
tumor associated with tinnitus and nerve deafness	*acoustic neuroma* [It is a benign tumor derived from Schwann cells that involves the eighth nerve. They arise in the cerebellopontine angle and may impinge on the fifth nerve, producing sensory changes on the face.]
microscopic findings in an acoustic neuroma (schwannoma, neurilemmoma)	*alternating dark areas* (Antoni A) *and light areas* (Antoni B), resembling zebra stripes [They are always benign.]

Table continued on following page

Table 20–4. CENTRAL NERVOUS SYSTEM TUMORS,
CENTRAL AND PERIPHERAL NERVOUS SYSTEM
DISORDERS IN ACQUIRED IMMUNODEFICIENCY
SYNDROME, PERIPHERAL NERVOUS SYSTEM
DISORDERS, EYE AND EAR DISORDERS *Continued*

Most Common...	Answer and Explanation
tumor associated with paralysis of upward gaze (Parinaud's syndrome)	*pinealoma* [It is a malignant, midline, germ cell tumor arising in the pineal gland.]
cancer in the CNS	*metastatic cancer* [It most commonly occurs from a primary site in the lungs.]
CNS manifestations of AIDS	**AIDS dementia complex** [It involves all cell lines and has characteristic multinucleated microglial cells, which are the reservoir of HIV in the CNS. *Others:* aseptic meningitis, vacuolar myelopathy resembling subacute combined degeneration in B_{12} deficiency, peripheral neuropathy resembling Guillain-Barré syndrome]
causes of CNS calcifications	**calcified pineal gland in old age** [Other causes: *congenital CMV, toxoplasmosis, and HSV; AV malformation; oligodendroglioma, meningioma, craniopharyngioma; tuberous sclerosis; primary hypoparathyroidism* (basal ganglia); *cysticercosis*]
causes of distal sensorimotor peripheral neuropathy	**DM** [*Other causes:* alcohol, lead poisoning, vincristine, isoniazid, thiamine deficiency]
cause of acute peripheral neuropathy	*Guillain-Barré syndrome* [It is an autoimmune demyelinating disease destroying the myelin sheath of spinal and cranial nerves.]
CSF findings in Guillain-Barré syndrome	*increased protein, lymphocytes, normal glucose*
causes of Bell's facial palsy	**HSV-1** [*Others:* Lyme disease]
S/S of Bell's palsy	*facial muscle weakness, ptosis of the eyelid, drooling, hyperacusis*

Table 20–4. CENTRAL NERVOUS SYSTEM TUMORS,
CENTRAL AND PERIPHERAL NERVOUS SYSTEM
DISORDERS IN ACQUIRED IMMUNODEFICIENCY
SYNDROME, PERIPHERAL NERVOUS SYSTEM
DISORDERS, EYE AND EAR DISORDERS *Continued*

Most Common...	Answer and Explanation
genetic cause of peripheral neuropathy	*Charcot-Marie-Tooth disease* [It is an AD disease that involves the peroneal nerve and produces atrophy of the muscles of the lower legs ("inverted bottle" appearance).]
cause of xanthelasmas	*CH deposition in the eyelid* [It may or may not indicate an underlying hypercholesterolemia.]
cause of a stye on the eyelid	*Staphylococcus aureus*
granulomatous infection involving the eyelid	*chalazion* [It involves the meibomian gland.]
causes of acute bacterial conjunctivitis	*S. aureus, group A Streptococcus, Streptococcus pneumoniae, Haemophilus influenzae (pink eye)*
causes of viral conjunctivitis	**adenovirus,** *HSV-1* (keratoconjunctivitis with dendritic ulcers noted with fluorescein staining)
cause of preauricular lymphadenopathy	*viral conjunctivitis*
cause of conjunctivitis in newborns within 24–48 hours	*chemical conjunctivitis from erythromycin* (protects against *Neisseria gonorrhoeae* and *Chlamydia trachomatis*) or *silver nitrate* (protects against *N. gonorrhoeae*) drops
cause of bilateral conjunctivitis in newborns within 3–5 days	*N. gonorrhoeae*
cause of bilateral conjunctivitis in newborns after 7 days	*C. trachomatis*

Table continued on following page

Table 20–4. CENTRAL NERVOUS SYSTEM TUMORS, CENTRAL AND PERIPHERAL NERVOUS SYSTEM DISORDERS IN ACQUIRED IMMUNODEFICIENCY SYNDROME, PERIPHERAL NERVOUS SYSTEM DISORDERS, EYE AND EAR DISORDERS *Continued*

Most Common...	Answer and Explanation
cause of severe keratoconjunctivitis in patients who do not clean their contact lenses properly	*Acanthamoeba*
disease associated with autoimmune destruction of the lacrimal glands	*Sjögren's syndrome*
seasonal cause of pruritic conjunctivitis	*allergic conjunctivitis*
cause of arcus senilis	*CH deposition in the outer margin of the cornea, which may or may not be associated with a hyperlipidemia*
cause of cataracts	*old age* (age-dependent disorder)
cause of glaucoma	*defect in the canal of Schlemm that impedes the drainage of aqueous humor*
S/S of glaucoma	**increased intraocular pressure,** *pain, blurry vision, steamy cornea, pupil fixed in mid-dilated position, pupil nonreactive to light*
causes of sudden loss of vision in one eye	**optic neuritis** (common in MS), *central retinal artery or retinal vein occlusion, amaurosis fugax* (cholesterol embolus in the retinal vessel; "curtain down, curtain up")
cause of papilledema	*increased intracranial pressure*
metabolic cause of optic neuritis	*methyl alcohol poisoning* [The alcohol is converted into formic acid.]
causes of optic atrophy [absence of disk vessels; cupping of the disk margin]	**optic neuritis,** *glaucoma, methyl alcohol poisoning*

Table 20–4. CENTRAL NERVOUS SYSTEM TUMORS, CENTRAL AND PERIPHERAL NERVOUS SYSTEM DISORDERS IN ACQUIRED IMMUNODEFICIENCY SYNDROME, PERIPHERAL NERVOUS SYSTEM DISORDERS, EYE AND EAR DISORDERS Continued

Most Common...	Answer and Explanation
causes of uveitis [inflammation of uveal tract: iris, ciliary body, choroid]	*sarcoidosis, ankylosing spondylitis, juvenile rheumatoid arthritis*
S/S of uveitis	*pain, blurry vision, photophobia, meiotic pupil, poor light reflex, ciliary body vascular congestion, normal intraocular pressure*
primary tumor of the eye in children and adults	*retinoblastoma, melanoma* (arises from the choroid), respectively
cause of blindness in AIDS	*CMV retinitis* (cotton wool exudates), a very late manifestation of the disease
causes of external otitis ("swimmer's ear")	*Pseudomonas aeruginosa, S. aureus, Aspergillus species*
cause of malignant external otitis	*P. aeruginosa* in elderly diabetics
causes of otitis media in children	***S. pneumoniae,** H. influenzae, Moraxella catarrhalis*
complication of otitis media	*conduction hearing loss*
cause of conduction hearing loss in the elderly	*otosclerosis* (fusion of the middle ear bones) [It is an age-dependent finding.]
cause of sensorineural loss in the elderly	*presbycusis*
sign of a conduction hearing loss	*Weber test* (tuning fork placed on the midforehead) *lateralizes to the abnormal ear and the Rinne test* (tuning fork placed on the mastoid bone) *reveals that bone conduction is greater than air conduction* (usually air conduction is longer than bone conduction)

Table continued on following page

Table 20–4. CENTRAL NERVOUS SYSTEM TUMORS, CENTRAL AND PERIPHERAL NERVOUS SYSTEM DISORDERS IN ACQUIRED IMMUNODEFICIENCY SYNDROME, PERIPHERAL NERVOUS SYSTEM DISORDERS, EYE AND EAR DISORDERS *Continued*

Most Common...	Answer and Explanation
sign of a sensorineural hearing loss	*Weber test lateralizes to the normal ear and air conduction is longer than bone conduction in the normal ear and the contralateral ear, which is the one that is affected*
cause of Meniere's disease	*increased endolymph in the inner ear*
S/S of Meniere's disease	*acute labyrinthitis resulting in a unilateral hearing loss and vertigo*

Question: Which of the following CNS disorders are more common in children than adults? **SELECT 2**
- (A) GBM
- (B) Medulloblastoma
- (C) Cerebellar astrocytoma
- (D) Ependymoma of the cauda equina
- (E) Primary CNS lymphoma
- (F) Acoustic neuroma
- (G) Meningioma
- (H) Oligodendroglioma

Answers: (B), (C): Choices A, D, E, F, G, and H are more common in adults. Ependymomas in children are more common in the fourth ventricle.

AD = autosomal dominant, AIDS = acquired immunodeficiency syndrome, AR = autosomal recessive, AV = arteriovenous, CH = cholesterol, CMV = cytomegalovirus, CNS = central nervous system, CSF = cerebral spinal fluid, DM = diabetes mellitus, EBV = Epstein-Barr virus, GBM = glioblastoma multiforme, G/M = gross and microscopic, HIV = human immunodeficiency virus, HSV = herpes simplex virus, MS = multiple sclerosis, S/S = signs and symptoms.

■ INDEX

Aspirin *(Continued)*
for gout, 401
for thrombosis, 101
AST, elevated blood level of, vs.
hemolysis, 4
in liver function testing, 313–315
Asthma, bronchial, 238, 239
Astrocytes, disorders of, 430
functions of, 430
in gliosis, 25
Astrocytoma, 156, 450
Ataxia, Friedreich's, 442
vitamin deficiencies and, 109, 110
Ataxia-telangiectasia, 36
lymphoma with, 171
Atelectasis, 223, 226–228
Atherosclerosis, 184–186
and claudication, 175
and stroke, 438, 443
dietary fat and, 115
in diabetes mellitus, 395
in hypertension, 197
of coronary arteries, 207
Atopic dermatitis, 416
in newborn, 51
Atrial fibrillation, heart sounds
in, 177
Atrial natriuretic peptide, 66
Atrial septal defect, 204, 206
Atrioventricular regurgitation,
with aortic coarctation, 206
Atrioventricular septal defect, in
Down syndrome, 204
Atrium, left, enlargement of, in
mitral stenosis, 213
Atrophy, cellular, 15
Auer rods, in acute myelogenous
leukemia, 267
Auscultation, of heart, sites for,
176
Austin-Flint murmur, 215
Autoantibodies, increased level
of, in elderly, 5
Autografts, 48
Autoimmunity, 54–59
and hemolytic anemia, 256,
260, 261
and hepatitis, 324
in celiac disease, 302
in Guillain-Barré syndrome,
446

Autoimmunity *(Continued)*
in Hashimoto's thyroiditis, 54,
384
in thrombocytopenia, 93
in vitiligo, 424
Automobile accidents, 141
Autosomal disorders, dominant,
121, 123
recessive, 122, 123
Autosplenectomy, in sickle cell
disease, 276
Avascular necrosis, of bone, 407
Avidin, and biotin deficiency, 110
Axillary lymph nodes, metastatic
cancer of, from breast, 376,
377
Azidothymidine, for HIV
infection, 39, 42
Azotemia, and oliguria, 346
prerenal, creatinine in, 336
in heart failure, 201
AZT, for HIV infection, 39, 42

B

B cells. See *Lymphocytes, B.*
Babesiosis, 403
Bacillus cereus, and diarrhea, 304
Bacterial infection, and
conjunctivitis, 447
and lymphangitis, 195
and meningitis, 434, 436
white blood cell response to,
in cerebral spinal fluid,
430
and neutrophilic leukocytosis,
261
and thyroiditis, 383
and tonsillitis, 290–291
and vasculitis, 187
in AIDS, 40–42
in granulomatous disease, 21
inflammatory response to, neutrophils in, 20
Bacteroides fragilis, and
vasculitis, 187
Bagassosis, 236
Barbiturates, and cytochrome
system enhancement, 4
Baroreceptors, in volume
regulation, 65
Barr bodies, in Klinefelter's
syndrome, 120, 121